New Advances in the Management of Voice Disorders

New Advances in the Management of Voice Disorders

Guest Editor

Ben Barsties v. Latoszek

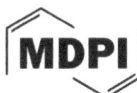

Basel • Beijing • Wuhan • Barcelona • Belgrade • Novi Sad • Cluj • Manchester

Guest Editor
Ben Barsties v. Latoszek
School of Health, Education
and Social Sciences
SRH University of Applied
Sciences Heidelberg
Düsseldorf
Germany

Editorial Office
MDPI AG
Grosspeteranlage 5
4052 Basel, Switzerland

This is a reprint of the Special Issue, published open access by the journal *Journal of Clinical Medicine* (ISSN 2077-0383), freely accessible at: https://www.mdpi.com/journal/jcm/special_issues/ZTWR37544F.

For citation purposes, cite each article independently as indicated on the article page online and as indicated below:

Lastname, A.A.; Lastname, B.B. Article Title. *Journal Name* **Year**, *Volume Number*, Page Range.

ISBN 978-3-7258-4319-0 (Hbk)
ISBN 978-3-7258-4320-6 (PDF)
https://doi.org/10.3390/books978-3-7258-4320-6

© 2025 by the authors. Articles in this book are Open Access and distributed under the Creative Commons Attribution (CC BY) license. The book as a whole is distributed by MDPI under the terms and conditions of the Creative Commons Attribution-NonCommercial-NoDerivs (CC BY-NC-ND) license (https://creativecommons.org/licenses/by-nc-nd/4.0/).

Contents

Ben Barsties v. Latoszek, Jörg Mayer, Christopher R. Watts and Bernhard Lehnert
Advances in Clinical Voice Quality Analysis with VOXplot
Reprinted from: *J. Clin. Med.* **2023**, *12*, 4644, https://doi.org/10.3390/jcm12144644 1

Elina Kankare and Anne-Maria Laukkanen
Validation of the Acoustic Breathiness Index in Speakers of Finnish Language
Reprinted from: *J. Clin. Med.* **2023**, *12*, 7607, https://doi.org/10.3390/jcm12247607 11

Virgilijus Uloza, Kipras Pribuišis, Nora Ulozaite-Staniene, Tadas Petrauskas, Robertas Damaševičius and Rytis Maskeliūnas
Accuracy Analysis of the Multiparametric Acoustic Voice Indices, the VWI, AVQI, ABI, and DSI Measures, in Differentiating between Normal and Dysphonic Voices
Reprinted from: *J. Clin. Med.* **2024**, *13*, 99, https://doi.org/10.3390/jcm13010099 22

Virgilijus Uloza, Nora Ulozaitė-Stanienė, Tadas Petrauskas, Kipras Pribuišis, Tomas Blažauskas, Robertas Damaševičius and Rytis Maskeliūnas
Reliability of Universal-Platform-Based *Voice Screen* Application in AVQI Measurements Captured with Different Smartphones
Reprinted from: *J. Clin. Med.* **2023**, *12*, 4119, https://doi.org/10.3390/jcm12124119 34

Alejandro Klein-Rodríguez, Irma Cabo-Varela, Francisco Vázquez-de la Iglesia, Carlos M. Chiesa-Estomba and Miguel Mayo-Yáñez
Comparison of TEVA vs. PRAAT in the Acoustic Characterization of the Tracheoesophageal Voice in Laryngectomized Patients
Reprinted from: *J. Clin. Med.* **2024**, *13*, 3748, https://doi.org/10.3390/jcm13133748 46

Calvin Peter Baker, Suzanne C. Purdy, Te Oti Rakena and Stefano Bonnini
It Sounds like It Feels: Preliminary Exploration of an Aeroacoustic Diagnostic Protocol for Singers
Reprinted from: *J. Clin. Med.* **2023**, *12*, 5130, https://doi.org/10.3390/jcm12155130 57

Joanna Hoffman, Magda Barańska, Ewa Niebudek-Bogusz and Wioletta Pietruszewska
Comparative Evaluation of High-Speed Videoendoscopy and Laryngovideostroboscopy for Functional Laryngeal Assessment in Clinical Practice
Reprinted from: *J. Clin. Med.* **2025**, *14*, 1723, https://doi.org/10.3390/jcm14051723 73

Dominika Valášková, Jitka Vydrová and Jan G. Švec
Determining the Mouth-to-Microphone Distance in Rigid Laryngoscopy: A Simple Solution Based on the Newly Measured Values of the Depth of Endoscope Insertion into the Mouth
Reprinted from: *J. Clin. Med.* **2023**, *12*, 7560, https://doi.org/10.3390/jcm12247560 95

Arianna Di Stadio, Jake Sossamon, Pietro De Luca, Iole Indovina, Giovanni Motta, Massimo Ralli, et al.
"Do You Hear What I Hear?" Speech and Voice Alterations in Hearing Loss: A Systematic Review
Reprinted from: *J. Clin. Med.* **2025**, *14*, 1428, https://doi.org/10.3390/jcm14051428 111

Ben Barsties v. Latoszek, Viktoria Jansen, Christopher R. Watts and Svetlana Hetjens
The Impact of Protective Face Coverings on Acoustic Markers in Voice: A Systematic Review and Meta-Analysis
Reprinted from: *J. Clin. Med.* **2023**, *12*, 5922, https://doi.org/ 123

Christopher R. Watts, Zoë Thijs, Adam King, Joshua C. Carr and Ryan Porter
A Pilot Study of the Effect of a Non-Contact Boxing Exercise Intervention on Respiratory Pressure and Phonation Aerodynamics in People with Parkinson's Disease
Reprinted from: *J. Clin. Med.* **2023**, *12*, 4806, https://doi.org/10.3390/jcm12144806 . . . . **134**

Ben Barsties v. Latoszek, Christopher R. Watts, Svetlana Hetjens and Katrin Neumann
The Efficacy of Different Voice Treatments for Vocal Fold Polyps: A Systematic Review and Meta-Analysis
Reprinted from: *J. Clin. Med.* **2023**, *12*, 3451, https://doi.org/10.3390/jcm12103451 . . . . **143**

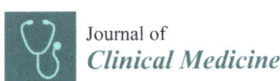

Article

Advances in Clinical Voice Quality Analysis with VOXplot

Ben Barsties v. Latoszek [1,*], Jörg Mayer [2], Christopher R. Watts [3] and Bernhard Lehnert [4]

1. Speech-Language Pathology, SRH University of Applied Health Sciences, 40210 Düsseldorf, Germany
2. Institute for Natural Language Processing, University of Stuttgart, 70049 Stuttgart, Germany; jmayer@lingphon.net
3. Harris College of Nursing & Health Sciences, Texas Christian University, Fort Worth, TX 76109, USA
4. Department of Oto-Rhino-Laryngology, Phoniatrics and Pedaudiology Division, University Medicine Greifswald, 17475 Greifswald, Germany
* Correspondence: benjamin.barstiesvonlatoszek@srh.de

Abstract: Background: The assessment of voice quality can be evaluated perceptually with standard clinical practice, also including acoustic evaluation of digital voice recordings to validate and further interpret perceptual judgments. The goal of the present study was to determine the strongest acoustic voice quality parameters for perceived hoarseness and breathiness when analyzing the sustained vowel [a:] using a new clinical acoustic tool, the VOXplot software. Methods: A total of 218 voice samples of individuals with and without voice disorders were applied to perceptual and acoustic analyses. Overall, 13 single acoustic parameters were included to determine validity aspects in relation to perceptions of hoarseness and breathiness. Results: Four single acoustic measures could be clearly associated with perceptions of hoarseness or breathiness. For hoarseness, the harmonics-to-noise ratio (HNR) and pitch perturbation quotient with a smoothing factor of five periods (PPQ5), and, for breathiness, the smoothed cepstral peak prominence (CPPS) and the glottal-to-noise excitation ratio (GNE) were shown to be highly valid, with a significant difference being demonstrated for each of the other perceptual voice quality aspects. Conclusions: Two acoustic measures, the HNR and the PPQ5, were both strongly associated with perceptions of hoarseness and were able to discriminate hoarseness from breathiness with good confidence. Two other acoustic measures, the CPPS and the GNE, were both strongly associated with perceptions of breathiness and were able to discriminate breathiness from hoarseness with good confidence.

Keywords: voice quality analysis; voice diagnostic; acoustic measures; hoarseness; breathiness

1. Introduction

Standard clinical practice for the evaluation of voice disorders includes a battery of multidimensional assessments (e.g., visual analysis, auditory-perceptual judgment, aerodynamic analysis, acoustic analysis, and self-assessment [1]) aimed to describe and diagnose the voice complaint. Voice disorders affect quality, volume, pitch, resonance, flexibility, and/or stamina. These vocal changes are the manifestation of disordered respiratory, laryngeal, and vocal tract functions, which might result, in many cases, from heterogeneous local etiologies [2]. Many voice disorders are associated with abnormal oscillation patterns of the vocal folds. The resulting voiced energy can vary as a function of vibrational changes at different vocal fold areas, but especially at the free vocal fold margin. Furthermore, the more a critical region of one vocal fold or both vocal folds are affected by laryngeal pathology, the more variation in vocal sound energy and subsequent perceptions of voice quality severity can be expected [3].

Although voice quality is not a clearly defined term, there are two general approaches to evaluation [4]. First, the subjective approach of listening to the patient's voice and assigning a score to different perceptual domains is considered a gold standard approach for perceptual voice analysis. Second, the use of an objective instrumental approach can be used, in which a specific computer algorithm is applied to recorded voice signals. Examples of instrumental assessment of voice quality include analysis of the acoustic voice sound signal and the inverse-filtered oral airflow signal or its derivative. Although many different terms have been used to describe voice quality, a wide acceptance has been acknowledged for terms such as hoarseness or overall voice quality, and major subtypes of the general anomalies in voice quality such as breathiness, roughness, and strain [4,5].

An objective acoustic analysis of voice signals is the most commonly used instrumental tool in clinical practice and research for objectively characterizing voice disorders [6]. Voice signals can be analyzed acoustically in the domains of time, frequency, amplitude, and quefrency. A large number of acoustic measures have been introduced and described to objectively predict dysphonia types and severities. This is illustrated in a taxonomy by Buder [6] with 15 signal-processing-based categories. The reliable and valid use of objective acoustic analysis in research or clinical practice depends on specific requirements (e.g., hardware, software, and examination circumstances) to enable voice analysis with high accuracy and reliability [4,7].

The quantification of voice quality with acoustic methods has traditionally been analyzed on sustained vowels. Although the assessment of voice quality based on sustained vowels (SV) does not necessarily correspond to that of continuous speech (CS) [8,9], acoustic measures from sustained vowels are ubiquitous in research and clinical practice. Acoustic parameters that correlate strongly with auditory-perceptual judgments are included in two examples of multiparametric acoustic indices: the acoustic voice quality index (AVQI) for the evaluation of hoarseness, and the acoustic breathiness index (ABI), which assesses the hoarseness subtype, breathiness [10]. Both AVQI and ABI have been used with wide international acceptance for research and clinical practice for a number of reasons: (a) their multivariate constructs based on linear regression analysis that combines relevant acoustic markers; (b) the inclusion of both continuous speech and sustained vowels in the acoustic analysis; (c), signal processing that uses algorithms of the freeware Praat; and (d) a single score ranging from 0 to 10 for the entire recording being analyzed (i.e., the higher AVQI or ABI score, the more severe the related anomaly of voice quality, and vice versa) [10].

The acoustic measures of AVQI and ABI include smoothed cepstral peak prominence (CPPS); harmonics-to-noise ratio (HNR); shimmer percentage; shimmer dB; general slope of the spectrum (Slope); and tilt of the regression line through the spectrum (Tilt); jitter local; glottal-to-noise excitation ratio with a maximum frequency of 4500 Hz (GNE); relative level of high-frequency noise between energy from 0 to 6 kHz and energy from 6 to 10 kHz (HF Noise); HNR by Dejonckere (HNR-D), which analyses the harmonic shape of the spectral display by using the frequency bandwidth between 500 and 1500 Hz and a cepstrum to determine F0, and thus locate the harmonic structure in the long-term average of the spectrum; differences between the amplitude of the first and second harmonics in the spectrum (H1H2); and period standard deviation (PSD).

Next to AVQI and ABI, a third multivariate index with a long tradition in the evaluation of overall voice quality on sustained vowels is the dysphonia severity index (DSI) [11,12]. The DSI includes four voice parameters (jitter local; highest frequency and lowest intensity of a voice range profile; and maximum phonation time), in which jitter local is the only acoustic single parameter directly associated with voice quality. To use the DSI with Praat algorithms for signal processing the pitch perturbation quotient was considered in place of jitter local [13].

VOXplot (Lingphon, Straubenhardt, Germany; https://voxplot.lingphon.com, accessed on 11 June 2023) is a new freeware application for acoustic voice quality analysis based on the Praat algorithms for signal processing. Whereas Praat is a versatile and correspondingly complex software for acoustic analysis of arbitrary signals, VOXplot is specifically tailored to the analysis of voice quality. With Praat, only the algorithms are used, while the user interface of VOXplot is designed to meet the demands of standardized and intuitive ease of use for clinicians and researchers. VOXplot covers the entire workflow of acoustic voice quality assessment: recording and recording quality assessment, acoustic voice quality analysis, and generation of a concise PDF (or JPEG/PNG) sheet with the analysis results. The core analysis of VOXplot is the voice quality analyses of continuous speech and sustained vowels with AVQI and ABI. VOXplot is currently available in 12 analysis languages for AVQI and ABI, which are based on more than one decade of research knowledge [14,15]. The validation results of both indices relate only to an objective evaluation of the hoarseness and breathiness levels for heterogeneous voice disorders in comparison with vocally healthy volunteers with no further specification of a specific disorder or vocal symptom. The usability of VOXplot is currently available in three interface languages. Further details of sustained vowels can be analyzed qualitatively with the narrowband spectrogram and quantitatively with single acoustic parameters.

As mentioned before, AVQI, ABI, and DSI are used in combination with highly sensitive acoustic markers for the evaluation of hoarseness and breathiness. However, a direct comparison of these objective metrics using the VOXplot application with perceptual ratings of hoarseness or breathiness is missing. Therefore, the aim of this study was to compare the concurrent validity and diagnostic validity outcomes of 13 single acoustic voice quality measures between hoarseness and breathiness aspects on sustained vowels.

2. Materials and Methods

2.1. Participants

In the present study, the voice recordings and auditory-perceptual judgment of hoarseness and breathiness acquired in a previous study [16] were applied to new analyses. The group of dysphonic participants consisted of 175 patients with various organic and nonorganic voice disorders and various degrees of dysphonia severity. The control group of 43 vocally healthy volunteers reported no voice complaints, history of voice, speech, or hearing problems, and no impact of voice problems as measured with the voice handicap index [17].

Table 1 summarizes the demographic data and the types of dysphonia for the two groups. For further details regarding the data and recording acquisition, and inclusion and exclusion criteria, we refer to Barsties v. Latoszek et al. (2020) [16].

Table 1. Demographic data and types of voice disorders of the dysphonia and control groups.

Group	Type of Dysphonia	Number	Gender		Age in Years	
			Female	Male	Mean	SD
Dysphonia Group	Carcinoma of head and neck	55	13	42	61.25	10.18
	Functional dysphonia	38	26	12	52.11	16.48
	Larynx carcinoma	28	1	27	69.96	9.05
	Paralyses	25	14	11	63.36	16.09
	Nodules	8	5	3	33.25	19.43
	Reflux laryngitis	4	4	0	54.50	5.45
	Cancer of unknown primary syndrome	4	2	2	61.00	8.21
	Mutational falsetto	3	0	3	15.67	3.06
	Leukoplakia	2	0	2	57.00	8.49
	Granuloma	2	0	2	42.00	11.31
	Laryngitis	2	1	1	39.50	12.02
	Parkinson's	2	0	2	74.00	11.31
	Polyp	1	0	1	60.00	-
	Laryngeal trauma	1	0	1	78.00	-
Control group	None	43	23	20	26.79	7.06

Abbreviation. SD = standard deviation.

All the participants gave their informed consent for inclusion before they participated in the study. The study was conducted in accordance with the Declaration of Helsinki, and the protocol was approved by the Ethics Committee of Greifswald University (BB072/16).

2.2. Auditory-Perceptual Judgment

For the auditory-perceptual judgment ratings, a panel of three male experts specialized in voice disorders with experience ranging from 8 to 31 years was used. The GRBAS scale was used for data collection. Each listener rated ordinally on a four-point scale the hoarseness level, which is represented in the G-parameter (Grade), and the breathiness severity, which is represented in the B-parameter (which represents the degree of the extent of air leakage through the glottis).

For further details regarding the rating scale, rating procedure, anchor voices, reliability results of the raters, and deviation of the rating level results from the expert panel for hoarseness and breathiness, we refer to Barsties v. Latoszek et al. (2020) [16].

2.3. Acoustic Measurements

The acoustic analyses were conducted only on recordings of the sustained vowel [a:] across 3 s of the mid-vowel segment from a single trial. The [a:] vowel was used as a typical open front vowel for the clinical and scientific acoustic tasks, which is easily recognized regardless of the native language, linguistic competence, or individual health problems (e.g., hearing disorders) from the test person in comparison to other vowels [18,19]. These sound files were applied to a new analysis using VOXplot. In total, 13 single voice quality parameters were acquired from each recording, which are listed in Table 2.

Table 2. List of 13 acoustic measures for the voice quality evaluation.

Category	Acoustic Measures	Abbreviation
Fourier and linear prediction coefficient spectra	Smoothed cepstral peak prominence is the distance between the first harmonic peak and the point with equal quefrency on the regression line through the smoothed cepstrum.	CPPS (dB)
	Differences between the amplitudes of the first and second harmonics in the spectrum. To localize the first harmonic peak, a cepstrum was performed for F0 determination.	H1H2 (dB)
	Relative level of high-frequency noise between energy from 0 to 6 kHz and energy from 6 to 10 kHz.	HF-Noise (dB)
	Harmonics-to-noise ratio is the base 10 logarithm of the ratio between the periodic energy and the noise energy, multiplied by 10 HNR.	HNR (dB)
	Harmonics-to-noise ratio from Dejonckere and Lebacq, which analyzes the harmonic emergence of the spectral display comprised within the frequency bandwidth between 500 Hz and 1500 Hz. A cepstrum was performed to determine F0 and thus to localize the harmonic structure in the long-term average spectrum.	HNR-D (dB)
	General slope of the spectrum is defined as the difference between the energy within 0–1000 Hz and the energy within 1000–10,000 Hz of the long-term average spectrum.	Slope (dB)
	Tilt of the regression line through the spectrum is the difference between the energy within 0–1000 Hz and the energy within 1000–10,000 Hz of the trendline through the long-term average spectrum.	Tilt (dB)

Table 2. *Cont.*

Category	Acoustic Measures	Abbreviation
Frequency of short-term perturbation measures	Period standard deviation is the variation in the standard deviation of periods in which the length of the sample is important for a valid computation of the standard deviation.	PSD (ms)
Frequency of short-term perturbation measures	Two jitter variations: Jitter local is the average difference between successive periods, divided by the average period.	Jitter local (%)
	Jitter of the five-point period perturbation quotient is the average absolute difference between a period and the average of it and its four closest neighbors, divided by the average period.	PPQ5 (%)
Amplitude of short-term perturbations measures	Two shimmer variations: Shimmer local is the absolute mean difference between the amplitudes of successive periods, divided by the average amplitude.	Shimmer (%)
	Shimmer local dB is the base 10 logarithm of the difference between the amplitudes of successive periods, multiplied by 20.	Shimmer (dB)
Combines spectral and perturbation features	The glottal-to-noise-excitation (GNE) ratio with a maximum frequency of 4500 Hz.	GNE

2.4. Statistics

The association of the 13 acoustic parameters with the two auditory-perceptual evaluations of hoarseness and breathiness from 218 recorded voice samples was investigated by calculating Spearman's rank correlation coefficients. An absolute correlation score of ≥ 0.70 is marked as a high relationship for the concurrent validity aspect between the acoustic parameter and the perceived voice quality evaluation [20].

The Fisher r-to-z transformation was used to assess the statistical significance of the two correlation coefficients from the outcomes of the acoustic parameter and perceived hoarseness vs. perceived breathiness levels.

A receiver operating characteristic (ROC) curve was then generated in order to analyze the diagnostic accuracy of the 13 acoustic metrics according to sensitivity (results of the participants with hoarseness or breathiness) and specificity (results of participants without hoarseness or breathiness). The power of the acoustic markers to discriminate between the absence and presence of hoarseness or breathiness was estimated using the area under the ROC curve (A_{ROC}). An A_{ROC} of >0.90 is considered to be exceptionally good; an A_{ROC} of <0.70 is considered to be low, and an A_{ROC} of ≤ 0.50 corresponds to a chance level of diagnostic accuracy [21]. In order to find the optimal threshold value that best differentiates between without and with hoarseness or breathiness, the Youden index (a measure that uses a receiver operating characteristic to determine which threshold value is best suited to distinguish two groups in a measurement) was calculated as sensitivity + specificity − 1.

The significant differences between the two ROC curves (calculated for hoarseness and breathiness) of the acoustic measures were determined by the difference between the areas under the curves [22].

The statistical analyses were performed using SPSS, version 23, for Windows (IBM Corp., Armonk, NY, USA). The tests of significance between the two correlation coefficients and between the areas under two independent ROC curves were analyzed on VassarStats (R. Lowry, Vassar College, NY, USA, 1998–2023; http://vassarstats.net/, accessed on 11 June 2023). Results were considered statistically significant at $p \leq 0.05$.

3. Results

Table 3 presents the validation outcomes for the 13 single acoustic voice quality parameters in direct comparison to the auditory-perceptual ratings of hoarseness and breathiness. The thresholds with sensitivity and specificity, based on the ROC statistics and the Youden Index, are also listed in Table 3.

Table 3. Validation results of the 13 single acoustic voice quality parameters of the sustained vowel phonation [a:].

Voice Quality Parameters	Validation Parameters	Hoarseness	Breathiness
CPPS (dB)	Correlation	−0.76 *	−0.81 *
	A_{ROC}	0.823 *	0.915 **
	Threshold	15.02 dB	14.47 dB
	Sensitivity	84.7%	88.1%
	Specificity	71.2%	81.7%
GNE	Correlation	−0.70	−0.78 *
	A_{ROC}	0.798 *	0.886 *
	Threshold	0.91	0.89
	Sensitivity	88.9%	91.7%
	Specificity	62.3%	74.3%
H1H2 (dB)	Correlation	0.03	0.12
	A_{ROC}	0.448	0.584
	Threshold	Chance−level based on A_{ROC}	6.39 dB
	Sensitivity	Chance−level based on A_{ROC}	40.4%
	Specificity	Chance−level based on A_{ROC}	82.6%
HNR (dB)	Correlation	−0.71 *	−0.56
	A_{ROC}	0.812 *	0.794 *
	Threshold	23.34 dB	23.34 dB
	Sensitivity	90.3%	78.9%
	Specificity	62.9%	68.5%
HNR-D (dB)	Correlation	−0.57	−0.38
	A_{ROC}	0.760 *	0.701 *
	Threshold	31.77 dB	24.23 dB
	Sensitivity	61.1%	77.1%
	Specificity	80.8%	53.2%
HF noise (dB)	Correlation	−0.48	−0.49
	A_{ROC}	0.698	0.728 *
	Threshold	2.28 dB	2.29 dB
	Sensitivity	80.6%	77.1%
	Specificity	54.1%	62.4%
Jitter local (%)	Correlation	0.68	0.57
	A_{ROC}	0.839 *	0.808 *
	Threshold	0.50%	0.57%
	Sensitivity	70.8%	71.0%
	Specificity	84.7%	78.0%
PPQ5 (%)	Correlation	0.71 *	0.55
	A_{ROC}	0.833 *	0.799 *
	Threshold	0.29%	0.32%
	Sensitivity	67.2%	67.0%
	Specificity	84.5%	75.9%
PSD (ms)	Correlation	0.59	0.41
	A_{ROC}	0.802 *	0.730 *
	Threshold	0.00012 ms	0.00018 ms
	Sensitivity	65.3%	50.5%
	Specificity	81.9%	88.1%
Shimmer (%)	Correlation	0.65	0.53
	A_{ROC}	0.773 *	0.780 *
	Threshold	3.08%	3.58
	Sensitivity	53.5%	57.0%
	Specificity	91.7%	90.8%

Table 3. Cont.

Voice Quality Parameters	Validation Parameters	Hoarseness	Breathiness
Shimmer (dB)	Correlation	0.66	0.55
	A$_{ROC}$	0.783 *	0.786 *
	Threshold	0.27 dB	0.33 dB
	Sensitivity	54.9%	57.9%
	Specificity	91.7%	91.7%
Slope (dB)	Correlation	−0.09	−0.11
	A$_{ROC}$	0.617	0.602
	Threshold	−25.08 dB	−25.34 dB
	Sensitivity	81.9%	80.7%
	Specificity	39.7%	43.1%
Tilt (dB)	Correlation	0.30	0.43
	A$_{ROC}$	0.592	0.673
	Threshold	−10.32 dB	−11.73 dB
	Sensitivity	34.9%	81.7%
	Specificity	86.1%	46.8%

* High correlation or high A$_{ROC}$ indicating a marked relationship in concurrent validity or sufficient diagnostic accuracy; ** exceptionally good diagnostic accuracy level. Darker grey boxes indicate nonsignificant differences of $p > 0.05$ (corresponding to Fisher r-to-z transformation for correlation results and/or significant differences in ROC results of A$_{ROC}$).

For hoarseness, a strong correlation was present for CPPS, HNR, and PPQ5. No acoustic parameter reached an exceptionally good level of A$_{ROC}$, and 4 of the 13 acoustic parameters revealed a low level of A$_{ROC}$, in which one of them was characterized by a chance level in diagnostic accuracy (H1H2).

For breathiness, a strong correlation was present for CPPS and GNE. However, GNE reached an exceptionally good A$_{ROC}$ result, and 9 of the remaining 12 acoustic parameters had a strong level of diagnostic accuracy.

To assign a single acoustic voice quality parameter with high validity to a type of voice abnormality, (a) the absolute correlation value and the A$_{ROC}$ had to be >0.70, and (b) significant differences in validity performances between hoarseness and breathiness must be obtained in the correlation results or the A$_{ROC}$ outcomes. According to the results listed in Table 3 for hoarseness, two acoustic parameters could be identified as highly valid (HNR and PPQ5) in comparison to breathiness. For breathiness, two acoustic metrics (CPPS and GNE) were also revealed to have outstanding validity results in comparison to hoarseness.

4. Discussion

The aim of the present study was to investigate the validity of single acoustic parameters representing voice quality characteristics of hoarseness or breathiness in a direct comparison of the auditory-perceptual voice quality ratings of those domains from sustained vowel [a:] phonation. Although multiparametric models are preferred in highly valid evaluations of hoarseness or breathiness [4,9,23,24], single acoustic parameters are mostly used in clinical practice and recommended protocols for instrumental assessment of voice [7]. The present study attempted to reveal the most relevant acoustic markers for hoarseness and breathiness from a pool of metrics, which are already part of relevant multiparametric models in the evaluation of voice quality, such as DSI, AVQI, and ABI.

In general, the results from the initial AVQI and ABI studies were confirmed by the present study, with comparable results to the correlation coefficients for hoarseness and breathiness [9,24]. Although continuous speech was also considered in the voice quality evaluation for AVQI and ABI, CPPS and HNR showed high agreement for hoarseness, and CPPS and GNE presented the strongest results for breathiness. Because perceptions of breathiness are associated with high irregularity in the acoustic spectrum (e.g., a lot of spectral aperiodicity or noise), while perceptions of hoarseness can be associated with multidimensional acoustic factors other than spectral aperiodicity, it was logical that the discriminative ability of CPPS (which measures the periodicity in the acoustic spectrum) for breathiness was significantly higher than for hoarseness in this study. Originally, CPPS was developed for the vocal quality abnormality of breathiness [25], in which breathiness is a main subtype of hoarseness [24]. Just like GNE, which was also developed for the evaluation of breathiness [26], the present study confirmed its strength in the evaluation of this voice quality aspect with significantly higher concurrent validity and diagnostic accuracy.

A clearer unique identifier for hoarseness versus breathiness was shown in this study by the two parameters HNR and PPQ5. In the case of HNR, it is the second most important acoustic parameter in the AVQI formula after CPPS, which is supported by the results of this study [9]. The findings of this study suggest that HNR is a general parameter that does not necessarily correspond to other strong breathiness measures such as CPPS or GNE. Only PPQ5 achieved a sufficiently high agreement with hoarseness and was significantly differentiated from breathiness in the current study. This result was contrary to the results of the original study on AVQI by Maryn et al. (2010) [9]. Furthermore, in a meta-analysis on the evaluation of hoarseness, jitter parameters generally ranked significantly lower than spectral or cepstral parameters and some shimmer markers [27], but, according to the present results, PPQ5 seems to be robust enough to assess hoarseness in the evaluation of sustained vowels, which may explain why this parameter is included in the DSI formula.

The new developments based on the present study were updated in VOXplot and are available from version 2.0 (see Figure 1).

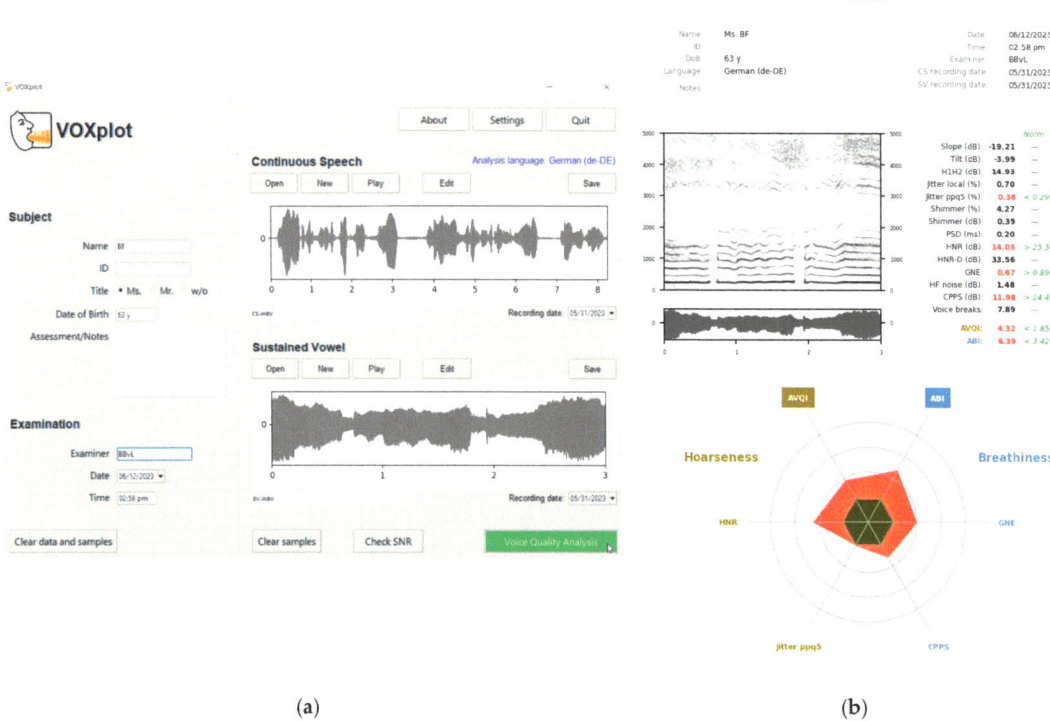

Figure 1. VOXplot version 2.0: (**a**) the user interface for preparing the acoustic analysis of continuous speech and/or sustained vowels selected in the English language with the analysis language German for the thresholds evaluations of AVQI and ABI; (**b**) the outcome of the main voice quality parameters in VOXplot, which are evaluated quantitatively and/or qualitatively for hoarseness and breathiness.

5. Conclusions

For the voice quality evaluation on the sustained vowel HNR and PPQ5 (for hoarseness), and CPPS and GNE (for breathiness) yielded the highest significant validity results compared to each of the other voice quality aspect." These four acoustic parameters should have priority in the evaluation of hoarseness and breathiness and are prominently included in VOXplot (e.g., in the voice quality circle plot).

Author Contributions: Conceptualization, B.B.v.L., B.L., C.R.W. and J.M.; methodology, B.B.v.L., C.R.W. and B.L.; software, J.M.; validation, B.B.v.L. and B.L.; formal analysis, B.B.v.L.; resources, B.L. and B.B.v.L.; data curation, B.L.; writing—original draft preparation, B.B.v.L. and J.M.; writing—review and editing, C.R.W. and B.L. All authors have read and agreed to the published version of the manuscript.

Funding: This research received no external funding.

Institutional Review Board Statement: The study was conducted in accordance with the Declaration of Helsinki and approved by the Ethics Committee of Greifswald University (protocol code: BB072/16 and date of approval: 05-04-2016).

Informed Consent Statement: Informed consent was obtained from all the subjects involved in the study.

Data Availability Statement: The original contributions presented in the study are included in the article; further inquiries can be directed to the corresponding author.

Conflicts of Interest: J.M. is the developer of the software, VOXplot, and the owner of the company lingphon.de (Straubenhardt, Germany). B.B.v.L. created the ABI and contributed to the development of AVQI v.03. He also acts as a scientific advisor in the creation of the VOXplot software.

References

1. Dejonckere, P.H.; Bradley, P.; Clemente, P.; Cornut, G.; Crevier-Buchman, L.; Friedrich, G.; Van De Heyning, P.; Remacle, M.; Woisard, V.; Committee on Phoniatrics of the European Laryngological Society (ELS). A basic protocol for functional assessment of voice pathology, especially for investigating the efficacy of (phonosurgical) treatments and evaluating new assessment techniques. Guideline elaborated by the Committee on Phoniatrics of the European Laryngological Society (ELS). *Eur. Arch. Otorhinolaryngol.* **2001**, *258*, 77–82. [CrossRef] [PubMed]
2. Verdolini, K.; Rosen, C.A.; Branski, R.C. Classification manual for voice disorders-I. In *Special Interest Division 3, Voice and Voice Disorders, American Speech-Language-Hearing Association*; Lawrence Erlbaum Associates, Inc.: Mahwah, NJ, USA, 2006.
3. Fleischer, S.; Hess, M. The significance of videostroboscopy in laryngological practice. *HNO* **2006**, *54*, 628–634. [CrossRef] [PubMed]
4. Barsties, B.; De Bodt, M. Assessment of voice quality: Current state-of-the-art. *Auris Nasus Larynx* **2015**, *42*, 183–188. [CrossRef] [PubMed]
5. Shrivastav, R. Evaluating voice quality. In *Handbook of Voice Assessments*; Ma, E.P.M., Yiu, E.M.L., Eds.; Singular Publishing Group: San Diego, CA, USA, 2011; pp. 305–318.
6. Buder, E.H. Acoustic analysis of voice quality: A tabulation of algorithms 1902–1990. In *Voice Quality Measurement*; Kent, R.D., Ball, M.J., Eds.; Singular Publishing Group: San Diego, CA, USA, 2000; pp. 119–244.
7. Patel, R.R.; Awan, S.N.; Barkmeier-Kraemer, J.; Courey, M.; Deliyski, D.; Eadie, T.; Paul, D.; Švec, J.G.; Hillman, R. Recommended protocols for instrumental assessment of voice: American Speech-Language-Hearing Association expert panel to develop a protocol for instrumental assessment of vocal function. *Am. J. Speech Lang. Pathol.* **2018**, *27*, 887–905. [CrossRef]
8. Maryn, Y.; Roy, N. Sustained vowels and continuous speech in the auditory-perceptual evaluation of dysphonia severity. *J. Soc. Bras. Fonoaudiol.* **2012**, *24*, 107–112. [CrossRef] [PubMed]
9. Maryn, Y.; Corthals, P.; Van Cauwenberge, P.; Roy, N.; De Bodt, M. Toward improved ecological validity in the acoustic measurement of overall voice quality: Combining continuous speech and sustained vowels. *J. Voice* **2010**, *24*, 540–555. [CrossRef]
10. Barsties v. Latoszek, B.; Mathmann, P.; Neumann, K. The cepstral spectral index of dysphonia, the acoustic voice quality index and the acoustic breathiness index as novel multiparametric indices for acoustic assessment of voice quality. *Curr. Opin. Otolaryngol. Head Neck Surg.* **2021**, *29*, 451–457. [CrossRef]
11. Sobol, M.; Sielska-Badurek, E.M. The Dysphonia Severity Index (DSI)-normative values. Systematic review and meta-analysis. *J. Voice* **2022**, *36*, 143.e9–143.e13. [CrossRef]
12. Uloza, V.; Barsties, V.; Latoszek, B.; Ulozaite-Staniene, N.; Petrauskas, T.; Maryn, Y. A comparison of Dysphonia Severity Index and Acoustic Voice Quality Index measures in differentiating normal and dysphonic voices. *Eur. Arch. Otorhinolaryngol.* **2018**, *275*, 949–958. [CrossRef]

13. Maryn, Y.; Morsomme, D.; De Bodt, M. Measuring the Dysphonia Severity Index (DSI) in the program Praat. *J. Voice* **2017**, *31*, 644.e29–644.e40. [CrossRef]
14. Batthyany, C.; Barsties, V.; Latoszek, B.; Maryn, Y. Meta-Analysis on the Validity of the Acoustic Voice Quality Index. *J. Voice* **2022**, in press. [CrossRef] [PubMed]
15. Barsties v. Latoszek, B.; Kim, G.H.; Delgado Hernandez, J.; Hosokawa, K.; Englert, M.; Neumann, K.; Hetjens, S. The validity of the Acoustic Breathiness Index in the evaluation of breathy voice quality: A Meta-Analysis. *Clin. Otolaryngol.* **2021**, *46*, 31–40. [CrossRef] [PubMed]
16. Barsties v. Latoszek, B.; Lehnert, B.; Janotte, B. Validation of the Acoustic Voice Quality Index Version 03.01 and Acoustic Breathiness Index in German. *J. Voice* **2020**, *34*, 157.e17–157.e25. [CrossRef] [PubMed]
17. Nawka, T.; Wiesmann, U.; Gonnermann, U. Validation of the German version of the Voice Handicap Index. *HNO* **2003**, *51*, 921–930. [CrossRef]
18. Franca, M.C. Acoustic comparison of vowel sounds among adult females. *J. Voice.* **2012**, *26*, 671.e9–671.e17. [CrossRef]
19. Brockmann, M.; Drinnan, M.J.; Storck, C.; Carding, P.N. Reliable jitter and shimmer measurements in voice clinics: The relevance of vowel, gender, vocal intensity, and fundamental frequency effects in a typical clinical task. *J. Voice.* **2011**, *25*, 44–53. [CrossRef]
20. Frey, L.R.; Botan, C.H.; Friedman, P.G.K.G. *Investigating Communication: An Introduction to Research Methods*; Prentice-Hall: Englewood Cliffs, NJ, USA, 1991.
21. Hosmer, D.W.; Lemeshow, S. *Applied Logistic Regression*, 2nd ed.; John Wiley & Sons: Hoboken, NJ, USA, 2000; pp. 156–164.
22. Hanley, J.A.; McNeil, B.J. The meaning and use of the area under a receiver operating characteristic (ROC) curve. *Radiology* **1982**, *143*, 29–36. [CrossRef] [PubMed]
23. Jayakumar, T.; Benoy, J.J. Acoustic Voice Quality Index (AVQI) in the measurement of voice quality: A systematic review and meta-analysis. *J. Voice* **2022**, in press. [CrossRef]
24. Barsties v. Latoszek, B.; Maryn, Y.; Gerrits, E.; De Bodt, M. The Acoustic Breathiness Index (ABI): A Multivariate Acoustic Model for Breathiness. *J. Voice* **2017**, *31*, 511.e11–511.e27. [CrossRef]
25. Hillenbrand, J.; Houde, R.A. Acoustic correlates of breathy vocal quality: Dysphonic voices and continuous speech. *J. Speech Hear. Res.* **1996**, *39*, 311–321. [CrossRef]
26. Michaelis, D.; Gramss, T.; Strube, H.W. Glottal-to-Noise Excitation Ratio—A New Measure for Describing Pathological Voices. *Acustica* **1997**, *83*, 700–706.
27. Maryn, Y.; Roy, N.; De Bodt, M.; Van Cauwenberge, P.; Corthals, P. Acoustic measurement of overall voice quality: A meta-analysis. *J. Acoust. Soc. Am.* **2009**, *126*, 2619–2634. [CrossRef] [PubMed]

Disclaimer/Publisher's Note: The statements, opinions and data contained in all publications are solely those of the individual author(s) and contributor(s) and not of MDPI and/or the editor(s). MDPI and/or the editor(s) disclaim responsibility for any injury to people or property resulting from any ideas, methods, instructions or products referred to in the content.

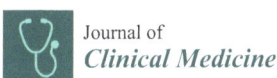

Article

Validation of the Acoustic Breathiness Index in Speakers of Finnish Language

Elina Kankare [1,*] and Anne-Maria Laukkanen [2]

[1] Department of Rehabilitation and Psychosocial Support, Logopedics, Phoniatrics, Tampere University Hospital, 33520 Tampere, Finland
[2] Speech and Voice Research Laboratory, Tampere University, 33100 Tampere, Finland; anne-maria.laukkanen@tuni.fi
* Correspondence: eliina.kankare@pirha.fi; Tel.: +358-444-729-792

Abstract: Breathiness (perception of turbulence noise in the voice) is one of the major components of hoarseness in dysphonic voices. This study aims to validate a multiparameter analysis tool, the Acoustic Breathiness Index (ABI), for quantification of breathiness in the speaking voice, including both sustained vowels and continuous speech. One hundred and eight speakers with dysphonia (28 M, 80 F, mean age 50, SD 15.4 years) and 87 non-dysphonic controls (18 M, 69 F, mean age 42, SD 14 years) volunteered as participants. They read a standard text and sustained vowel /a:/. Acoustic recordings were made using a head-mounted microphone. Acoustic samples were evaluated perceptually by nine voice experts of different backgrounds (speech therapists, vocologists and laryngologists). Breathiness (B) from the GRBAS scale was rated. Headphones were used in the perceptual analysis. The dysphonic and non-dysphonic speakers differed significantly from each other in the auditory perceptual evaluation of breathiness. A significant difference was also found for ABI, which had a mean value of 2.26 (SD 1.15) for non-dysphonic and 3.07 (SD 1.75) for dysphonic speakers. ABI correlated strongly with B (r_s = 0.823, p = 0.01). ABI's power to distinguish the groups was high (88.6%). The highest sensitivity and specificity of ABI (80%) was obtained at threshold value 2.68. ABI is a valid tool for differentiating breathiness in non-dysphonic and dysphonic speakers of Finnish.

Keywords: dysphonia; hoarseness; GRBAS; acoustic noise detection

1. Introduction

1.1. What Is Breathiness

Breathiness is a characteristic in many disordered voices [1,2]. It occurs in organic voice disorders as well as in functional or neurological voice disorders [1,3]. Some breathiness can also be heard in the softly produced healthy voice, especially in women [4,5]. Breathiness refers to the auditory perception of air turbulence and is caused by air leakage from the glottis [6–8].

1.2. Perceptual Tools to Detect Breathiness

Many auditory perceptual tools have been developed to evaluate voice quality and at the same time breathiness in the voice. These tools include, for example, the GRBAS scale [6], the Australian Perceptual Voice Profile [9], the Swedish Stockholm Voice Evaluation [10], the CAPE-V (Consensus Auditory Perceptual Evaluation of Voice) [8] and the Danish Dysphonia Assessment [11]. Although an experienced listener can estimate the amount of breathiness in the voice by perceptual analysis, this is a subjective estimation [12]. An objective measure to evaluate voice quality and the amount of breathiness is needed, especially in clinical work and in the rehabilitation of patients with varying voice disorders [13,14].

1.3. Acoustic Tools to Detect Breathiness

Various signal analysis methods have been applied to predict perceived breathiness from acoustic characteristics. All of the methods aim to measure the amount of periodic and non-periodic components in a sound signal. These methods include, e.g., harmonic-to-noise ratio (HNR) [15], noise-to-harmonic ratio (NHR), voice turbulence index and soft phonation index [16,17], signal periodicity, first harmonic amplitude and spectral tilt and cepstral peak prominence (CPP and its smoothed version CPPS) [1,18]. Periodicity or, rather, reduced periodicity with increased jitter and shimmer (i.e., irregular variation in period duration or amplitude, respectively) has been found to predict well perceived breathiness both in non-dysphonic and in dysphonic voices [1,18]. On the other hand, jitter and shimmer are characteristics that are related to irregular vocal fold vibration, whose main perceptual correlate is "roughness" [6]. Furthermore, jitter, shimmer and spectrum based measures of noise, like HNR, are affected by the pitch and intensity of the voice, which impairs their reliability in dysphonia detection [19–21]. CPPS, which is based on the spectrum of the logarithmic spectrum [18], is independent of pitch and intensity. It has been found to show highest correlations with perceived hoarseness, roughness and breathiness [22,23]. Thus, there seemed to be a need to develop an index that would be able to focus more on the acoustic characteristics of breathiness rather than those of roughness which refers to irregular vocal fold vibration, and to distinguish non-dysphonic and dysphonic breathiness. The Acoustic Breathiness Index (ABI) has been developed to meet these needs [12,24].

1.4. What Is ABI?

The ABI is a multidimensional method with nine separate acoustic measures for detecting breathiness in the voice. Measures used in the ABI are smoothed cepstral peak prominence (CPPs), jitter local (Jit), glottal-to-noise excitation ratio (GNE), high frequency noise of 6000 Hz (Hfno), harmonic-to-noise ratio of Dejonckere (HNR-D), the amplitude difference between the first two harmonics (H1-H2), two measures of shimmer (Shim dB and Shim%) and period standard deviation (PSD) [12]. CPPs is the distance between the cepstral peak that corresponds to the first harmonic and the point with equal quefrency (inverse of frequency) on the regression line through the smoothed cepstrum [12]. The higher the value of CPPs, the more periodic, i.e., the clearer and more noiseless, the sound is in terms of auditory perception. CPPs is affected by both turbulence noise and signal perturbation (jitter and shimmer). Jit, i.e., jitter local, is the mean difference between successive periods, divided by the average period length. GNE [25] indicates whether a voice signal originates from vocal fold vibrations or from turbulent noise. GNE is independent of jitter and shimmer. A clear, nonbreathy voice results in high GNE. Hfno (up to 6000 Hz) indicates the spectral level difference between the ranges of 0–6 kHz and 6–10 kHz. A breathy voice with more noise in the high-frequency range has a smaller Hfno. HNR-D from Dejonckere and Lebacq [26] analyses the harmonic structure against noise in the long-term average spectrum in the formant zone between 500 Hz and 1500 Hz. A cepstrum is calculated to determine F0. A higher value of HNR-D indicates a less breathy voice. H1–H2, i.e., the difference in level between the first two harmonics, is greater in breathy voices. Shimmer measures the amplitude perturbation through the difference between successive periods divided by the mean amplitude. The value is calculated both in dB and in percentages. PSD is a perturbation measure revealing the variation in the standard deviation of periods [12].

Since the ABI is calculated from both sustained vowels and continuous speech, it needs to be validated in different languages [24]. The ABI has so far been validated in eight different languages, Dutch [12], German [24], Japanese [27], Korean [28], Brazilian Portuguese [29], Spanish [30], South Indian [31] and Persian [32].

1.5. Aim and Research Questions of the Present Study

The present article introduces a study where we aimed to validate the ABI in a Finnish speaking population. In this study, we sought an answer to two main questions:

(1) Is the ABI a valid robust method to distinguish dysphonic breathy voice quality in a Finnish speaking population? (2) What is the best threshold value for ABI analysis in a Finnish speaking population?

2. Materials and Methods

2.1. Participants

The present study applied the ABI and auditory perceptual evaluation of breathiness to 195 Finnish speaking participants. The voice material of this study is the same as in the validation study of the Acoustic Voice Quality Index version 03.01 in Finnish.

2.2. Dysphonic Participants

One hundred and eight dysphonic participants were volunteer patients in the phoniatric department in the university hospital. Twenty-eight of the patients were males (mean age 51 years, SD 13.8, range 19–75). Eighty of the patients were females (mean age 51 years, SD 16.2, range 19–84). Table 1 shows the diagnoses of the participants.

Table 1. Number of dysphonic participants and their diagnoses.

Diagnosis	Number
Functional dysphonia	30
Paralysis/paresis of vocal fold	23
Laryngeal dystonia	23
Other diseases of vocal fold or larynx/other undefined dysphonia	10
Chronic laryngitis	9
Nodules	5
Larynx irritable with voice symptoms	2
Cough with voice symptoms	1
Polyp of vocal cord	1
Laryngeal spasm	1
Dysphagia with voice symptoms	1
Ehlers–Danlos syndrome	1
Larynx trauma	1
Total	108

2.3. Non-Dysphonic Controls

Eighty-seven vocally healthy persons with no diagnosis of dysphonia participated as controls. Eighteen of the participants were males (mean age 49 years, SD 9.9, range 32–60), and 69 were females (mean age 40 years, SD 14.5, range 19–67). Seventy-nine of the healthy participants scored under 38 points on the VAPP questionnaire (Voice Activity and Participation Profile) [33] and eight of them scored over 38 which has been considered the threshold value for voice disorder [34]. However, all participants considered themselves to be vocally healthy.

2.4. Recordings

All voice samples were recorded with an AKG C544L (AKG, Vienna, Austria) head-mounted condenser microphone with the Focusrite iTrack Solo (Focusrite PLC, High Wycombe, England) audio interface and using Praat software (version 6.2.23) in the computer. The recording used a sampling frequency of 44.1 kHz and the amplitude resolution was 16 bits. The distance of the microphone was 4 cm from the right side of the corner of the mouth at an angle of 45 degrees. The distance and position of the microphone were checked for each participant by measuring the distance from the corner of the mouth with a ruler.

The voice material for the study was collected for patients and 49 vocally healthy participants in a quiet treatment room at Tampere University Hospital. Thirty-eight of the healthy voices were recorded in studio conditions at Tampere University. The mean signal-to-noise ratio of the recordings (i.e., the difference in level between the sample and that of the background noise level) was 39.8 dB (SD 5.6 dB). In all samples the SNR was well over the recommended norm of SNR > 30 dB, so it can be confirmed that the recording conditions were acceptable.

2.5. Voice Samples

As voice samples, the standard text "Pohjantuuli ja aurinko" (North wind and the sun) was read aloud and a sustained vowels [a:] was produced three times. The participants were asked to use a voice pitch and intensity that suited them best, and the length of the sustained vowel was suggested to be five seconds. The participants were asked to produce the vowel in a spoken manner rather than singing.

For the ABI analysis the first 31 syllables from the read text and three seconds from the middle of the second sustained vowel were used. In the Finnish AVQI validation study, it was confirmed that 31 syllables of Finnish language text readings correspond on average to three-second long vowels [35]. The confirmation of the 31 syllables was executed for Finnish language the same way as described when finding out the syllable count of the Dutch sample [36]. Therefore, the index to be obtained would consist of a balanced duration of speech and sustained vowel phonation. For the analysis, connected speech sample was marked "cs" and the three-second sustained vowel sample "sv". The ABI analysis was executed with VOXplot Acoustic Voice Quality Analysis software, version 2.0.0 [12,37]. The equation to calculate the ABI in the VOXplot software was the one presented by Barsties v. Latoszek et al. 2017 [12]: ABI = (5.0447740915 − [0.172 × CPPs] − [0.193 × Jit] − [1.283 × GNEmax − 4500 Hz] − [0.396 × Hno − 6000 Hz] + [0.01 × HNR −D] + [0.017 × H1 − H2] + [1.473 × Shim − dB] − [0.088 × Shim] − [68.295 × PSD]) × 2.9257400394. The ABI analysis gives the result of an index value between 0 and 10, a value of 0 meaning that there is no breathy sound in the voice and the higher the index number, the breathier sound there is in the voice sample.

2.6. Auditory–Perceptual Analysis

In order to validate the ABI analysis of the Finnish language, a listening analysis was performed. Nine voice experts in the field of voice (three phoniatrician/otolaryngologists, three speech therapists and three vocologists) listened to the voice samples and gave their evaluation of B from the GRBAS scale [6]. The scale is from 0 to 3, 0 signifying "no breathiness at all" and 3 signifying "very much breathiness" in the voice. The listening samples consisted of 31 syllables of continuous speech from the beginning of the text reading and three seconds of a sustained vowel. The length of one sample was thus six seconds and there was a total of 220 samples. For the intra-rater reliability analysis, 25 samples were rated twice. Before the listening test, listeners' ears were calibrated with the anchor voice samples [38,39]. In the calibration, there were two anchor voice samples for each category of the degree of breathiness 0–3, i.e., there were in total eight anchor samples. The anchor voice samples were selected from the voice material of the present study by one experienced speech therapist and one experienced vocologist. The listening test was conducted on each listener's own computer with around-ear headphones. Listeners received the voice material and instructions for the listening analysis on a memory stick. They were asked to make a judgement from a combination of continuous speech and sustained vowel phonation and mark the results in an Excel table. During the listening analysis the raters were able to listen to the samples as many times as they felt necessary; moreover, they were asked to listen to the anchor voice samples at least once after every 32 samples. This was carried out to prevent the listeners from losing focus and straining their hearing too much. Reminders about the anchors were marked in the Excel table as was the instruction to take a short break after listening to 128 samples, about halfway through the task. The interval for listening to the anchors was chosen on the basis of previous listening analyses. The listening analysis took on average from two to three hours.

2.7. Statistical Analysis

The statistical analysis was conducted using SPSS for Windows version 26 (IBM Corp., Armonk, NY, USA). All the results were considered statistically significant at $p \leq 0.05$. In the Finnish validation of the ABI, first the intra-rater reliability of the perceptual raters was analysed with the Cohen kappa ($C\kappa$) and secondly the raters' inter-rater reliability was analysed with the Fleiss kappa ($F\kappa$) [40]. Raters with intra-rater reliability $C\kappa \geq 0.41$ were selected for inclusion in the study. The inter-rater reliability between the perceptual rates was defined to be at least ≥ 0.41 [40]. Next in the validation process, the relationship between the mean values of ABI and the mean values of the perceptual evaluation of breathiness were tested with the Spearman's rank order correlation coefficient (r_s, r^2). Finally, the diagnostic accuracy of the ABI was evaluated with ROC (receiver operating characteristic) curve. The diagnostic accuracy was evaluated according to the sensitivity of the ABI to distinguish between disordered voice and heathy voice, and specificity to detect voices without breathiness. A nonbreathy voice was defined as a voice that received a perceptual mean rating of B 0–0.49. Additionally, the ability of the ABI to distinguish between normal and dysphonic breathiness was evaluated by the area under ROC curve (A_{ROC}). The ROC curve and the Youden index were used to differentiate the best threshold level for the ABI to differentiate healthy and dysphonic voices in the Finnish language. Likelihood ratios (LR+ and LR−) were used to differentiate the probability of persons with breathy voice having ABI value above the threshold level (LR+) or persons with nonbreathy voice having ABI value below the threshold level. To define the optimal threshold level, both the positive and negative likelihood ratio and the sensitivity/(1 − specificity) and (1 − sensitivity/specificity were used).

3. Results
3.1. Reliability of the Perceptual Evaluation

The intra-rater reliability of the listening analysis of the breathiness in $C\kappa$ was between 0.395 and 0.809. One rater, however, presented a $C\kappa$ value lower than the acceptable 0.41 and was excluded from the analysis. The remaining eight raters reported $C\kappa$ values between 0.451 and 0.809. This group of eight raters showed reasonable inter-rater reliability ($F\kappa = 0.435$) and therefore the mean of their listening analysis represents the auditory assessment of breathiness in this study. The mean distribution of the auditory perceptual rating is seen in Figure 1. It is possible to deduce from Figure 1 that some breathiness was also heard in some of the non-dysphonic voices.

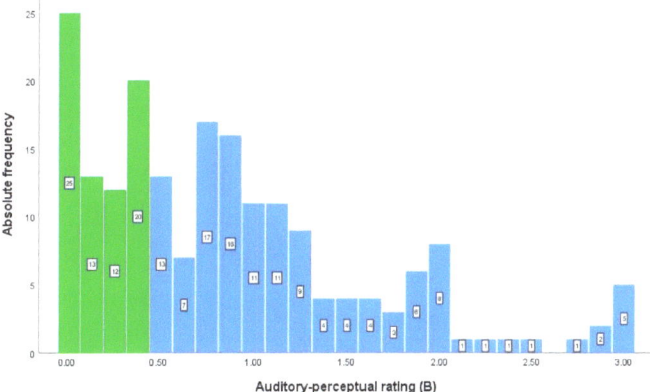

Figure 1. Frequency distribution of the mean breathiness by eight raters. Green colour on the graph indicates those participants who did not have breathiness (mean 0–0.49) in their voices and blue indicates those who were rated to have breathy voice quality (mean 0.50–3).

The listeners in this study represented three different occupational groups: phoniatrician/otolaryngologists, speech therapists and vocologists. The vocologists' evaluation differed significantly from that of the other two groups (Mann–Whitney U test, phoniatrician/otolaryngologists vs. vocologists $p = 0.002$, speech therapists vs. vocologists $p = 0.000$). Vocologists rated more breathiness in the voice than the raters in the other groups.

3.2. Results for the ABI and Perceptual Evaluation of Breathiness

ABI results correlated strongly with auditory perceptual rating of breathy voice quality (Spearman's rho 0.823, $p = 0.01$) (Figure 2). Non-dysphonic and dysphonic groups differed significantly from each other in both ABI and perceptual results (Mann–Whitney test, $p < 0.001$) (Table 2).

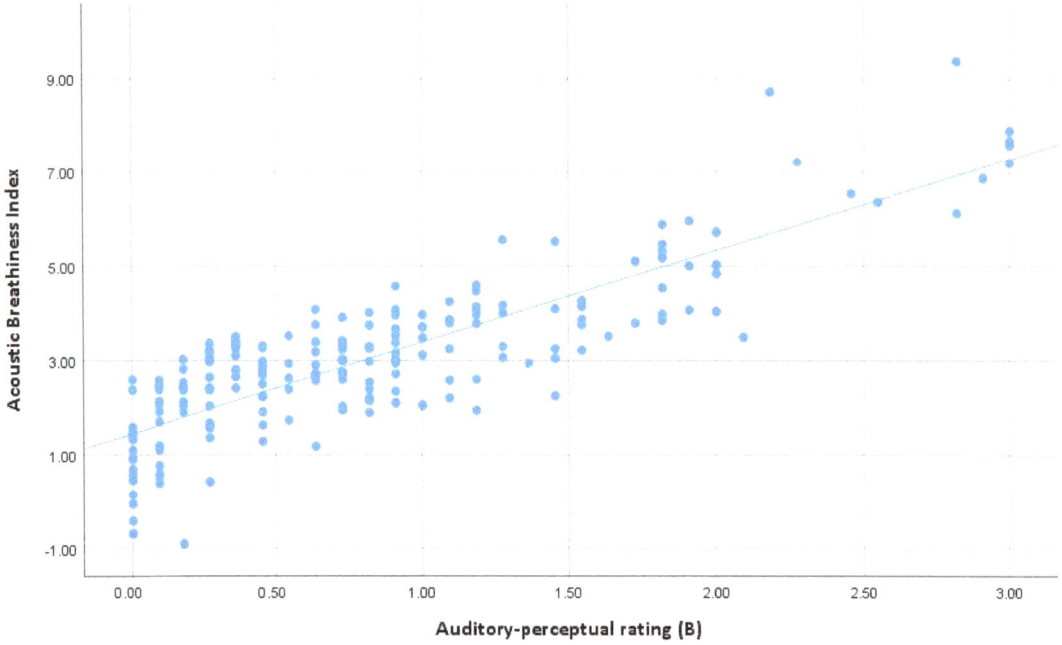

Figure 2. Scatter plot and the linear regression line between auditory–perceptual rating and ABI results.

Table 2. Mean values of ABI and perceptual rating of breathiness in non-dysphonic (participants with no diagnosis of dysphonia) and dysphonic groups (participants with diagnosis of dysphonia). Comparison of the groups using Mann–Whitney U test.

	N	Mean	SD	Min	Max	p-Value
ABI						
Non-dysphonic	87	2.26	1.15	−0.70	4.58	<0.001
Dysphonic	108	3.07	1.75	−0.91	9.38	
Perceptually assessed B Non-dysphonic	87	0.37	0.35	0	1.25	<0.001
Dysphonic	108	1.26	0.74	0	3	

3.3. Sensitivity and Specificity of ABI

The ability of the ABI to distinguish between breathy and nonbreathy voices was evaluated with ROC analysis. $A_{ROC} = 0.886$ (i.e., 88.6%) showed high discriminatory power to distinguish nonbreathy voices from breathy voices (Figure 3). The highest Youden's index was 0.60, where the best sensitivity of 80% and specificity of 80% were obtained at the cut point value 2.68. In the likelihood ratio the statistical guideline values were not reached (likelihood ratios LR+ 4.00 and LR− 0.25). Table 3 shows the threshold values of the eight previous ABI validation studies and the cut-point value of the Finnish validation study, as well as the statistical values of sensitivity, specificity, likelihood ratios, and the correlations between the ABI and the perceptual evaluation.

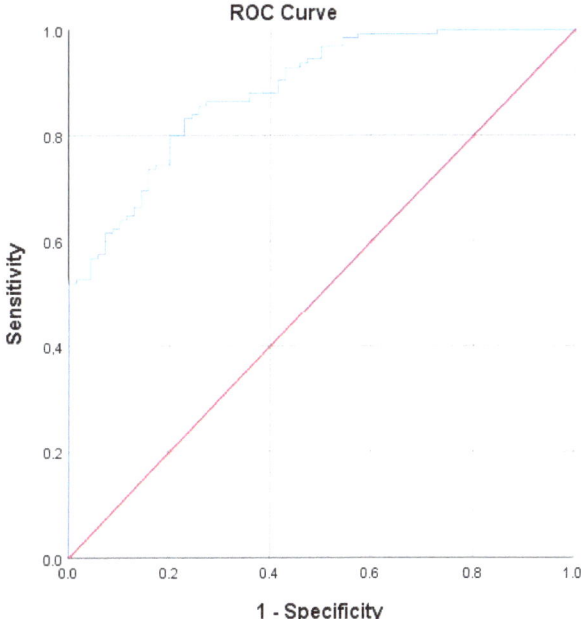

Figure 3. ROC curve analysis illustrating the diagnostic accuracy of ABI, area under ROC curve = 88.6% (A_{ROC} line blue, reference line red).

Table 3. The results of nine ABI-validated languages showing ABI thresholds, sensitivities, specificities, likelihood ratios, and correlation values r_s between the ABI and perceptual evaluation of breathiness (B).

Language	ABI Cut-Off Value	Sensitivity %	Specificity %	LR+	LR−	Correlation r_s between ABI and B
Dutch	3.44	82	93	11.63	0.19	0.84
German	3.42	72	90	7.40	0.31	0.86
Japanese	3.44	76	94	8.09	0.13	0.89
Korean	3.69	88	86	6.47	0.14	0.87
Brazilian Portuguese	3.13	88	91	−0.03	0.13	0.87
Spanish	3.40	74	95	16.02	0.27	0.83
South Indian	3.66	62	95	12.19	2.48	0.76
Persian	2.97	70	87	5.44	0.35	0.74
Finnish	2.68	80	80	4.00	0.25	0.82

4. Discussion

This study aimed to investigate whether the acoustic breathiness index (ABI) is a valid and robust method to distinguish dysphonic breathiness from healthy voices in a Finnish speaking population, and, if so, what the best threshold value for ABI would be. These research questions are important; while breathiness is one of the main characteristics in dysphonia and the first component of hoarseness [41], it is also frequently found in the non-dysphonic population. This requires a more focused, multi-parameter tool for the detection of true breathiness and to be able to distinguish dysphonic breathiness. Breathiness appears to be perceived better in females' voices but reduced loudness of voice increases its presence in both genders [42]. It has been found to be related to perceptions of femininity and attractiveness in female voice quality [5,43], and it may also be related to attractiveness in male voices [44], although voice characteristics evoke different evaluations in different cultures [45,46].

Some breathiness was perceived in some of the healthy voices in the present study. This is to be expected, as breathiness is also a cultural characteristic. In particular, vocologists who work with normal and supranormal (trained) voices were more sensitive than clinicians (phoniatrician/otolaryngologists and speech therapists) in rating breathiness. The main reason for including raters from different professional groups was to get a larger distribution of evaluations, which would also take into account the existence of some breathiness in normal voices. Furthermore, breathiness was the only characteristic that was rated in the present study; thus, the raters had to focus on this particular characteristic, which the acoustic tool was also specifically developed to measure.

The results of the present study show that the dysphonic voices scored significantly higher both on perceived breathiness and ABI, although the dysphonic group included patients with very different diagnoses and thus with different acoustic characteristics. This suggests that ABI measures what it is intended to measure. Perceived breathiness correlated strongly with ABI (r_s 0.823, p 0.01) suggesting the ecological validity of the index. The discriminatory power of the ABI was high (88.6), showing that the method successfully differentiated between the dysphonic and non-dysphonic groups. The highest sensitivity (80%) and specificity (80%) in differentiation was obtained at ABI = 2.68. This can be thus used as a threshold for the clinical analysis of breathiness in a Finnish speaking population. Other studies [12,24,27–32] have reported slightly higher threshold values than what was found in the present study (Table 3). The reason may be related to language and cultural differences [29]. The Finnish language has a high prevalence of vowels, and a lack of linguistically breathy vowels that occur for instance in Gujarati, Mon-Khmer and Jalapa Mazatec [47], or sonorous fricatives. Finns may be more sensitive in perceiving breathiness. It may be speculated whether there could be a connection to some earlier findings where breathy voice quality seemed to convey an impression of emotional instability and implausibility of the speaker among Finnish listeners [46,48].

The mean age in the dysphonic group of the present study was somewhat higher than that of the non-dysphonic group and, in both groups, females were in the majority. These characteristics reflect the clinical reality that dysphonic patients are typically not very young and that females form the majority of voice patients [49–51]. However, earlier findings have shown that the ABI is not significantly dependent on age or sex [22,27].

The use of only one perceptual variable in the listening evaluation may be seen as a limitation in the study since then the presence of other potential characteristics of hoarseness remain unknown. This is, however, the policy that other ABI validation studies have adopted [12,24,28,30,32]. Further study of the average ABI results for different diagnostic groups is warranted. This would require larger numbers of participants in different diagnostic groups. Such a study should also address further the capability of listeners and ABI to differentiate between breathiness and other components of dysphonia by including other perceptual variables than merely the B.

5. Conclusions

The present study showed that the ABI is a robust and valid tool for use with a Finnish-speaking population. It distinguishes well between healthy and dysphonic voices. The threshold value for breathiness in Finnish healthy and dysphonic voices was 2.68.

Author Contributions: E.K. and A.-M.L. contributed equally to the study and the article. All authors have read and agreed to the published version of the manuscript.

Funding: This research received no external funding.

Institutional Review Board Statement: The study was conducted in accordance with the Declaration of Helsinki and approved by the Ethics Committee of Tampere University Hospital (R15014) 15 January 2015.

Informed Consent Statement: Informed consent was obtained from all subjects involved in the study.

Data Availability Statement: The data presented in this study are available on request from the corresponding author. The data are not publicly available due to privacy or ethical restrictions.

Conflicts of Interest: The authors declare no conflict of interest. No funder had any role in the design of the study; in the collection, analyses, or interpretation of data; in the writing of the manuscript; or in the decision to publish the results.

References

1. Hillenbrand, J.M.; Houde, R.A. Acoustic Correlates of Breathy Vocal Quality: Dysphonic Voices and Continuous Speech. *J. Speech Hear Res.* **1996**, *39*, 311–321. [CrossRef] [PubMed]
2. Colton, R.H.; Casper, J.K.; Leonard, R. *Understanding Voice Problems: A Physiological Perspective for Diagnosis and Treatment.*; Lippincott Williams & Wilkins: Baltimore, MD, USA, 2006.
3. Dejonckere, P.H.; Obbens, C.; De Moor, G.M.; Wieneke, G.H. Perceptual Evaluation of Dysphonia: Reliability and Relevance. *Folia Phoniatr. Logop.* **1993**, *45*, 76–83. [CrossRef] [PubMed]
4. Mendoza, E.; Valencia, N.; Muñoz, J.; Trujillo, H. Differences in Voice Quality between Men and Women: Use of the Long-Term Average Spectrum (LTAS). *J. Voice* **1996**, *10*, 59–66. [CrossRef] [PubMed]
5. Van Borsel, J.; Janssens, J.; De Bodt, M. Breathiness as a Feminine Voice Characteristic: A Perceptual Approach. *J. Voice* **2009**, *23*, 291–294. [CrossRef] [PubMed]
6. Hirano, M. Psycho-Acoustic Evaluation of Voice. In *Book Disorders of Human Communication 5. Clinical Examination of Voice*; Hirano, M., Arnold, G.E., Winckel, F., Wyke, B.D., Eds.; Springer: Vienna, Austria, 1981.
7. Dejonckere, P.H.; Wieneke, G.H. Cepstra of Normal and Pathological Voices: Correlation with Acoustic, Aerodynamic and Perceptual Data. *Adv. Clin. Phon.* **1996**, *6*, 217–226.
8. Kempster, G.B.; Verdolini Abbott, K.; Barkmeier-Kraemer, J.; Hillman, R. Consensus Auditory-Perceptual Evaluation of Voice: Development of a Standardized Clinical Protocol. *Am. J. Speech Lang. Pathol.* **2009**, *8*, 124–132. [CrossRef]
9. Oates, J.; Russell, A. Learning Voice Analysis Using an Interactive Multi-Media Package: Development and Preliminary Evaluation. *J. Voice* **1998**, *12*, 500–512. [CrossRef]
10. Hammarberg, B. Voice Research and Clinical Needs. *Folia Phoniatr. Logop.* **2000**, *52*, 93–102. [CrossRef]
11. Iwarsson, J.; Bingen-Jakobsen, A.; Johansen, D.S.; Kølle, I.E.; Pedersen, S.G.; Thorsen, S.L.; Petersen, N.R. Auditory-Perceptual Evaluation of Dysphonia: A Comparison Between Narrow and Broad Terminology Systems. *J. Voice* **2018**, *32*, 428–436. [CrossRef]
12. Latoszek, B.B.v.; Maryn, Y.; Gerrits, E.; De Bodt, M. The Acoustic Breathiness Index (ABI): A Multivariate Acoustic Model for Breathiness. *J. Voice* **2017**, *31*, 511.e11–511.e27. [CrossRef]
13. Penido, F.A.; Gama, A.C.C. Accuracy Analysis of the Multiparametric Acoustic Indices AVQI, ABI, and DSI for Speech-Language Pathologist Decision-Making. *J. Voice*, 2023, in press. [CrossRef]
14. Kankare, E.; Latoszek, B.B.v.; Maryn, Y.; Asikainen, M.; Rorarius, E.; Vilpas, S.; Rantala, L.; Laukkanen, A.M. The Acoustic Voice Quality Index Version 02.02 in the Finnish-Speaking Population. *Logoped. Phoniatr. Vocol.* **2020**, *45*, 49–56. [CrossRef]
15. De Krom, G. A Cepstrum-Based Technique for Determining a Harmonics-to-Noise Ratio in Speech Signals. *J. Speech Lang. Hear. Res.* **1993**, *36*, 254–266. [CrossRef] [PubMed]
16. Deliyski, D. Acoustic Model and Evaluation of Pathological Voice Production. In Proceedings of the Third European Conference on Speech Communication and Technology Eurospeech, Berlin, Germany, 22–25 September 1993; pp. 1969–1972.
17. Bhuta, T.; Patrick, L.; Garnett, J.D. Perceptual Evaluation of Voice Quality and Its Correlation with Acoustic Measurements. *J. Voice* **2004**, *18*, 299–304. [CrossRef]
18. Hillenbrand, J.M.; Cleveland, R.A.; Erickson, R.L. Acoustic Correlates of Breathy Vocal Quality. *J. Speech Hear Res.* **1994**, *37*, 769–778. [CrossRef] [PubMed]
19. Glaze, L.E.; Bless, D.M.; Susser, R.D. Acoustic Analysis of Vowel and Loudness Differences in Children's Voice. *J. Voice* **1990**, *4*, 37–44. [CrossRef]

20. Orlikoff, R.F.; Kahane, J.C. Influence of Mean Sound Pressure Level on Jitter and Shimmer Measures. *J. Voice* **1991**, *5*, 113–119. [CrossRef]
21. Brockmann-Bauser, M.; Bohlender, J.E.; Mehta, D.D. Acoustic Perturbation Measures Improve with Increasing Vocal Intensity in Individuals with and without Voice Disorders. *J. Voice* **2018**, *32*, 162–168. [CrossRef]
22. Latoszek, B.B.v.; Maryn, Y.; Gerrits, E.; De Bodt, M. A Meta-Analysis: Acoustic Measurement of Roughness and Breathiness. *J. Speech Lang. Hear Res.* **2018**, *61*, 298–323. [CrossRef]
23. Maryn, Y.; Roy, N.; De Bolt, M.; Van Cauwenberge, P.; Corthals, P. Acoustic Measurement of Overall Voice Quality: A Meta-Analysis. *J. Acoust. Soc. Am.* **2009**, *126*, 2619–2634. [CrossRef]
24. Latoszek, B.B.v.; Lehnert, B.; Janotte, B. Validation of the Acoustic Voice Quality Index Version 03.01 and Acoustic Breathiness Index in German. *J. Voice* **2020**, *34*, 157.e17–157.e25. [CrossRef]
25. Michaelis, D.; Gramss, T.; Strube, H.W. Glottal-to-Noise Excitation Ratio—A New Measure for Describing Pathological Voices. *Acta Acust. United Acust.* **1997**, *83*, 700–706.
26. Dejonckere, P.H.; Lebacq, J. Harmonic Emergence in Formant Zone of a Sustained [a] as a Parameter for Evaluating Hoarseness. *Acta Otorhinolaryngol. Belg.* **1987**, *41*, 988–996. [PubMed]
27. Hosokawa, K.; von Latoszek, B.B.; Ferrer-Riesgo, C.A.; Iwahashi, T.; Iwahashi, M.; Iwaki, S.; Kato, C.; Yoshida, M.; Umatani, M.; Miyauchi, A.; et al. Acoustic Breathiness Index for the Japanese-Speaking Population: Validation Study and Exploration of Affecting Factors. *J. Speech Lang. Hear Res.* **2019**, *62*, 2617–2631. [CrossRef] [PubMed]
28. Kim, G.-H.; von Latoszek, B.B.; Lee, Y.-W. Validation of Acoustic Voice Quality Index Version 3.01 and Acoustic Breathiness Index in Korean Population. *J. Voice* **2021**, *35*, 660.e9–660.e18. [CrossRef] [PubMed]
29. Englert, M.; Lima, L.; Behlau, M. Acoustic Voice Quality Index and Acoustic Breathiness Index: Analysis With Different Speech Material in the Brazilian Portuguese. *J. Voice* **2020**, *34*, 810.e11–810.e17. [CrossRef]
30. Delgado Hernández, J.; León Gómez, N.M.; Jiménez, A.; Izquierdo, L.M.; Latoszek, B.B.v. Validation of the Acoustic Voice Quality Index Version 03.01 and the Acoustic Breathiness Index in the Spanish Language. *Annal. Otol. Rhinol. Laryngol.* **2018**, *127*, 317–326. [CrossRef] [PubMed]
31. Jayakumar, T.; Benoy, J. Validation of Acoustic Breathiness Index (ABI) in the South Indian Population. *J. Voice*, **2022**, *in press*. [CrossRef] [PubMed]
32. Aghajanzadeh, M.; Saeedi, S.; Jalaie, S.; Esarian, K.; Latoszek, B.B.v. Validation of the Acoustic Voice Quality Index and the Acoustic Breathiness Index in the Persian Language. *J. Voice*, **2023**, *in press*. [CrossRef]
33. Ma, E.P.-M.; Yiu, E.M.-L. Voice Activity and Participation Profile: Assessing the Impact of Voice Disorders on Daily Activities. *J. Speech Lang. Hear Res.* **2001**, *44*, 511–524. [CrossRef]
34. Kleemola, L.; Helminen, M.; Rorarius, E.; Isotalo, E.; Sihvo, M. Voice Activity and Participation Profile in Assessing the Effects of Voice Disorders on Quality of Life: Estimation of the Validity, Reliability and Responsiveness of the Finnish Version. *Folia Phoniatr. Logop.* **2010**, *63*, 113–121. [CrossRef]
35. Kankare, E.; Rantala, L.; Ikävalko, T.; Latoszek, B.B.v.; Laukkanen, A.-M. Akustisen Äänenlaatuindeksin (AVQI) Version 03.01 Validointi Suomenkielisille Puhujille. *Puhe Kieli* **2020**, *40*, 165–182. [CrossRef]
36. Barsties, B.; Maryn, Y. The Improvement of Internal Consistency of the Acoustic Voice Quality Index. *Am. J. Otolaryngol.* **2015**, *36*, 647–656. [CrossRef] [PubMed]
37. Gierlich, J.; Latoszek, B.B.v. Test-Retest Reliability of the Acoustic Voice Quality Index and the Acoustic Breathiness Index. *J. Voice*, **2023**, *in press*. [CrossRef] [PubMed]
38. Brinca, L.; Batista, A.P.; Tavares, A.I.; Pinto, P.N.; Araújo, L. The Effect of Anchors and Training on the Reliability of Voice Quality Ratings for Different Types of Speech Stimuli. *J. Voice* **2015**, *29*, 776.e7–776.e14. [CrossRef] [PubMed]
39. dos Santos, P.C.M.; Vieira, M.N.; Sansão, J.P.H.; Gama, A.C.C. Effect of Auditory-Perceptual Training With Natural Voice Anchors on Vocal Quality Evaluation. *J. Voice* **2019**, *33*, 220–225. [CrossRef]
40. Landis, J.R.; Koch, G. The Measurement of Observer Agreement for Categorical Data. *Biometrics* **1977**, *33*, 159–174. [CrossRef]
41. Dejonckere, P.H.; Lebacq, J. Acoustic, Perceptual, Aero-Dynamic and Anatomical Correlations Invoice Pathology. *J. Oto-Rhino-Laryngol. Relat. Specialt.* **1996**, *58*, 326–332. [CrossRef]
42. Södersten, M.; Lindestad, P.-Å. Glottal Closure and Perceived Breathiness During Phonation in Normally Speaking Subjects. *J. Speech Lang. Hear Res.* **1990**, *33*, 601–611. [CrossRef]
43. Liu, X.; Xu, Y. What Makes a Female Voice Attractive? In Proceedings of the Proceedings of ICPhS XVII, Hong Kong, China, 17–21 August 2011; pp. 1274–1277.
44. Šebesta, P.; Kleisner, K.; Tureček, P.; Kočnar, T.; Akoko, R.M.; Třebický, V.; Havlíček, J. Voices of Africa: Acoustic Predictors of Human Male Vocal Attractiveness. *Anim. Behav.* **2017**, *127*, 205–211. [CrossRef]
45. Giles, H. Ethnicity Markers in Speech. In *Book Social Markers in Speech*; Scherer, K.R., Giles, H., Eds.; Cambridge University Press: Cambridge, UK, 1979.
46. Waaramaa, T.; Lukkarila, P.; Järvinen, K.; Geneid, A.; Laukkanen, A.-M. Impressions of Personality from Intentional Voice Quality in Arabic-Speaking and Native Finnish-Speaking Listeners. *J. Voice* **2021**, *35*, 326.e21–326.e28. [CrossRef]
47. Ladefoged, P.; Maddieson, I. Vowels of the World's Languages. *J. Phon.* **1990**, *18*, 93–122. [CrossRef]
48. Lukkarila, P.; Laukkanen, A.M.; Palo, P. Influence of the Intentional Voice Quality on the Impression of Female Speaker. *Logoped. Phoniatr. Vocol.* **2012**, *37*, 158–166. [CrossRef]

49. De Bodt, M.; Van den Steen, L.; Mertens, F.; Raes, J.; Van Bel, L.; Heylen, L.; Pattyn, J.; Gordts, F.; van de Heyning, P. Characteristics of a Dysphonic Population Referred for Voice Assessment and/or Voice Therapy. *Folia Phoniatr. Logop.* **2016**, *67*, 178–186. [CrossRef]
50. Mozzanica, F.; Ginocchio, D.; Barillari, R.; Barozzi, S.; Maruzzi, P.; Ottaviani, F.; Schindler, A. Prevalence and Voice Characteristics of Laryngeal Pathology in an Italian Voice Therapy-Seeking Population. *J. Voice* **2016**, *30*, 774.e13–774.e21. [CrossRef] [PubMed]
51. Remacle, A.; Petitfils, C.; Flinck, C.; Morsomme, D. Description of Patients Consulting the Voice Clinic Regarding Gender, Age, Occupational Status, and Diagnosis. *Eur. Arch. Otorhinolaryngol.* **2017**, *274*, 1567–1576. [CrossRef] [PubMed]

Disclaimer/Publisher's Note: The statements, opinions and data contained in all publications are solely those of the individual author(s) and contributor(s) and not of MDPI and/or the editor(s). MDPI and/or the editor(s) disclaim responsibility for any injury to people or property resulting from any ideas, methods, instructions or products referred to in the content.

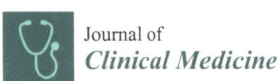 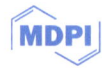

Article

Accuracy Analysis of the Multiparametric Acoustic Voice Indices, the VWI, AVQI, ABI, and DSI Measures, in Differentiating between Normal and Dysphonic Voices

Virgilijus Uloza [1], Kipras Pribuišis [1], Nora Ulozaite-Staniene [1,*], Tadas Petrauskas [1], Robertas Damaševičius [2] and Rytis Maskeliūnas [2]

[1] Department of Otorhinolaryngology, Lithuanian University of Health Sciences, 50061 Kaunas, Lithuania; virgilijus.ulozas@lsmuni.lt (V.U.); kipras.pribuisis@lsmuni.lt (K.P.); tadas@petrauskas.co.uk (T.P.)
[2] Faculty of Informatics, Kaunas University of Technology, 51368 Kaunas, Lithuania
* Correspondence: nora.ulozaite@lsmuni.lt

Abstract: The study aimed to investigate and compare the accuracy and robustness of the multiparametric acoustic voice indices (MAVIs), namely the Dysphonia Severity Index (DSI), Acoustic Voice Quality Index (AVQI), Acoustic Breathiness Index (ABI), and Voice Wellness Index (VWI) measures in differentiating normal and dysphonic voices. The study group consisted of 129 adult individuals including 49 with normal voices and 80 patients with pathological voices. The diagnostic accuracy of the investigated MAVI in differentiating between normal and pathological voices was assessed using receiver operating characteristics (ROC). Moderate to strong positive linear correlations were observed between different MAVIs. The ROC statistical analysis revealed that all used measurements manifested in a high level of accuracy (area under the curve (AUC) of 0.80 and greater) and an acceptable level of sensitivity and specificity in discriminating between normal and pathological voices. However, with AUC 0.99, the VWI demonstrated the highest diagnostic accuracy. The highest Youden index equaled 0.93, revealing that a VWI cut-off of 4.45 corresponds with highly acceptable sensitivity (97.50%) and specificity (95.92%). In conclusion, the VWI was found to be beneficial in describing differences in voice quality status and discriminating between normal and dysphonic voices based on clinical diagnosis, i.e., dysphonia type, implying the VWI's reliable voice screening potential.

Keywords: acoustic voice analysis; screening; DSI; AVQI; ABI; VWI

1. Introduction

A multidimensional approach is used in clinical practice to diagnose laryngeal/voice abnormalities. This approach includes subjective evaluation of a voice both by the medical professional and the patient, objective measurement of voice acoustics and voice aerodynamics, and visualizing the larynx using video laryngostroboscopy (VLS) [1].

In this context, acoustic voice analysis plays a crucial role in the assessment of vocal function and diagnostics in phoniatrics and laryngology [2]. Voice acoustic data are noninvasive, reasonably easy-to-capture, and accurate biomarkers that also offer workable and trustworthy options for dysphonia screening and monitoring. Therefore, measurement of acoustic voice signals represents the most commonly used instrumental tool in clinical practice and research for objectively and quantitative characterizing voice quality [3,4].

In the last decades, numerous acoustic analysis algorithms were developed to measure the pitch, amplitude and waveform perturbation, and spectral and cepstral characteristics of sound waves [2,5]. In order to address the limiting validity of a single acoustic parameter in comparison to the multidimensionality of voice signals, researchers have created several multiparametric acoustic voice indices (MAVIs) during the past few decades. These indices assess and fuse multiple acoustic voice parameters based on the domains of time, frequency, amplitude, and quefrency while taking into consideration both sustained phonation and connected speech and provide a single score that measures voice quality [6–8].

Nowadays, several MAVI models based on sustained vowels and continuous speech have been introduced in research and clinical practice for the evaluation of voice quality: the Dysphonia Severity Index (DSI), the Acoustic Voice Quality Index (AVQI), the Acoustic Breathiness Index (ABI), and the Voice Wellness Index (VWI).

Wuyts et al.'s DSI model, presented in 2000, is a multivariate model that provides an objective and quantitative indicator of overall voice quality by incorporating acoustic (jitter, and the lowest intensity and highest fundamental frequency in the vocal range profile) and aerodynamic (maximum phonation time of the vowel [a:]) markers [9]. DSI has been regarded as a valuable and viable assessment for assessing overall voice quality, voice treatment, vocal training, and phonosurgery results [10–17]. Additional research found connections between the DSI and auditory-perceptual judgment and quality of life evaluation, establishing the DSI as a valid approach for evaluating dysphonia severity [13–15,18–20]. The findings of the comparison research revealed that the DSI and AVQI's performances were comparable with an elevated degree of accuracy in distinguishing among normal and dysphonic voices [21].

The DSI is originally scored from −5 to +5, in which an average subject with a normal healthy voice has a score of +5, and −5 indicates a severely disordered voice [9]. However, it should be noticed that the DSI value might vary across different geographic regions, age, vocal performance, and ethnic groups [19,22–24]. In meta-analysis performed on a group of healthy adult participants, the mean normative value of the DSI was +3.05 (the confidence level was 2.13–3.98) [25].

The AVQI is a six-variable acoustic model developed by Maryn et al. in 2010 [26] for the multiparametric measurement of voice quality concatenating both the sustained vowel [a:] and the voiced parts of a continuous speech fragment. The equation of the AVQI includes acoustic markers from time, frequency, and quefrency domains, and it is a multidimensional representation of the dysphonia severity. The AVQI scores may range from 0 to 10 points with a higher score indicating more severe dysphonia. Numerous studies have confirmed the remarkable features of the AVQI, including its high consistency, concurrent validity, test-retest reliability, high sensitivity to changes in voice quality brought about by voice therapy, usefulness in differentiating between dysphonia severity levels perceptually, and adequate diagnostic accuracy between normal and pathological voices with good discriminatory power [27–30]. The AVQI values are independent of age and gender, which expands the possibilities for the further generalization of this tool for potential voice-screening applications [24]. In consequence, the AVQI is currently regarded as a globally recognized multiparametric voice quality assessment instrument for clinical and research applications [31–33].

The ABI is a multiparametric, nine-variable acoustic measure based on concatenated samples of continuous speech and the sustained vowel /a/ to quantify the degree of breathiness with a single score, and was developed by Barsties v Latoszek in 2017 [34]. The ABI score ranges from 0 to 10, and the higher an ABI score, the more severe the breathiness, and vice versa.

The ABI revealed highly reliable results in a test-retest measurement of vocally healthy subjects [35]. The results of several studies confirmed the ABI as a robust and valid objective measure for evaluating breathiness because ABI scores and perceived breathiness ratings were shown to be strongly correlated; however, neither age and gender nor roughness significantly affected the ABI in the evaluation of natural voices [4,36]. In addition, the ABI also indicates highly sensitive therapy-related voice quality changes and, therefore, is useful for therapy studies in order to more accurately characterize differences in voice quality before and after treatment [4,37]. Also, the ABI appears to be relatively robust to phonetic inter-language differences [38]. The diagnostic accuracy of the ABI in distinguishing between normal and pathological voices revealed in different validation studies showed high to very high results in terms of both sensitivity and specificity [37].

The VWI integrates the voice-related data from two different information sources (i.e., acoustic voice analysis, such as the AVQI and Glottal Function Questionnaire (GFI), as patient-reported outcome measures) and supports the concept that the voice assessment process should consider the multidimensionality involved in the manifestation of voice disorders. The VWI is the equalizing proportion summation of the AVQI and GFI scores [39]. The VWI scores may range from 0 to 20 points with a higher score indicating more severe dysphonia. The results of the recent study showed that VWI application represents an accurate and reliable tool for voice quality measurement and normal versus pathological voice screening, manifesting in excellent diagnostic accuracy (AUC = 0.972) and the best balance between sensitivity (94.15%) and specificity (95.72%) [39].

The GFI questionnaire was developed by Bach et al. in 2005 [40]. It can be used as a compounding part of the VWI and represents a concise (four-item) and reliable symptom-based self-administered tool, which is focused on the functional aspects of voice disorder and easily comprehensible. Its purpose is to assess the extent of vocal dysfunction in adults. The GFI scores may range from 0 to 20 points with a higher score indicating more severe vocal dysfunction. The later studies revealed the GFI cut-off score of >3.0 points distinguishing dysphonic patients from healthy normal voice controls with a high level of sensitivity and specificity [41]. Additionally, the dysphonia screening potential of GFI was revealed by merging separate acoustic voice parameters with responses to GFI questions and combining AVQI and GFI measurements [42].

The examination of comparison research data indicated equal findings for the DSI and AVQI in terms of identifying normal and dysphonic voice, although the AVQI had greater validity features. Based on auditory-perceptual judgment, the research team concluded that the AVQI appears to be useful in defining variations in vocal quality state and distinguishing between normal and dysphonic voices [21]. However, the consequent study yielded that both these MAVIs can also differentiate between vocally healthy and voice-disordered subjects in comparison with the dysphonia classification based on the diagnosis of laryngeal disorder, thus enabling the quantification of abnormality [43]. In 2023, Penido et al. evaluated the AVQI, ABI, and DSI for speech–language pathologist decision-making in the assessment of teachers' voice complications. The findings of their study revealed that the AVQI, ABI, and DSI are measures that may provide substantial voice information and assist vocal healthcare providers in deciding on whether instructors should be professionally limited in their vocal activities [30].

However, the comparison of the MAVI in respect to the voice screening problem has not been tested before. Therefore, the aim of the study was to investigate and compare the accuracy and robustness of the multiparametric acoustic voice indices, the VWI, AVQI, ABI, and DSI measures in differentiating between normal and dysphonic voices.

2. Materials and Methods

The examinations of study participants took place at the Department of Otolaryngology, Lithuanian University of Health Sciences, Kaunas, Lithuania. All data from individuals with voice disorders were collected before any treatment, constituting the baseline. Informed consent was obtained from all the participants before their involvement in the study.

The inclusion criteria for the normal voice subgroup were as follows: (a) self-perceived normal voice with no voiced-related complaints, (b) absence of chronic laryngeal diseases or voice disorders history, (c) absence of pathological laryngeal alterations based on video videolaryngostroboscopy (VLS), and (d) evaluation of voice samples as normal by a laryngologist.

The pathological voice subgroup included a variety of laryngeal diseases and voice disturbances, notably benign and malignant mass lesions of the vocal folds and unilateral vocal fold paralysis. The inclusion criteria for this subgroup were: (a) complaints of voice disorders, (b) voice assessed as pathological by a laryngologist, (c) presence of laryngoscopically positive signs, and (d) histologically verified diagnosis in cases of mass lesions of the vocal folds.

The diagnosis of voice disorders relied on clinical examination (complaints and history), VLS, and histological verification of excised mass lesions of the vocal folds. Positive laryngoscopic findings comprised vocal fold hypertrophy, paralysis, and benign and malignant mass lesions of the vocal folds. Endolaryngeal microsurgical interventions were performed on subjects with mass lesions, and the diagnosis was verified by histological evaluation of the excised tissue. The final diagnosis was used to assess the diagnostic accuracy of the investigated MAVI in distinguishing among normal and pathological voice participants.

2.1. Glottal Function Index Questionnaire

Each participant of the study (normal and pathological voice subgroups) filled in the GFI questionnaire at the baseline, i.e., pre-treatment, along with voice recordings.

2.2. Voice Recordings

Voice recordings from the research participants were collected using a studio oral cardioid AKG Perception 220 microphone (AKG Acoustics, Vienna, Austria) in a T-series soundproof room for auditory assessment (T-room, CATegner AB, Bromma, Sweden). The microphone was set 10.0 cm away from the lips, maintaining a 90° microphone-to-mouth angle. Every individual was assigned two voice tasks that were recorded digitally. The challenges included phonating the vowel sound [a:] for at least 4 s and reciting a phonetically balanced text fragment in Lithuanian "Turėjo senelė žilą ožełį" ("The granny had a small grey goat"). The respondents were told to execute both voice activities at their personal volume and pitch. These narrations were recorded using the Audacity audio recording application (https://www.audacityteam.org/, accessed on 11 October 2023), at a sampling rate of 44.1 kHz and saved for storage on the computer's hard disk drive in a 16-bit resolution uncompressed "wav" audio file format.

2.3. DSI Estimation

The DSI was calculated using the Voice Diagnostic Center (VDS) (lingWAVES software, version 2.5, WEVOSYS, Forchheim, Germany). Firstly, the jitter percentage was calculated using a sustained vowel [a:] of no less than 2 s. Secondly, following maximal inhalation, maximal phonation duration was determined for vowel [a:] sustained for as long as feasible at a usual pitch and loudness. Thirdly, the individuals' voice range profiles were established. Only the lowest intensity (Ilow) and highest frequency (Fhigh) of the vocal range profiles were used to calculate the DSI. Lastly, the DSI was determined using lingWaves VDC Vospector analysis depending on the weighted combination of the highest frequency in Hz (FoHigh), lowest intensity in dBA (I-low), maximum phonation time in seconds (MPT), and jitter percentage.

2.4. AVQI Estimation

The Praat application (version 5.3.57; https://www.fon.hum.uva.nl/praat/, accessed on 11 October 2023) was used for processing the speech recordings for AVQI estimations. The speech recordings were combined in the following sequence: text segment, 2 s pause, 3 s sustained vowel/a/segment. The AVQI script version 02.02 designed for the Praat application was utilized for the acoustic analysis https://www.vvl.be/documenten-en-paginas/praat-script-avqi-v0203?download=AcousticVoiceQualityIndexv.02.03.txt, accessed 11 October 2023 [6].

2.5. ABI Estimation

For ABI calculations, the signal processing of the voice samples was conducted using the Praat software (version 5.4.22; https://www.fon.hum.uva.nl/praat/, accessed on 11 October 2023). The voice samples were analyzed using the ABI script developed for the Praat program (version 5.4.22): https://www.jvoice.org/cms/10.1016/j.jvoice.2016.11.017/attachment/c1 56729a-af1a-4973-b77d-940ccb085145/mmc1.docx, accessed on 11 October 2023 [4].

2.6. VWI Estimation

The "Voice Wellness Index" application for use both with iOS and Android operating devices was utilized for WVI estimation [39]. This application allows voice recording, automatically extracting acoustic voice features consisting of the AVQI, the GFI measures, and displaying the VWI result alongside a recommendation to the user.

2.7. Statistical Analysis

The statistical analysis was conducted using IBM SPSS Statistics for Windows, version 28.0.1.1 (Armonk, NY, USA: IBM Corp.) and MedCalc Version 20.118 (Ostend, Belgium, BE: MedCalc Software Ltd.). The chosen level of statistical significance was set at 0.05.

To assess the data distribution, the normality law was examined using the Shapiro–Wilk test of normality, along with the calculation of coefficients of skewness and kurtosis. In cases of normally distributed data, a Student's *t*-test was employed to test the equality of means. An analysis of variance (ANOVA) was utilized to ascertain significant differences among the multiple means of independent groups [44].

The linear relationship between variables obtained from continuous scales was evaluated using Pearson's correlation coefficient. To evaluate optimum sensitivity and specificity at appropriate cut-off values, receiver operating characteristic (ROC) curves were constructed. To assess discriminatory accuracy, the "area under the ROC curve" (AUC) was used. An AUC of more than 0.90 was deemed excellent, an AUC of less than 0.70 was considered low, and an AUC of less than 0.50 showed chance-level accuracy for diagnosis.

A pairwise analysis, as reported by De Long et al., was used to determine whether there were statistically significant variations among two or more factors when defining normal/pathological voices [45].

3. Results

3.1. Study Group

The research cohort comprised 129 adults, with 58 men and 71 women. The average age of the participants was 42.32 years (SD 14.83). Within the study, a subgroup of normal voices comprised 49 healthy volunteers (16 men and 33 women) with an average age of 31.69 years (SD 9.89). Conversely, the pathological voice subgroup consisted of 80 patients (42 men and 38 women) with an average age of 48.83 years (standard deviation 13.6). This subgroup presented a range of laryngeal diseases and associated voice disruptions, including benign and malignant mass lesions of the vocal folds and unilateral paralysis of the vocal folds.

The demographic data of the study group and diagnoses of the pathological voice subgroup are presented in Table 1.

Findings from prior research indicated no significant correlations between the subjects' age, sex, AVQI, and ABI measurements [31,36]. However, DSI values were found to be unrelated to sex but showed a slight correlation with age [43]. Consequently, in the current study, the control and patient groups were deemed appropriate for analyzing the investigated MAVI data, even though these groups were not matched in terms of sex and age.

Table 1. Demographic data of the study group.

Diagnosis	n	Age	
		Mean	SD
Normal voice	49	31.69	9.89
Mass lesions of the vocal folds (vocal fold polyp, nodules, cyst, granuloma)	49	44.39	12.4

Table 1. Cont.

Diagnosis	n	Age	
		Mean	SD
Vocal fold cancer (T1-2N0M0)	11	65.09	7.71
Chronic hyperplastic laryngitis	10	55.9	7.34
Unilateral vocal fold paralysis	6	40.83	12.77
Bilateral vocal fold paralysis	4	52.75	12.61
Total	129	42.32	14.83

Abbreviation: SD—standard deviation.

3.2. MAVI Evaluation Outcomes

The statistical analysis of the mean MAVI scores demonstrated significant differences ($p = 0.001$) between the normal and pathological voice groups. The specific details regarding the mean scores for various MAVIs are presented in Table 2.

Table 2. Mean MAVI scores in normal and pathological voice groups.

MAVI	Voice Group	n	F	Mean	Std. Deviation	p
Acoustic Breathiness Index	Normal voice	49	18.59	3.28	1.17	0.01
	Pathological	80		5.33	2.08	
Dysphonia Severity Index	Normal	49	0.03	6.28	2.22	0.01
	Pathological	80		−0.49	5.83	
Acoustic Voice Quality Index	Normal	49	30.78	2.09	0.77	0.01
	Pathological	80		4.26	1.80	
Voice Wellness Index	Normal	49	35.41	2.53	1.14	0.01
	Pathological	80		9.29	3.01	

Abbreviations: MAVI—Multiparametric Acoustic Voice Index; F—degrees of freedom.

Table 2 demonstrates the separate MAVI scores for the normal and pathological voice groups. The findings indicate that the normal voice group exhibited statistically significantly lower mean scores when compared to the pathological voice group.

Moderate to strong positive linear correlations were observed between different MAVIs. Pearson's correlation coefficients ranged from 0.446 to 0.881 and can be observed in Table 3.

Table 3. Correlations between different MAVI scores.

MAVI	Acoustic Breathiness Index	Dysphonia Severity Index	Acoustic Voice Quality Index	Voice Wellness Index
Acoustic Breathiness Index	1	0.45 *	0.88 *	0.72 *
Dysphonia Severity Index	0.45 *	1	0.56 *	0.54 *
Acoustic Voice Quality Index	0.88 *	0.56 *	1	0.76 *
Voice Wellness Index	0.72 *	0.54 *	0.76 *	1

*—Correlations are significant at the 0.01 level (2-tailed), Abbreviation: MAVI—Multiparametric Acoustic Voice Index.

3.3. Normal vs. Pathological Voice Diagnostic Accuracy of the Investigated MAVI

The ROC analysis was employed to assess the diagnostic accuracy of the investigated MAVI in distinguishing between normal and pathological voices. The ROC curves were visually examined to identify the optimal cut-off scores based on general interpretation guidelines [46]. Figure 1 displays the ROC curves for reference.

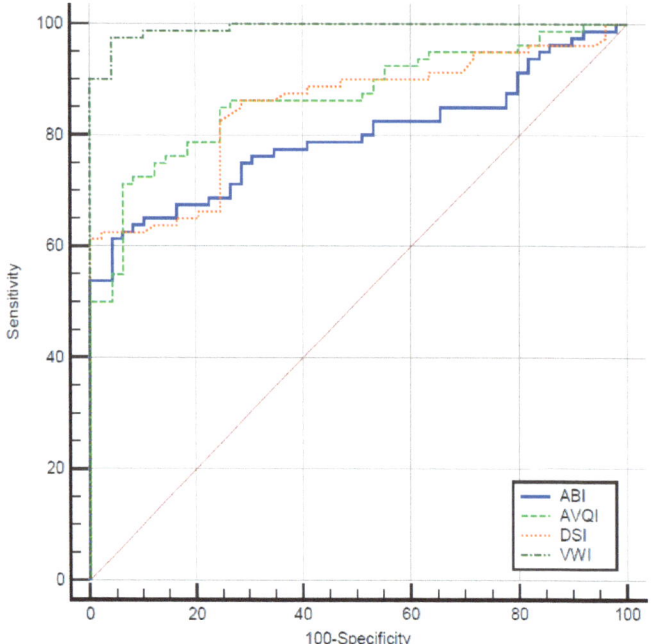

Figure 1. ROC curves illustrating the diagnostic accuracy of the Acoustic Breathiness Index (ABI), Acoustic Voice Quality Index (AVQI), Dysphonia Severity Index (DSI), and Voice Wellness Index (VWI) in discriminating between normal/pathological voices.

As depicted in Figure 1, the ROC curves generated from various MAVI values predominantly occupy the upper portion of the graph, surpassing the middle reference line. This observation distinctly underscores the commendable capability of the investigated MAVI in effectively distinguishing between normal and pathological voices. Notably, the VWI scores exhibited the largest area under the curve, indicating a higher predictive value and greater accuracy of this index in discerning between the normal and pathological voice groups.

The results of the detailed comparative ROC statistical analysis and the descriptive outcomes of the MAVI between normal and pathological voice groups are presented in Table 4.

Table 4. ROC statistics illustrating the accuracy of the different MAVIs in differentiating between normal and pathological voices.

MAVI	AUC	Cut-off	Sensitivity %	Specificity %	Youden-Index J
Acoustic Breathiness Index	0.80	4.87	61.25	95.92	0.57
Dysphonia Severity Index	0.85	−4.3	61.25	100	0.61
Acoustic Voice Quality Index	0.87	3.27	71.25	93.88	0.65
Voice Wellness Index	0.99	4.45	97.50	95.92	0.93

Abbreviations: ROC—Receiver Operating Curve; MAVI—Multiparametric Acoustic Voice Index; AUC—area under the curve.

Table 4 provides an overview of the statistics concerning the MAVI's ability to effectively differentiate between normal and pathological voice groups, yielding the following outcomes. The ROC statistical analysis indicated that all employed measurements exhibited a high accuracy (AUC of 0.80 and greater) and an acceptable balance of sensitivity and specificity in distinguishing between normal and pathological voices. The VWI, with an AUC of 0.99, demonstrated the highest diagnostic accuracy based on clinical diagnosis, specifically the dysphonia type. The highest Youden index, reaching 0.93, indicated a VWI cut-off of 4.45 corresponds to highly acceptable sensitivity (97.50%) and specificity (95.92%). Other MAVIs displayed AUCs ranging from 0.80 to 0.87, sensitivities from 61.25% to 71.25%, specificities from 95.92% to 100%, and Youden indices from 0.57 to 0.65, respectively. A further pairwise comparison of the AUC differences of separate MAVIs in discriminating between normal and pathological voices is presented in Table 5.

Table 5. A pairwise comparison of the AUC's differences of separate MAVIs in discriminating between normal and pathological voices.

MAVI	Acoustic Breathiness Index	Dysphonia Severity Index	Acoustic Voice Quality Index	Voice Wellness Index
Acoustic Breathiness Index	-	0.053	0.073 *	0.198 *
Dysphonia Severity Index	0.053	-	0.02	0.145 *
Acoustic Voice Quality Index	0.073 *	0.02	-	0.125 *
Voice Wellness Index	0.198 *	0.145 *	0.125 *	-

*—Significance level $p < 0.01$ level, Abbreviation: MAVI—Multiparametric Acoustic Voice Index.

As demonstrated in Table 5, the pairwise comparison of the significance of the differences between the AUCs of separate MAVIs, as described by DeLong et al., revealed that considering the AUCs, the VWI showed the statistically significantly highest difference when compared to the other MAVIs used in this study.

4. Discussion

For the very first time in a single research project and for exactly the same cohort of participants, the reliability of the multiparametric acoustic voice indices, the VWI, AVQI, ABI, and DSI measures in discriminating between normal and diseased voices was investigated in this study. Clinical evaluation, i.e., the findings of the examination of complaints, history, subjective voice assessment, laryngeal imaging, and histological research, was used to identify a p pathological voice. Strict standards for a normal voice were established. As a result, although diverse kinds of dysphonia were addressed, correct categorization between vocally healthy and voice-disordered participants was evaluated in the current investigation.

The results of this study, related to the ROC analysis, indicated that all four investigated indices, the VWI, AVQI, ABI, and DSI, revealed good discrimination between individuals with normal and pathological voices as determined via the clinical diagnosis of laryngeal disorder. However, among the four investigated indices, the VWI achieved an AUC of 0.99, sensitivity of 97.50%, and specificity of 95.92%, which showed greater power for reaching this goal. Thus, the comparative analysis of the results of the present study highlighted the significantly higher level of accuracy of the VWI in differentiating between normal and pathological voices, suggesting the reliable voice screening potential of the VWI.

These outcomes, to some extent, can be considered as predictable and comprehensible. The current findings are consistent with the statement in the literature that amalgamating acoustic voice analysis and the results of a patient's self-assessment provides complementary information that increases the strength, and reinforces the importance, of multidimensional assessment, thereby investigating different aspects of a voice disorder [33,42,47].

The results of the present study demonstrated the significantly higher power of the VWI obtained from voice recordings using a studio microphone to discriminate between normal and pathological voices compared to that of the DSI. The DSI is primarily regarded as an indicator of vocal function, and it is assumed to more accurately represent the capabilities or limits in vocal functioning, and it can be used as a universal measure of vocal performance and/or voice dysfunction [30]. The DSI includes just one acoustic parameter linked to voice quality (jitter percentage), and three other variables relating to voice performance and functionality: maximum phonation time, softest magnitude, and a higher frequency. The AVQI relies on six acoustic voice quality indicators and is regarded as being a superior indicator of overall voice quality [6], whereas the ABI relies on nine acoustic voice quality indicators and is better suited to identifying breathiness in voice quality, especially in cases of vocal fold nodules, paralysis, or paresis of the recurrent laryngeal nerve, and vocal fold bowing corresponding to presbyphonia [38].

In clinical practice, it is probable that people with or without laryngoscopic abnormalities cannot always be accurately classified by using auditory perceptual assessment or using acoustic parameters that have been validated as measures of perceived dysphonia severity. However, it is widely recognized from clinical experience that individuals exhibiting laryngoscopically aberrant symptoms can, in turn, produce a perceptually "normal" voice, and vice versa. This may be explained by the observation that the existence of a mass lesion or other structural variation in the vocal folds does not always result in dysphonia as perceived or as measured by acoustics, particularly if the lesion's location has little bearing on the vocal folds' vibratory characteristics. The VWI, which incorporates two sources of data known as the AVQI and GFI, guarantees that both of these modalities give related but distinct kinds of discriminating information useful for differentiating between healthy and pathological voices and boosts classification performance.

It is important to note that, despite the relative ease and consistency of DSI registration, this technique necessitates the assistance of a professionally qualified speech therapist or phoniatrician. As a result, DSI estimation cannot be automated and completed as a vocal "self-assessment" by a person. As a result, despite a lengthy tradition of evaluating the overall quality of a voice based on sustained vowels, this DSI registration peculiarity reduces the DSI's potential utility for voice pathology screening purposes. The multivariate structures of the VWI, AVQI, and ABI, on the other hand, depend on a linear regression model which incorporates pertinent acoustic parameters; they consist of both continuous speech and sustained vowel sounds in the acoustic evaluation, and the processing of signals employs freeware Praat algorithms, and can thus be standardized and made automated. This has already been realized in several applications available for AVQI estimation: VoiceEvalU8 [48], A Comprehensive Application for Grading Severity of Voice [29], VoiceScreen, version 4.4.22 [49], and ABI assessment: VOXplot, version 2.0 [50]. As a result, the registration of the AVQI, ABI, and VWI as an "ecologically valid" MAVI may be readily accomplished using specific programs, even without the presence of trained staff, allowing individuals to self-assess their voice quality. Consequently, these MAVIs suggest reliable voice screening options. Moreover, the VWI application provides recommendations to users based on the test results.

Merging the data from the two information sources has additional benefits for the VWI as the suitable method for differentiating between voice quality groups with and without disorders. The significant aspect of the VWI is its relatively high discrimination power based on the GFI data. Therefore, this sensor-independent data source with such a strong discrimination strength lessens the possibility of acoustic parameter-dependent variances resulting from variations in smartphone microphones and balances the effects of the two compounding parts (AVQI and GFI) on the VWI score. When using various voice recording devices, like various cellphones or other mobile communication devices, this capability is crucial.

Several of the current study's limitations must be taken into account. The study group of individuals with clinically discriminative organic laryngeal diseases and voice disorders served as the basis for the current study's findings. In order to maximize the comparability of various MAVIs, more research is needed of a broad range of vocal disorders, including functional voice disorders. The voice recordings for the current investigation were made in a soundproof room. Nevertheless, in actual clinical settings with background noise, the omnidirectional inbuilt microphones in cellphones might produce different outcomes.

Therefore, additional research is needed to assess how well the various MAVI applications work with various cellphones in a real-world clinical scenario, as well as the effects of the microphone's peculiarities and the speech recording environment.

5. Conclusions

All MAVIs used in this study, namely the DSI, AVQI, ABI, and VWI, displayed good accuracy in distinguishing between normal and dysphonic voices. The VWI, on the other hand, yielded greater validity characteristics. As a result, the VWI appears to be useful in defining changes in voice quality status and distinguishing between normal and dysphonic voices based on clinical diagnosis, i.e., the dysphonia type, implying the VWI's trustworthy voice screening capability.

Author Contributions: Conceptualization, V.U. and R.M.; methodology, R.D.; software, T.P.; validation, K.P., N.U.-S. and T.P.; formal analysis, K.P.; investigation, N.U.-S. and T.P.; resources, V.U.; data curation, T.P.; writing—original draft preparation, V.U.; writing—review and editing, R.M. and R.D.; supervision, V.U.; project administration, R.M.; funding acquisition, V.U. and R.M. All authors have read and agreed to the published version of the manuscript.

Funding: This project has received funding from the European Regional Development Fund (project No 13.1.1-LMT-K-718-05-0027) under a grant agreement with the Research Council of Lithuania (LMTLT). Funded as the European Union's measure in response to the COVID-19 pandemic and No. S-MIP-23-46.

Institutional Review Board Statement: The study was conducted in accordance with the Declaration of Helsinki of 1975, and the protocol was approved by the Kaunas Regional Ethics Committee for Biomedical Research (20 April 2022, No. BE-2-49).

Informed Consent Statement: Informed consent was obtained from all the subjects involved in the study.

Data Availability Statement: The data presented in this study are available on request from the corresponding author.

Conflicts of Interest: The authors declare no conflicts of interest.

References

1. Lechien, J.R.; Geneid, A.; Bohlender, J.E.; Cantarella, G.; Avellaneda, J.C.; Desuter, G.; Sjogren, E.V.; Finck, C.; Hans, S.; Hess, M.; et al. Consensus for voice quality assessment in clinical practice: Guidelines of the European Laryngological Society and Union of the European Phoniatricians. *Eur. Arch. Otorhinolaryngol.* **2023**, *280*, 5459–5473. [CrossRef] [PubMed]
2. Patel, R.R.; Awan, S.N.; Barkmeier-Kraemer, J.; Courey, M.; Deliyski, D.; Eadie, T.; Paul, D.; Švec, J.G.; Hillman, R. Recommended Protocols for Instrumental Assessment of Voice: American Speech-Language-Hearing Association Expert Panel to Develop a Protocol for Instrumental Assessment of Vocal Function. *Am. J. Speech Lang. Pathol.* **2018**, *27*, 887–905. [CrossRef] [PubMed]
3. Maryn, Y.; Roy, N.; De Bodt, M.; Van Cauwenberge, P.; Corthals, P. Acoustic measurement of overall voice quality: A meta-analysis. *J. Acoust. Soc. Am.* **2009**, *126*, 2619–2634. [CrossRef] [PubMed]
4. Latoszek, B.B.V.; Maryn, Y.; Gerrits, E.; De Bodt, M. A Meta-Analysis: Acoustic Measurement of Roughness and Breathiness. *J. Speech Lang. Hear. Res.* **2018**, *61*, 298–323. [CrossRef] [PubMed]
5. Narasimhan, S.V.; Rashmi, R. Multiparameter Voice Assessment in Dysphonics: Correlation Between Objective and Perceptual Parameters. *J. Voice* **2022**, *36*, 335–343. [CrossRef] [PubMed]
6. Maryn, Y.; Weenink, D. Objective dysphonia measures in the program Praat: Smoothed cepstral peak prominence and acoustic voice quality index. *J. Voice* **2015**, *29*, 35–43. [CrossRef] [PubMed]
7. Awan, S.N.; Roy, N.; Zhang, D.; Cohen, S.M. Validation of the Cepstral Spectral Index of Dysphonia (CSID) as a Screening Tool for Voice Disorders: Development of Clinical Cutoff Scores. *J. Voice* **2016**, *30*, 130–144. [CrossRef] [PubMed]
8. Murton, O.; Hillman, R.; Mehta, D. Cepstral Peak Prominence Values for Clinical Voice Evaluation. *Am. J. Speech Lang. Pathol.* **2020**, *29*, 1596–1607. [CrossRef]
9. Wuyts, F.L.; De Bodt, M.S.; Molenberghs, G.; Remacle, M.; Heylen, L.; Millet, B.; Van Lierde, K.; Raes, J.; Van de Heyning, P.H. The dysphonia severity index: An objective measure of vocal quality based on a multiparameter approach. *J. Speech Lang. Hear. Res.* **2000**, *43*, 796–809. [CrossRef]
10. Salmen, T.; Ermakova, T.; Möller, A.; Seipelt, M.; Weikert, S.; Rummich, J.; Gross, M.; Nawka, T.; Caffier, P.P. The Value of Vocal Extent Measure (VEM) Assessing Phonomicrosurgical Outcomes in Vocal Fold Polyps. *J. Voice* **2017**, *31*, 114.e7–114.e15. [CrossRef]

11. Song, W.; Caffier, F.; Nawka, T.; Ermakova, T.; Martin, A.; Mürbe, D.; Caffier, P.P. T1a Glottic Cancer: Advances in Vocal Outcome Assessment after Transoral CO_2-Laser Microsurgery Using the VEM. *J. Clin. Med.* **2021**, *10*, 1250. [CrossRef]
12. Wu, P.; Klein, L.; Rozema, Z.; Haderlein, N.; Cai, J.; Scholp, A.; Xu, X.; Jiang, J.J.; Zhuang, P. The Influence of Voice Training on Vocal Learner's Objective Acoustic Voice Components. *J. Voice* **2023**, *37*, 355–361. [CrossRef]
13. Aghadoost, S.; Jalaie, S.; Dabirmoghaddam, P.; Khoddami, S.M. Effect of Muscle Tension Dysphonia on Self-perceived Voice Handicap and Multiparametric Measurement and Their Relation in Female Teachers. *J. Voice* **2022**, *36*, 68–75. [CrossRef]
14. Ataee, E.; Khoramshahi, H.; Naderifar, E.; Dastoorpour, M. Relation Between Dysphonia Severity Index (DSI) and Consensus Auditory-Perceptual Evaluation of Voice (CAPE-V). *J. Voice* **2022**, *36*, 435.e1–435.e14. [CrossRef]
15. Graf, S.; Kirschstein, L.; Knopf, A.; Mansour, N.; Jeleff-Wölfler, O.; Buchberger, A.M.S.; Hofauer, B. Systematic evaluation of laryngeal impairment in Sjögren's syndrome. *Eur. Arch. Otorhinolaryngol.* **2021**, *278*, 2421–2428. [CrossRef]
16. Nasrin, S.; Ali, D.; Jamshid, J.; Hamed, G.; Bashir, R.; Hamide, G. The effects of Cricothyroid Visor Maneuver (CVM) therapy on the voice characteristics of patients with muscular tension dysphonia: A Case Series Study. *J. Voice* **2022**, in press. [CrossRef]
17. D'haeseleer, E.; Papeleu, T.; Leyns, C.; Adriaansen, A.; Meerschman, I.; Tomassen, P. Voice Outcome of Glottoplasty in Trans Women. *J. Voice* **2023**, in press. [CrossRef]
18. Hussein Gaber, A.G.; Liang, F.; Yang, J.; Wang, Y.; Zheng, Y. Correlation among the dysphonia severity index (DSI), the RBH voice perceptual evaluation, and minimum glottal area in female patients with vocal fold nodules. *J. Voice* **2014**, *28*, 20–23. [CrossRef]
19. Nemr, K.; Simões-Zenari, M.; de Souza, G.S.; Hachiya, A.; Tsuji, D.H. Correlation of the Dysphonia Severity Index (DSI), Consensus Auditory-Perceptual Evaluation of Voice (CAPE-V), and Gender in Brazilians with and Without Voice Disorders. *J. Voice* **2016**, *30*, 765.e7–765.e11. [CrossRef]
20. Mansouri, Y.; Naderifar, E.; Hajiyakhchali, A.; Moradi, N. The Relationship Between Dysphonia Severity Index and Voice-Related Quality of Life in the Elementary School Teachers with Voice Complaint. *J. Voice* **2023**, *37*, 466.e35–466.e39. [CrossRef]
21. Uloza, V.; Barsties VL, B.; Ulozaite, N.; Petrauskas, T.; Maryn, Y. A comparison of Dysphonia Severity Index and Acoustic Voice Quality Index measures in differentiating normal and dysphonic voices. *Eur. Arch. Otorhinolaryngol.* **2018**, *275*, 949–958. [CrossRef]
22. Goy, H.; Fernandes, D.N.; Pichora-Fuller, M.K.; van Lieshout, P. Normative voice data for younger and older adults. *J. Voice* **2013**, *27*, 545–555. [CrossRef] [PubMed]
23. Maruthy, S.; Ravibabu, P. Comparison of dysphonia severity index between younger and older carnatic classical singers and nonsingers. *J. Voice* **2015**, *29*, 65–70. [CrossRef] [PubMed]
24. Barsties V Latoszek, B.; Ulozaitė-Stanienė, N.; Maryn, Y.; Petrauskas, T.; Uloza, V. The Influence of Gender and Age on the Acoustic Voice Quality Index and Dysphonia Severity Index: A Normative Study. *J. Voice* **2019**, *33*, 340–345. [CrossRef] [PubMed]
25. Sobol, M.; Sielska-Badurek, E.M. The Dysphonia Severity Index (DSI)-Normative Values. Systematic Review and Meta-Analysis. *J. Voice* **2022**, *36*, 143.e9–143.e13. [CrossRef]
26. Maryn, Y.; De Bodt, M.; Roy, N. The Acoustic Voice Quality Index: Toward improved treatment outcomes assessment in voice disorders. *J. Commun. Disord.* **2010**, *43*, 161–174. [CrossRef]
27. Kankare, E.; Barsties V Latoszek, B.; Maryn, Y.; Asikainen, M.; Rorarius, E.; Vilpas, S.; Ilomäki, I.; Tyrmi, J.; Rantala, L.; Laukkanen, A. The acoustic voice quality index version 02.02 in the Finnish-speaking population. *Logoped. Phoniatr. Vocol.* **2020**, *45*, 49–56. [CrossRef]
28. Lehnert, B.; Herold, J.; Blaurock, M.; Busch, C. Reliability of the Acoustic Voice Quality Index AVQI and the Acoustic Breathiness Index (ABI) when wearing CoViD-19 protective masks. *Eur. Arch. Otorhinolaryngol.* **2022**, *279*, 4617–4621. [CrossRef]
29. Shabnam, S.; Pushpavathi, M.; Gopi Sankar, R.; Sridharan, K.V.; Vasanthalakshmi, M.S. A Comprehensive Application for Grading Severity of Voice Based on Acoustic Voice Quality Index v.03. *J. Voice* **2022**, in press. [CrossRef]
30. Penido, F.A.; Gama, A.C.C. Accuracy Analysis of the Multiparametric Acoustic Indices AVQI, ABI, and DSI for Speech-Language Pathologist Decision-Making. *J. Voice* **2023**, in press. [CrossRef]
31. Jayakumar, T.; Benoy, J.J.; Yasin, H.M. Effect of Age and Gender on Acoustic Voice Quality Index Across Lifespan: A Cross-sectional Study in Indian Population. *J. Voice* **2022**, *36*, 436.e1–436.e8. [CrossRef]
32. Batthyany, C.; Latoszek, B.B.V.; Maryn, Y. Meta-Analysis on the Validity of the Acoustic Voice Quality Index. *J. Voice* **2022**, in press. [CrossRef] [PubMed]
33. Saeedi, S.; Aghajanzadeh, M.; Khatoonabadi, A.R. A Literature Review of Voice Indices Available for Voice Assessment. *J. Rehabil. Sci. Res.* **2022**, *9*, 151–155. [CrossRef]
34. Barsties V Latoszek, B.; Maryn, Y.; Gerrits, E.; De Bodt, M. The Acoustic Breathiness Index (ABI): A Multivariate Acoustic Model for Breathiness. *J. Voice* **2017**, *31*, 511.e11–511.e27. [CrossRef] [PubMed]
35. Gierlich, J.; Latoszek, B.B.V. Test-Retest Reliability of the Acoustic Voice Quality Index and the Acoustic Breathiness Index. *J. Voice* **2023**, in press. [CrossRef] [PubMed]
36. Hosokawa, K.; Barsties, V.; Latoszek, B.; Ferrer-Riesgo, C.A.; Iwahashi, M.; Iwaki, S.; Kato, C.; Yoshida, M.; Umatani, M.; Miyauchi, A.; et al. Acoustic Breathiness Index for the Japanese-Speaking Population: Validation Study and Exploration of Affecting Factors. *J. Speech Lang. Hear. Res.* **2019**, *62*, 2617–2631. [CrossRef] [PubMed]
37. Latoszek, B.B.V.; Mathmann, P.; Neumann, K. The cepstral spectral index of dysphonia, the acoustic voice quality index and the acoustic breathiness index as novel multiparametric indices for acoustic assessment of voice quality. *Curr. Opin. Otolaryngol. Head Neck Surg.* **2021**, *29*, 451–457. [CrossRef] [PubMed]

38. Barsties V Latoszek, B.; Kim, G.; Delgado Hernández, J.; Hosokawa, K.; Englert, M.; Neumann, K.; Hetjens, S. The validity of the Acoustic Breathiness Index in the evaluation of breathy voice quality: A Meta-Analysis. *Clin. Otolaryngol.* **2021**, *46*, 31–40. [CrossRef] [PubMed]
39. Uloza, V.; Ulozaite-Staniene, N.; Pertrauskas, T.; Uloziene, I.; Pribuisis, K.; Blažauskas, T.; Damaševičius, R.; Maskeliūnas, R. Smartphone-based Voice Wellness Index application for dysphonia screening and assessment: Development and reliability. *J. Voice* **2023**, *in press*. [CrossRef]
40. Bach, K.K.; Belafsky, P.C.; Wasylik, K.; Postma, G.N.; Koufman, J.A. Validity and reliability of the glottal function index. *Arch. Otolaryngol. Head Neck Surg.* **2005**, *131*, 961–964. [CrossRef]
41. Cohen, J.T.; Oestreicher-Kedem, Y.; Fliss, D.M.; DeRowe, A. Glottal function index: A predictor of glottal disorders in children. *Ann. Otol. Rhinol. Laryngol.* **2007**, *116*, 81–84. [CrossRef]
42. Ulozaite-Staniene, N.; Petrauskas, T.; Šaferis, V.; Uloza, V. Exploring the feasibility of the combination of acoustic voice quality index and glottal function index for voice pathology screening. *Eur. Arch. Otorhinolaryngol.* **2019**, *276*, 1737–1745. [CrossRef]
43. Barsties V Latoszek, B.; Ulozaitė-Stanienė, N.; Petrauskas, T.; Uloza, V.; Maryn, Y. Diagnostic Accuracy of Dysphonia Classification of DSI and AVQI. *Laryngoscope* **2019**, *129*, 692–698. [CrossRef]
44. McHugh, M.L. Multiple comparison analysis testing in ANOVA. *Biochem. Med.* **2011**, *21*, 203–209. [CrossRef]
45. Hanley, J.A.; McNeil, B.J. The meaning and use of the area under a receiver operating characteristic (ROC) curve. *Radiology* **1982**, *143*, 29–36. [CrossRef]
46. Dollaghan, C.A. *The Handbook for Evidence-Based Practice in Communication Disorders*; Paul H. Brookes Pub.: Baltimore, MD, USA, 2007. Available online: https://worldcat.org/title/608392915 (accessed on 11 October 2023).
47. Lopes, L.W.; da Silva, J.D.; Simões, L.B.; Evangelista, D.d.S.; Silva, P.O.C.; Almeida, A.A.; de Lima-Silva, M.F.B. Relationship Between Acoustic Measurements and Self-evaluation in Patients with Voice Disorders. *J. Voice* **2017**, *31*, 119.e1–119.e10. [CrossRef]
48. Grillo, E.U.; Wolfberg, J. An Assessment of Different Praat Versions for Acoustic Measures Analyzed Automatically by VoiceEvalU8 and Manually by Two Raters. *J. Voice* **2023**, *37*, 17–25. [CrossRef]
49. Uloza, V.; Ulozaite-Staniene, N.; Petrauskas, T. An iOS-based VoiceScreen application: Feasibility for use in clinical settings-a pilot study. *Eur. Arch. Otorhinolaryngol.* **2023**, *280*, 277–284. [CrossRef]
50. Barsties V Latoszek, B.; Mayer, J.; Watts, C.R.; Lehnert, B. Advances in Clinical Voice Quality Analysis with VOXplot. *J. Clin. Med.* **2023**, *12*, 4644. [CrossRef]

Disclaimer/Publisher's Note: The statements, opinions and data contained in all publications are solely those of the individual author(s) and contributor(s) and not of MDPI and/or the editor(s). MDPI and/or the editor(s) disclaim responsibility for any injury to people or property resulting from any ideas, methods, instructions or products referred to in the content.

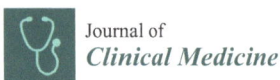

Article

Reliability of Universal-Platform-Based *Voice Screen* Application in AVQI Measurements Captured with Different Smartphones

Virgilijus Uloza [1], Nora Ulozaitė-Stanienė [1,*], Tadas Petrauskas [1], Kipras Pribuišis [1], Tomas Blažauskas [2], Robertas Damaševičius [2] and Rytis Maskeliūnas [2]

[1] Department of Otorhinolaryngology, Lithuanian University of Health Sciences, 50061 Kaunas, Lithuania; virgilijus.ulozas@lsmuni.lt (V.U.); tadas@petrauskas.co.uk (T.P.); kipras.pribuisis@lsmuni.lt (K.P.)
[2] Faculty of Informatics, Kaunas University of Technology, 51368 Kaunas, Lithuania; tomas.blazauskas@ktu.lt (T.B.); robertas.damasevicius@ktu.lt (R.D.); rytis.maskeliunas@ktu.lt (R.M.)
* Correspondence: nora.ulozaite@lsmuni.lt

Abstract: The aim of the study was to develop a universal-platform-based (UPB) application suitable for different smartphones for estimation of the Acoustic Voice Quality Index (AVQI) and evaluate its reliability in AVQI measurements and normal and pathological voice differentiation. Our study group consisted of 135 adult individuals, including 49 with normal voices and 86 patients with pathological voices. The developed UPB "*Voice Screen*" application installed on five iOS and Android smartphones was used for AVQI estimation. The AVQI measures calculated from voice recordings obtained from a reference studio microphone were compared with AVQI results obtained using smartphones. The diagnostic accuracy of differentiating normal and pathological voices was evaluated by applying receiver-operating characteristics. One-way ANOVA analysis did not detect statistically significant differences between mean AVQI scores revealed using a studio microphone and different smartphones (F = 0.759; p = 0.58). Almost perfect direct linear correlations (r = 0.991–0.987) were observed between the AVQI results obtained with a studio microphone and different smartphones. An acceptable level of precision of the AVQI in discriminating between normal and pathological voices was yielded, with areas under the curve (AUC) displaying 0.834–0.862. There were no statistically significant differences between the AUCs (p > 0.05) obtained from studio and smartphones' microphones. The significant difference revealed between the AUCs was only 0.028. The UPB "*Voice Screen*" application represented an accurate and robust tool for voice quality measurements and normal vs. pathological voice screening purposes, demonstrating the potential to be used by patients and clinicians for voice assessment, employing both iOS and Android smartphones.

Keywords: voice screen app; dysphonia screening; AVQI; smartphones

1. Introduction

Mobile communication devices such as smartphones or tablets are widely available to most of the global population, with the number of smartphone subscriptions expected to reach about 7145 billion by 2024 [1]. The increasing number of validated applications for smartphones in the field of general otorhinolaryngology and especially in a field related to voice assessment and management of voice disorders is permanently monitored in the literature [2–6]. Advances in smartphone technology and microphone quality offer an affordable and accessible alternative to studio microphones traditionally used for speech analysis, thus providing an effective tool for assessing, detecting, and caring for voice disorders [7–9].

The combination of variables in smartphone hardware and software may lead to differences between voice quality measures. Whether acoustic voice features recorded using smartphones sufficiently match the current gold standard for remote monitoring and clinical assessment with a studio microphone remains uncertain [7,10,11]. Some controversies on this matter in the literature still exist. Several studies found that smartphone-provided voice recordings and derived acoustic voice quality parameters are comparable to those derived using standard studio microphones [8,12–14]. Seung Jin Lee et al. found a significant correlation of several selected acoustic measures and no difference in the diagnostic ability between the Computerized Speech Lab and smartphone devices, although differences in several measures and higher cut-off scores of the smartphone were noted. Authors concluded that smartphones could be used as a screening tool for voice disorders [15]. On the other hand, using some other acoustic voice quality parameters could be discouraging [16]. Two recent studies found that none of the studied smartphones could replace the professional microphone in a voice recording to evaluate the six parameters analyzed, except for f_0 and jitter. Moreover, passing a voice signal through a telecom channel induced both filter and noise effects which significantly impacted common acoustic voice quality measures [17,18].

Nowadays, multiparametric models for voice quality assessment are generally accepted to be more reliable and valid than single-parameter measures because they demonstrate stronger correlations with auditory–perceptual voice evaluation and are more representative of daily use patterns. For example, the Acoustic Voice Quality Index (AVQI) is a six-variable acoustic model for the multiparametric measurement, evaluating both the voiced parts of a continuous speech fragment and a sustained vowel (a:), developed by Maryn et al. in 2010 [19,20].

Multiple studies across different languages have attested to the reliability of the AVQI as a clinical voice quality evaluation tool. High consistency, concurrent validity, test–retest reliability, high sensitivity to voice quality changes through voice therapy, utility in discriminating across the perceptual levels of dysphonia severity, and adequate diagnostic accuracy with good discriminatory power of the AVQI in differentiating between normal and abnormal voice qualities were observed [20–27]. It is noteworthy that several studies have reported that sex and age do not affect the overall AVQI value, thus proving the perspectives for further generalization of this objective and quantitative voice quality measurement [27–30]. Therefore, nowadays, AVQI is considered a recognized-around-the-globe multiparametric construct of voice quality assessment for its clinical and research applications [31–33].

Several previous studies have proved the suitability of using smartphone voice recordings performed both in acoustically treated sound-proof rooms or in ordinary users' environments to estimate the AVQI [4,9,11,14,27,34]. However, just a few studies in the literature provide data about AVQI realization using different applications for mobile communication devices [4,9,27]. The study by Grillo et al. in 2020 presented an application (*VoiceEvalU8*) that provided an automatic option for the reliable calculation of several acoustic voice measures and AVQIs on iOS and Android smartphones using the Praat source code and algorithms [4]. A user-friendly application/graphical user interface for the Kannada-speaking population was proposed by Shabnam et al. in 2022. The application provided a simplified output for AVQI cut-off values to depict the AVQI-based severity of dysphonia, which could be comprehendible by patients with voice disorders and health professionals [27]. The multilingual *"Voice Screen"* application developed by Uloza et al. allowed voice recording in clinical settings, automatically extracting acoustic voice features, estimating the AVQI result and displaying it alongside a recommendation to the user [9]. However, the *"Voice Screen"* application runs the iOS operating system, and that feature limits the usability only to iPhones, tablets, etc.

The results of the studies mentioned above enabled us to presume the feasibility of voice recordings captured with different smartphones for the estimation of AVQI. Consequently, the current research was designed to answer the following questions regarding the possibility of a smartphone-based *"Voice Screen"* application for AVQI estimation: (1) are the average AVQI values estimated by different smartphones consistent and comparable, and (2) are the diagnostic accuracy properties of different smartphone-estimated AVQIs relevant to differentiate normal and pathological voices? We hypothesize that using different smartphones for voice recordings and estimations of AVQI will be feasible for the quantitative voice assessment.

Therefore, the present study aimed to develop a universal-platform-based (UPB) application suitable for different smartphones for the estimation of AVQI and evaluate its reliability in AVQI measurements and normal/pathological voice differentiation.

2. Materials and Methods

All subjects gave their informed consent for inclusion before they participated in the study. The study was conducted in accordance with the Declaration of Helsinki of 1975, and the protocol was approved by the Kaunas Regional Ethics Committee for Biomedical Research (2022-04-20 No. BE-2-49).

The study group consisted of 135 adult individuals: 58 men and 77 women. The mean age of the study group was 42.9 (SD 15.26) years. They were all examined at the Department of Otolaryngology of the Lithuanian University of Health Sciences, Kaunas, Lithuania. The pathological voice subgroup consisted of 86 patients: 42 men and 44 women, with a mean age of 50.8 years (SD 14.3). They presented with a relatively common and clinically discriminative group of laryngeal diseases and related voice disturbances, i.e., benign and malignant mass lesions of the vocal folds and unilateral paralysis of the vocal fold. The normal voice subgroup consisted of 49 selected healthy volunteer individuals: 16 men and 33 women, mean age 31.69 (SD 9.89) years. This subgroup was collected following three criteria to define a vocally healthy subject: (1) all selected subjects considered their voice as normal and had no actual voice complaints and no history of chronic laryngeal diseases or voice disorders; (2) no pathological alterations in the larynx of the healthy subjects were found during video laryngoscopy; and (3) all these voice samples were evaluated as normal voices by otolaryngologists working in the field of voice. Demographic data of the study group and diagnoses of the pathological voice subgroup are presented in Table 1.

Table 1. Demographic data of the study group.

Diagnosis	n	Age	
		Mean	SD
Normal voice	49	31.69	9.89
Mass lesions of vocal folds	49	44.39	12.4
Vocal fold cancer	11	65.09	7.71
Chronic hyperplastic laryngitis	10	55.9	7.34
Unilateral vocal fold paralysis	6	40.83	12.77
Bilateral vocal folds paralysis	4	52.75	12.61
Functional dysphonia	2	39	24.04
Reflux laryngitis	2	57	15.56
Parkinson's disease	2	71.5	9.19
Total	135	42.92	15.26

Abbreviation: SD—standard deviation.

No correlations between the subject's age, sex, and AVQI measurements were found in the previous study [28]. Therefore, in the present study, the control and patient groups were considered suitable for AVQI-related data analysis, despite these groups not being matched by sex and age.

2.1. Original Voice Recordings

Voice samples from each subject were recorded in a T-series sound-proof room for hearing testing (T-room, CATegner AB, Bromma, Sweden) using a studio oral cardioid AKG Perception 220 microphone (AKG Acoustics, Vienna, Austria). The microphone was placed at a 10.0 cm distance from the mouth, keeping a 90° microphone-to-mouth angle. Each participant was asked to complete two vocal tasks, which were digitally recorded. The tasks consisted of (1) sustaining phonation of the vowel sound (a:) for at least 4 s duration and (2) reading a phonetically balanced text segment in Lithuanian "Turėjo senelė žilą oželį" ("The granny had a small grey goat"). The participants completed both vocal tasks at a personally comfortable loudness and pitch. All voice recordings were captured with Audacity recording software (https://www.audacityteam.org/, accessed on 30 May 2023) at a sampling frequency of 44.1 kHz and exported in a 16-bit depth lossless "wav" audio file format onto the computer's hard disk drive (HDD).

2.2. Auditory-Perceptual Evaluation

Five experienced physicians–laryngologists, who were all native Lithuanians, served as the rater panel. Blind to all relevant information regarding the subject (i.e., identity, age, gender, diagnosis, and disposition of the voice samples), they performed auditory–perceptual evaluations to quantify the vocal deviations, judging the voice samples into four ordinal severity classes of grade from the GRBAS scale (i.e., 0 = normal, 1 = slight, 2 = moderate, 3 = severe dysphonia) [35]. A detailed description of the auditory–perceptual evaluation is presented elsewhere [22].

2.3. Transmitting Studio Microphone Voice Recordings to Smartphones

The impact on voice recordings caused by technical differences in studio and smartphone microphones was averted by applying the filtration (equalization) of the already recorded flat frequency audio using the data from the smartphone frequency response curves. The filtered result would represent audio recorded with the selected smartphone. Using this method, the only variable affected was the frequency response, keeping other variables, i.e., room reflections, distance to the microphone, directionality, user loudness, and other variables, constant. Ableton DAW (digital audio workstation) was implemented as an editing environment, and the VST (virtual studio plugin) plugin MFreeformEqualizer by MeldaProduction (https://www.meldaproduction.com/MFreeformEqualizer/features, accessed on 4 June 2023) was used to import the frequency response datasets and equalize the frequencies according to the required frequency response. The MFreeformEqualizer filter quality was set to the extreme (highest available), with 0% curve smoothing. All the audio files were then re-exported as 44,100 Hz 16-bit wav files. With this method, the digital voice recordings obtained with a studio microphone were directly transmitted to different smartphones for analysis, avoiding not only the surrounding environment's impact but also ideally synchronizing all voice samples throughout all devices without the need for additional audio synchronization methods to ensure that the exact same parts of vowels and speech were used for each smartphone's analysis.

2.4. AVQI Estimation

For AVQI calculations, the signal processing of the voice samples was performed in the Praat software (version 5.3.57; https://www.fon.hum.uva.nl/praat/, accessed on 4 June 2023). Only voiced parts of the continuous speech were manually extracted and concatenated to the medial 3 s of the sustained (a) phonation. The voice samples were concatenated for auditory–perceptual judgment in the following order: text segment, a 2 s pause, followed by a 3 s sustained vowel /a/ segment. This chain of signals was used for acoustic analysis with the AVQI script version 02.02 developed for the program Praat https://www.vvl.be/documenten-en-paginas/praat-script-avqi-v0203?download=AcousticVoiceQualityIndexv.02.03.txt, accessed on 4 June 2023.

2.5. Development of a Universal-Platform-Based "Voice Screen" Application for Automated AVQI Estimation

The "*Voice Screen*" application for use with iOS operating devices was developed in the initial stage. Background noise monitoring, voice recording, and developed automated

AVQI calculations were implemented in the application. Consequently, the *"Voice Screen"* application allowed voice recording, automatically extracted acoustic voice features, and displayed the AVQI result alongside a recommendation to the user [9].

The upgraded UPB version of the *"Voice Screen"* application, suitable for iOS and Android devices, was elaborated in the next stage. In this case, the calculation of the AVQI and its characteristics was performed on the server; therefore, the computationally costly sound processing was not dependent on the user's device's computational capabilities. We used the Flutter framework (https://flutter.dev/, accessed on 4 June 2023) to create our client application. It allowed for compiling applications for different platforms (devices and their operating systems) from a single code base. The framework ensured that the same algorithms ran on different devices and that no new software errors were introduced while porting the application. Currently, our application works with both iOS and Android devices. Figure 1 shows the structure of the system. The numbers in the picture depict the flow of the operations.

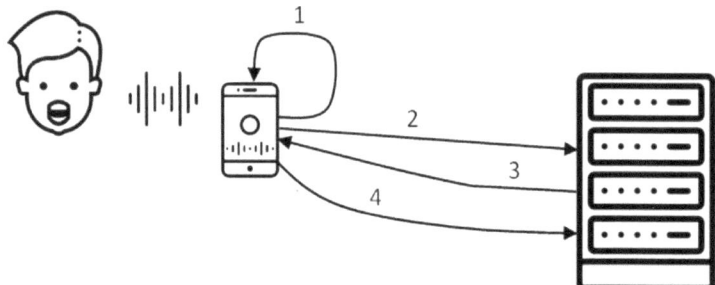

Figure 1. Structure of the system and flow of the operations.

In the first step, the given smartphone (iOS or Android) records sound waves acquired while saying given phrases aloud. The sound waves are preprocessed (see Step 1 in Figure 1) in real-time. The preprocessing aims to clean the sound waves from pauses and ensure the minimum amount of sound suitable for further analysis. Step 2 sends the preprocessed sound wave to the server for further analysis. The server runs a Linux operating system and provides web services for software in Python. That software is based on the Praat (https://www.fon.hum.uva.nl/praat/, accessed on 4 June 2023) application ported into a Python library by the Parselmouth project (https://parselmouth.readthedocs.io/, accessed on 4 June 2023). We use this library to calculate AVQI and other sound characteristics used in AVQI calculation. In Step 3, the AVQI index and the related data are returned to the smartphone and displayed to the user. Step 4 is optional. If the user chooses to save the results, the sound waves and calculated characteristics are saved into the server's database. No personal data relating to a specific person with the calculated AVQI and its parameters is saved on a server.

In the present study, the UPB *"Voice Screen"* application was installed on five different smartphones (namely, iPhone Pro Max 13, iPhone SE (iOS operating system), OnePlus 9 PRO, Samsung S22 Ultra, Huawei P50 pro (Android operating system)) used for AVQI estimation. The AVQI measures estimated with the *"Voice Screen"* application from voice recordings obtained from a flat frequency response studio microphone AKG Perception 220 were compared with AVQI results obtained using these smartphone devices.

2.6. Statistical Analysis

Statistical analysis was performed using IBM SPSS Statistics for Windows, version 20.0 (IBM Corp., Armonk, NY, USA) and MedCalc Version 20.118 (MedCalc Software Ltd., Ostend, Belgium). The chosen level of statistical significance was 0.05.

The data distribution was determined according to the normality law by applying the Shapiro–Wilk test of normality and calculating the coefficients of skewness and kurtosis. Student's *t*-test was used to test the equality of means in normally distributed data [36]. An analysis of variance (ANOVA) was employed to determine if there were significant differences between the multiple means of the independent groups [37]. Cronbach's alpha was used to measure the internal consistency of measures [38]. Pearson's correlation coefficient was applied to assess the linear relationship between variables obtained from continuous scales. Spearman's correlation coefficient was used to determine the relationship in ordinal results. Receiver operating characteristic (ROC) curves were used to obtain the optimal sensitivity and specificity at optimal AVQI cut-off points. The "area under the ROC curve" (AUC) served to calculate the possible discriminatory accuracy of AVQI performed with a studio microphone and different smartphones. A pairwise comparison of ROC curves, as described by De Long et al., was used to determine if there was a statistically significant difference between two or more variables when categorizing normal/pathological voices [39].

3. Results

3.1. Raters' Perceptual Evaluation Outcomes

The rater panel demonstrated excellent inter-rater agreement (Cronbach's $\alpha = 0.967$) with a mean intra-class correlation coefficient of 0.967 between five raters (from 0.961 to 0.973).

3.2. AVQI Evaluation Outcomes

An individual smartphone AVQI evaluation displayed excellent agreement by achieving a Cronbach's alpha of 0.984. The inter-smartphone AVQI measurements' reliability was excellent, with an average Intra-class Correlation Coefficient (ICC) of 0.983 (ranging from 0.979 to 0.987).

The mean AVQI scores provided by different smartphones and a studio microphone can be observed in Table 2.

Table 2. Comparison of the mean AVQI results obtained with different smartphones and studio microphone.

Microphone	n	Mean AVQI	Std. Deviation	F	p
AKG Perception 220		3.43	1.83		
iPhone SE		3.56	1.86		
iPhone Pro Max 13	135	3.16	1.83	0.759	0.58
Huawei P50 pro		3.37	1.96		
Samsung S22 Ultra		3.52	1.93		
OnePlus 9 PRO		3.42	1.86		

Abbreviation: AVQI—acoustic voice quality index.

As shown in Table 2, the one-way ANOVA analysis did not detect statistically significant differences between mean AVQI scores revealed using different smartphones ($F = 0.759$; $p = 0.58$). Further Bonferroni analysis reaffirmed the lack of difference between the AVQI scores obtained from different smartphones ($p = 1.0$, estimated Bonferroni's p for statistically significant difference $p = 0.01$). The mean AVQI differences ranged from 0.01 to 0.4 points when comparing different smartphones.

Almost perfect direct linear correlations were observed between the AVQI results obtained with a studio microphone and different smartphones. Pearson's correlation coefficients ranged from 0.991 to 0.987 and can be observed in Table 3.

The relationships between the AVQI scores obtained with a studio microphone and different smartphones are graphically presented in Figure 2.

Table 3. Correlations of AVQI scores obtained with studio microphone and different smartphones.

Microphones		iPhone SE	iPhone Pro Max 13	Huawei P50 pro	Samsung S22 Ultra	OnePlus 9 PRO
AKG Perception 220	r	0.991	0.987	0.970	0.979	0.992
	p	0.001	0.001	0.001	0.001	0.001
	n	135	135	135	135	135

Abbreviations: r—Pearsons's correlation coefficient; p—statistical significance.

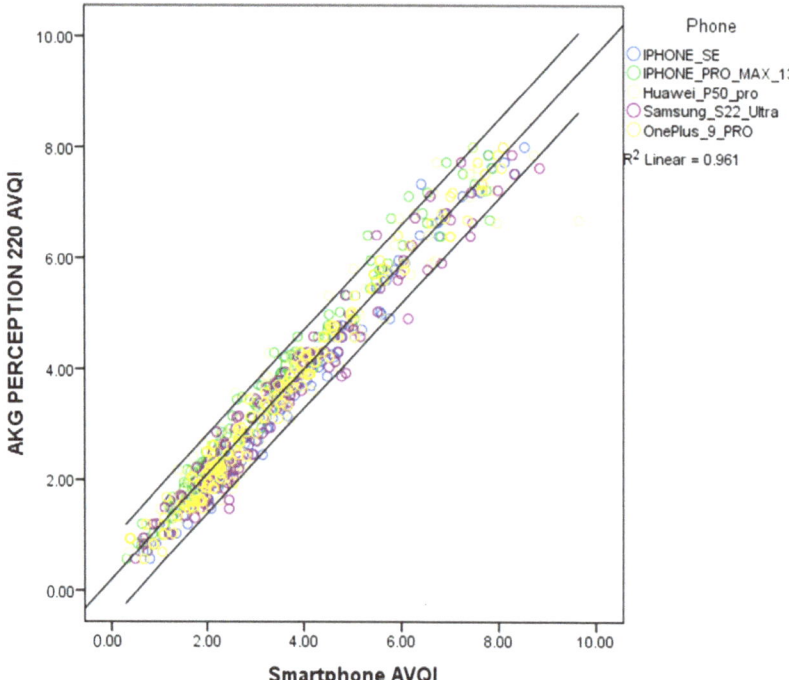

Figure 2. Scatterplot illustrating the correlation between the AVQI results obtained from the studio and different smartphones with a 95% confidence interval.

As demonstrated in Figure 2, it is evident that AVQI results obtained with different smartphones closely resemble the AVQI results obtained with a studio microphone, with very few data points outside of the 95% confidence interval ($R^2 = 0.961$). Therefore, it is safe to conclude that the AVQI scores obtained with smartphones are directly compatible with the ones obtained with the reference studio microphone.

3.3. The Normal vs. Pathological Voice Diagnostic Accuracy of the AVQI Using Different Smartphones

First, the ROC curves of AVQI obtained from a studio microphone and different smartphone voice recordings were inspected visually to identify optimum cut-off scores according to general interpretation guidelines [40]. All of the ROC curves were visually almost identical and occupied the largest part of the graph, clearly revealing their respectable power to discriminate between normal and pathological voices (Figure 3).

Second, as revealed by the AUC statistics analysis, a high level of precision of the AVQI in discriminating between normal and pathological voices was yielded with the suggested AUC = 0.800 threshold. The results of the ROC statistical analysis are presented in Table 4.

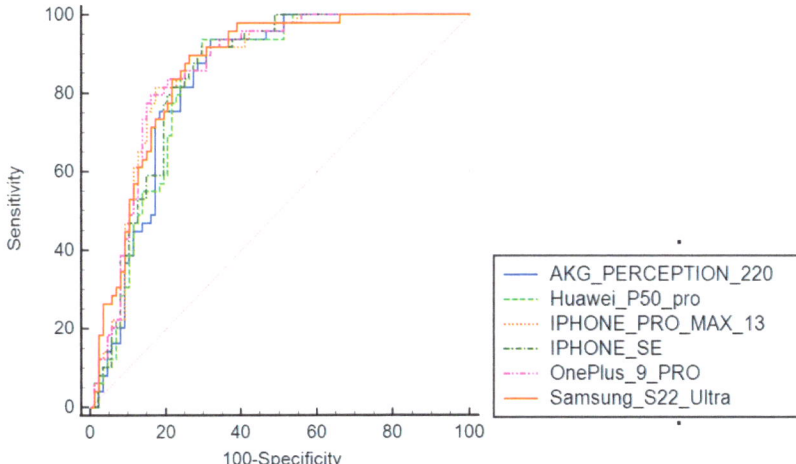

Figure 3. ROC curves illustrating the diagnostic accuracy of studio and different smartphone microphones in discriminating normal/pathological voices.

Table 4. Statistics illustrating the accuracy the AVQI differentiating normal and pathological voices recorded using studio and different smartphones' microphones.

AVQI	AUC	Cut-Off	Sensitivity %	Specificity %	Youden-Index J
AKG Perception 220	0.834	3.27	93.88	68.18	0.62
iPhone SE	0.844	3.23	91.84	70.45	0.62
iPhone Pro Max 13	0.858	2.14	81.63	82.95	0.65
Huawei P50 pro	0.835	3.08	93.88	70.45	0.64
Samsung S22 Ultra	0.862	2.93	89.8	73.86	0.64
OnePlus 9 PRO	0.86	2.3	79.59	84.09	0.64

Abbreviations: AVQI acoustic voice quality index, AUC area under the curve.

As demonstrated in Table 4, the ROC analysis determined the optimal AVQI cut-off values for distinguishing between normal and pathological voices for each smartphone. All employed microphones passed the proposed 0.8 AUC threshold and revealed an acceptable Youden-index value.

Third, a pairwise comparison of the significance of the differences between the AUCs revealed in the present study is presented in Table 5.

Table 5. A pairwise comparison of the significance of differences between the AUCs.

p	AKG Perception 220	iPhone SE	iPhone Pro Max 13	Huawei P50 Pro	Samsung S22 Ultra	OnePlus 9 Pro
AKG Perception 220	-	0.163	0.099	0.966	0.11	0.086
iPhone SE	0.163	-	0.367	0.579	0.282	0.863
iPhone Pro Max 13	0.099	0.367	-	0.268	0.718	0.863
Huawei P50 pro	0.966	0.579	0.268	-	0.223	0.256
Samsung S22 Ultra	0.11	0.282	0.718	0.223	-	0.863
OnePlus 9 PRO	0.086	0.863	0.863	0.256	0.863	-

Abbreviations: AUC area under the curve.

As shown in Table 5, a comparison of the AUCs-dependent ROC curves (AVQI measurements obtained from studio microphone and different smartphones), according to the test of DeLong et al., confirmed no statistically significant differences between the AUCs ($p > 0.05$). The most considerable observed difference between the AUCs was only 0.028. These results confirmed the compatible results of the AVQI's diagnostic accuracy in differentiating normal vs. pathological voices when using voice recordings from a studio microphone and different smartphones.

4. Discussion

In the present study, the novel UPB *"Voice Screen"* application for the estimation of AVQI and detection of voice deteriorations in patients with various voice disorders and healthy controls was tested for the first time simultaneously with different smartphones. The AVQI was chosen for voice quality assessment because of some essential favorable features of this multiparametric measurement: the less vulnerability of the AVQI to environmental noise compared to other complex acoustic markers and the robustness of the AVQI regarding the interaction between acoustic voice quality measurements and room acoustics; there were no significant differences within subjects for both women and men when comparing the AVQI across different voice analysis programs [11,14,41]. Another essential attribute of the AVQI is that Praat is the only freely available program that estimates the AVQI. That eliminates the impact of possible software differences on AVQI computation.

In the present study, the results of the ANOVA analysis did not detect statistically significant differences between mean AVQI scores revealed using different smartphones ($F = 0.759$; $p = 0.58$). Moreover, the mean AVQI differences ranged from 0.01 to 0.4 points when comparing AVQI estimated with different smartphones, thus establishing a low level of variability. This corresponded with a value of 0.54 for the absolute retest difference of AVQI values proposed by Barsties and Maryn in 2013 [20,42]. Consequently, these outcomes of AVQI measurements with different smartphones were considered neither statistically nor clinically significant, justifying the possibility of practical use of the UPB *"Voice Screen"* app.

The correlation analysis showed that all AVQI measurements were highly correlated (Pearson's r ranged from 0.991 to 0.987) across the devices used in the present study. This concurred with the literature data on the high correlation between acoustic voice features derived from studio microphones and smartphones and examined both for control participants and synthesized voice data [7,12–14].

Furthermore, analysis of the results revealed that the AVQI showed a remarkable ability to discriminate between normal and pathological voices as determined by auditory–perceptual judgment. The ROC analysis determined the optimal AVQI cut-off values for distinguishing between normal and pathological voices for each smartphone used. A remarkable precision of AVQI in discriminating between normal and pathological voices was yielded (AUC 0.834–0.862), resulting in an acceptable balance between sensitivity and specificity. These findings suggested that the AVQI was a reliable tool in differentiating normal/pathological voices independently of the voice recordings from tested studio microphones and different smartphones. The comparison of the AUC-dependent ROC curves (AVQI measurements obtained from studio microphone and different smartphones) demonstrated no statistically significant differences between the AUCs ($p > 0.05$), with the largest revealed difference between the AUCs of only 0.028. These results confirmed the compatible results of the AVQI diagnostic accuracy in differentiating normal vs. pathological voices when using voice recordings from studio microphone and different smartphones and presented remarkable importance from a practical point of view.

Several limitations of the present study have to be considered. Despite the encouraging results of the AVQI measurements, some individual discrepancies between AVQI results revealed with different smartphones still exist. Therefore, further research in a wide diversity of voice pathologies, including functional voice disorders, is needed to ensure the maximum comparability of acoustic voice features derived from voice recordings obtained with mobile communication devices and reference studio microphones. In the present study, the voice recordings were performed in a sound-proof room. However, in real clinical situations where environmental noise exists, the omni-directional built-in microphones of smartphones may induce different results. Therefore, further studies of the Voice Screen application's performance with different smartphones in a real clinical setting are required to evaluate both the impact of the voice recording environment and the peculiarities of the microphones on the AVQI estimation in real clinical situations by performing simultaneous voice recordings with different smartphones. The outcomes of further studies will potentially make possible the results and improvements to be employed in healthcare applications.

Summarizing the results of the previous and present studies allows for the presumption that the performance of the novel UPB "*Voice Screen*" app using different smartphones represents an adequate and compatible performance of AVQI estimation. However, it is important to note that due to existing differences in recording conditions, microphones, hardware, and software, the results of acoustic voice quality measures may differ between recording systems [11]. Therefore, using the UPB "*Voice Screen*" app with some caution is advisable. For voice screening purposes, it is more reliable to perform AVQI measurements using the same device, especially when performing repeated measurements. Moreover, these bits of advice should be considered when comparing data of acoustic voice analysis between different voice recording systems, i.e., different smartphones or other mobile communication devices, and when using them for diagnostic purposes or monitoring voice treatment outcomes.

5. Conclusions

The UPB "*Voice Screen*" app represents an accurate and robust tool for voice quality measurement and normal vs. pathological voice screening purposes, demonstrating the potential to be used by patients and clinicians for voice assessments, employing both iOS and Android smartphones.

Author Contributions: Conceptualization, V.U. and R.M.; methodology, R.D.; software, T.B. and T.P.; validation, K.P., N.U.-S. and T.P.; formal analysis, K.P.; investigation, N.U.-S. and T.P.; resources, V.U.; data curation, T.P.; writing—original draft preparation, V.U.; writing—review and editing, R.M. and R.D.; visualization, T.B.; supervision, V.U.; project administration, R.M.; funding acquisition, V.U. and R.M. All authors have read and agreed to the published version of the manuscript.

Funding: This project has received funding from European Regional Development Fund (project No. 13.1.1-LMT-K-718-05-0027) under grant agreement with the Research Council of Lithuania (LMTLT). Funded by the European Union's measures in response to the COVID-19 pandemic.

Institutional Review Board Statement: The study was conducted in accordance with the Declaration of Helsinki of 1975, and the protocol was approved by the Kaunas Regional Ethics Committee for Biomedical Research (2022-04-20 No. BE-2-49).

Informed Consent Statement: Informed consent was obtained from all subjects involved in the study.

Data Availability Statement: The data presented in this study are available on request from the corresponding author.

Conflicts of Interest: The authors declare no conflict of interest.

References

1. Mobile Network Subscriptions Worldwide. 2028. Available online: https://www.statista.com/statistics/330695/number-of-smartphone-users-worldwide/ (accessed on 3 April 2023).
2. Casale, M.; Costantino, A.; Rinaldi, V.; Forte, A.; Grimaldi, M.; Sabatino, L.; Oliveto, G.; Aloise, F.; Pontari, D.; Salvinelli, F. Mobile applications in otolaryngology for patients: An update. *Laryngoscope Investig. Otolaryngol.* **2018**, *3*, 434. [CrossRef]
3. Eleonora, M.C.T.; Lonigro, A.; Gelardi, M.; Kim, B.; Cassano, M. Mobile Applications in Otolaryngology: A Systematic Review of the Literature, Apple App Store and the Google Play Store. *Ann. Otol. Rhinol. Laryngol.* **2021**, *130*, 78–91. [CrossRef]
4. Grillo, E.U.; Wolfberg, J. An Assessment of Different Praat Versions for Acoustic Measures Analyzed Automatically by VoiceEvalU8 and Manually by Two Raters. *J. Voice* **2020**, *37*, 17–25. [CrossRef] [PubMed]

5. Boogers, L.S.; Chen, B.S.J.; Coerts, M.J.; Rinkel, R.N.P.M.; Hannema, S.E. Mobile Phone Applications Voice Tools and Voice Pitch Analyzer Validated with LingWAVES to Measure Voice Frequency. *J. Voice* **2022**. Available online: https://www.sciencedirect.com/science/article/pii/S0892199722003186 (accessed on 3 April 2023). [CrossRef]
6. Kojima, T.; Hasebe, K.; Fujimura, S.; Okanoue, Y.; Kagoshima, H.; Taguchi, A.; Yamamoto, H.; Shoji, K.; Hori, R. A New iPhone Application for Voice Quality Assessment Based on the GRBAS Scale. *Laryngoscope* **2021**, *131*, 580–582. [CrossRef]
7. Fahed, V.S.; Doheny, E.P.; Busse, M.; Hoblyn, J.; Lowery, M.M. Comparison of Acoustic Voice Features Derived from Mobile Devices and Studio Microphone Recordings. *J. Voice* **2022**. Available online: https://www.sciencedirect.com/science/article/pii/S0892199722003125 (accessed on 3 April 2023). [CrossRef] [PubMed]
8. Awan, S.N.; Shaikh, M.A.; Awan, J.A.; Abdalla, I.; Lim, K.O.; Misono, S. Smartphone Recordings are Comparable to "Gold Standard" Recordings for Acoustic Measurements of Voice. *J. Voice* **2023**. Available online: https://www.sciencedirect.com/science/article/pii/S0892199723000310 (accessed on 10 April 2023). [CrossRef]
9. Uloza, V.; Ulozaite-Staniene, N.; Petrauskas, T. An iOS-based VoiceScreen application: Feasibility for use in clinical settings-a pilot study. *Eur. Arch. Otorhinolaryngol.* **2023**, *280*, 277–284. [CrossRef]
10. Munnings, A.J. The Current State and Future Possibilities of Mobile Phone "Voice Analyser" Applications, in Relation to Otorhinolaryngology. *J. Voice* **2020**, *34*, 527–532. Available online: https://www.sciencedirect.com/science/article/pii/S0892199718302595 (accessed on 3 April 2023). [CrossRef] [PubMed]
11. Maryn, Y.; Ysenbaert, F.; Zarowski, A.; Vanspauwen, R. Mobile Communication Devices, Ambient Noise, and Acoustic Voice Measures. *J. Voice* **2017**, *31*, 248.e11–248.e23. Available online: https://www.sciencedirect.com/science/article/pii/S0892199716301965 (accessed on 10 April 2023). [CrossRef] [PubMed]
12. Kardous, C.A.; Shaw, P.B. Evaluation of smartphone sound measurement applications. *J. Acoust. Soc. Am.* **2014**, *135*, EL186–EL192. [CrossRef]
13. Manfredi, C.; Lebacq, J.; Cantarella, G.; Schoentgen, J.; Orlandi, S.; Bandini, A.; DeJonckere, P.H. Smartphones Offer New Opportunities in Clinical Voice Research. *J. Voice* **2017**, *31*, 111.e1–111.e7. Available online: https://www.sciencedirect.com/science/article/pii/S0892199716000059 (accessed on 10 April 2023). [CrossRef]
14. Grillo, E.U.; Brosious, J.N.; Sorrell, S.L.; Anand, S. Influence of Smartphones and Software on Acoustic Voice Measures. *Int. J. Telerehabil.* **2016**, *8*, 9–14. [CrossRef]
15. Lee, S.J.; Lee, K.Y.; Choi, H.; Lee, S.J.; Lee, K.Y.; Choi, H. Clinical Usefulness of Voice Recordings using a Smartphone as a Screening Tool for Voice Disorders. *Commun. Sci. Disord.* **2018**, *23*, 1065–1077. Available online: http://www.e-csd.org/journal/view.php?doi=10.12963/csd.18540 (accessed on 13 June 2023). [CrossRef]
16. Schaeffler, F.; Jannetts, S.; Beck, J.M. Reliability of clinical voice parameters captured with smartphones—Measurements of added noise and spectral tilt. In Proceedings of the 20th Annual Conference of the International Speech Communication Association INTERSPEECH 2019, Graz, Austria, 15–19 September 2019; pp. 2523–2527. Available online: https://eresearch.qmu.ac.uk/handle/20.500.12289/10013 (accessed on 3 April 2023). [CrossRef]
17. Marsano-Cornejo, M.; Roco-Videla, Á. Comparison of the Acoustic Parameters Obtained with Different Smartphones and a Professional Microphone. *Acta Otorrinolaringol. ESP* **2022**, *73*, 51–55. [CrossRef]
18. Pommée, T.; Morsomme, D. Voice Quality in Telephone Interviews: A preliminary Acoustic Investigation. *J. Voice* **2022**. Available online: https://www.sciencedirect.com/science/article/pii/S0892199722002685 (accessed on 10 April 2023). [CrossRef]
19. Maryn, Y.; De Bodt, M.; Roy, N. The Acoustic Voice Quality Index: Toward improved treatment outcomes assessment in voice disorders. *J. Commun. Disord.* **2010**, *43*, 161–174. Available online: https://www.sciencedirect.com/science/article/pii/S0021992409000884 (accessed on 12 December 2022). [CrossRef]
20. Barsties, B.; Maryn, Y. The Acoustic Voice Quality Index. Toward expanded measurement of dysphonia severity in German subjects. *HNO* **2012**, *60*, 715–720. [CrossRef]
21. Hosokawa, K.; Barsties, B.; Iwahashi, T.; Iwahashi, M.; Kato, C.; Iwaki, S.; Sasai, H.; Miyauchi, A.; Matsushiro, N.; Inohara, H.; et al. Validation of the Acoustic Voice Quality Index in the Japanese Language. *J. Voice* **2017**, *31*, 260.e1–260.e9. Available online: https://www.sciencedirect.com/science/article/pii/S0892199716300789 (accessed on 3 April 2023). [CrossRef]
22. Uloza, V.; Petrauskas, T.; Padervinskis, E.; Ulozaitė, N.; Barsties, B.; Maryn, Y. Validation of the Acoustic Voice Quality Index in the Lithuanian Language. *J. Voice* **2017**, *31*, 257.e1–257.e11. Available online: https://www.sciencedirect.com/science/article/pii/S0892199716300716 (accessed on 3 January 2023). [CrossRef] [PubMed]
23. Kankare, E.; Barsties, V.; Latoszek, B.; Maryn, Y.; Asikainen, M.; Rorarius, E.; Vilpas, S.; Ilomäki, I.; Tyrmi, J.; Rantala, L.; et al. The acoustic voice quality index version 02.02 in the Finnish-speaking population. *Logop. Phoniatr. Vocol.* **2020**, *45*, 49–56. [CrossRef] [PubMed]
24. Englert, M.; Lopes, L.; Vieira, V.; Behlau, M. Accuracy of Acoustic Voice Quality Index and Its Isolated Acoustic Measures to Discriminate the Severity of Voice Disorders. *J. Voice* **2022**, *36*, 582.e1–582.e10. Available online: https://www.sciencedirect.com/science/article/pii/S0892199720302939 (accessed on 3 April 2023). [CrossRef] [PubMed]
25. Yeşilli-Puzella, G.; Tadıhan-Özkan, E.; Maryn, Y. Validation and Test-Retest Reliability of Acoustic Voice Quality Index Version 02.06 in the Turkish Language. *J. Voice* **2022**, *36*, 736.e25–736.e32. Available online: https://www.sciencedirect.com/science/article/pii/S0892199720303222 (accessed on 10 April 2023). [CrossRef]

26. Englert, M.; Latoszek, B.B.V.; Behlau, M. Exploring the Validity of Acoustic Measurements and Other Voice Assessments. *J. Voice* **2022**. Available online: https://www.sciencedirect.com/science/article/pii/S0892199721004392 (accessed on 3 April 2023). [CrossRef]
27. Shabnam, S.; Pushpavathi, M.; Gopi Sankar, R.; Sridharan, K.V.; Vasanthalakshmi, M.S. A Comprehensive Application for Grading Severity of Voice Based on Acoustic Voice Quality Index v.02.03. *J. Voice* **2022**. Available online: https://www.sciencedirect.com/science/article/pii/S0892199722002454 (accessed on 3 April 2023). [CrossRef] [PubMed]
28. Latoszek, B.B.V.; Uloząitė-Stanienė, N.; Maryn, Y.; Petrauskas, T.; Uloza, V. The Influence of Gender and Age on the Acoustic Voice Quality Index and Dysphonia Severity Index: A Normative Study. *J. Voice* **2019**, *33*, 340–345. Available online: https://www.sciencedirect.com/science/article/pii/S089219971730468X (accessed on 3 April 2023). [CrossRef] [PubMed]
29. Batthyany, C.; Maryn, Y.; Trauwaen, I.; Caelenberghe, E.; van Dinther, J.; Zarowski, A.; Wuyts, F. A case of specificity: How does the acoustic voice quality index perform in normophonic subjects? *Appl. Sci.* **2019**, *9*, 2527. [CrossRef]
30. Jayakumar, T.; Benoy, J.J.; Yasin, H.M. Effect of Age and Gender on Acoustic Voice Quality Index Across Lifespan: A Cross-sectional Study in Indian Population. *J. Voice* **2022**, *36*, 436.e1–436.e8. Available online: https://www.sciencedirect.com/science/article/pii/S0892199720301995 (accessed on 10 April 2023). [CrossRef]
31. Jayakumar, T.; Benoy, J.J. Acoustic Voice Quality Index (AVQI) in the Measurement of Voice Quality: A Systematic Review and Meta-Analysis. *J. Voice* **2022**. Available online: https://www.sciencedirect.com/science/article/pii/S0892199722000844 (accessed on 3 April 2023). [CrossRef] [PubMed]
32. Batthyany, C.; Latoszek, B.B.V.; Maryn, Y. Meta-Analysis on the Validity of the Acoustic Voice Quality Index. *J. Voice* **2022**. [CrossRef] [PubMed]
33. Saeedi, S.; Aghajanzade, M.; Khatoonabadi, A.R. A Literature Review of Voice Indices Available for Voice Assessment. *JRSR* **2022**, *9*, 151–155. [CrossRef]
34. Uloza, V.; Uloząitė-Stanienė, N.; Petrauskas, T.; Kregždytė, R. Accuracy of Acoustic Voice Quality Index Captured with a Smartphone—Measurements with Added Ambient Noise. *J. Voice* **2021**, *37*, 465.e19–465.e26. [CrossRef]
35. Dejonckere, P.H.; Bradley, P.; Clemente, P.; Cornut, G.; Crevier-Buchman, L.; Friedrich, G.; Van De Heyning, P.; Remacle, M.; Woisard, V. A basic protocol for functional assessment of voice pathology, especially for investigating the efficacy of (phonosurgical) treatments and evaluating new assessment techniques. Guideline elaborated by the Committee on Phoniatrics of the European Laryngological Society (ELS). *Eur. Arch. Otorhinolaryngol.* **2001**, *258*, 77–82. [CrossRef]
36. Senn, S.; Richardson, W. The first *t*-test. *Stat. Med.* **1994**, *13*, 785–803. [CrossRef]
37. McHugh, M.L. Multiple comparison analysis testing in ANOVA. *Biochem. Med.* **2011**, *21*, 203–209. [CrossRef] [PubMed]
38. Cho, E. Making Reliability Reliable: A Systematic Approach to Reliability Coefficients. *Organ. Res. Methods* **2016**, *19*, 651–682. [CrossRef]
39. Hanley, J.A.; McNeil, B.J. The meaning and use of the area under a receiver operating characteristic (ROC) curve. *Radiology* **1982**, *143*, 29–36. [CrossRef]
40. Dollaghan, C.A. *The Handbook for Evidence-Based Practice in Communication Disorders*; Paul H. Brookes Publishing Co.: Baltimore, MD, USA, 2007.
41. Bottalico, P.; Codino, J.; Cantor-Cutiva, L.C.; Marks, K.; Nudelman, C.J.; Skeffington, J.; Shrivastav, R.; Jackson-Menaldi, M.C.; Hunter, E.J.; Rubin, A.D. Reproducibility of Voice Parameters: The Effect of Room Acoustics and Microphones. *J. Voice* **2020**, *34*, 320–334. Available online: https://www.sciencedirect.com/science/article/pii/S0892199718304338 (accessed on 10 April 2023). [CrossRef] [PubMed]
42. Lehnert, B.; Herold, J.; Blaurock, M.; Busch, C. Reliability of the Acoustic Voice Quality Index AVQI and the Acoustic Breathiness Index (ABI) when wearing COVID-19 protective masks. *Eur. Arch. Otorhinolaryngol.* **2022**, *279*, 4617–4621. [CrossRef] [PubMed]

Disclaimer/Publisher's Note: The statements, opinions and data contained in all publications are solely those of the individual author(s) and contributor(s) and not of MDPI and/or the editor(s). MDPI and/or the editor(s) disclaim responsibility for any injury to people or property resulting from any ideas, methods, instructions or products referred to in the content.

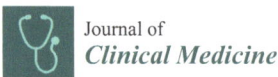

Article

Comparison of TEVA vs. PRAAT in the Acoustic Characterization of the Tracheoesophageal Voice in Laryngectomized Patients

Alejandro Klein-Rodríguez [1,2,3], Irma Cabo-Varela [1,2,3], Francisco Vázquez-de la Iglesia [1,2], Carlos M. Chiesa-Estomba [4] and Miguel Mayo-Yáñez [1,2,5,*]

1. Otorhinolaryngology—Head and Neck Surgery Department, Complexo Hospitalario Universitario (A Coruña (CHUAC), 15006 A Coruña, Spain; alejandro.klein.rodriguez@sergas.es (A.K.-R.); irma.cabo.varela@sergas.es (I.C.-V.); francisco.vazquez.de.la.iglesia@sergas.es (F.V.-d.l.I.)
2. Otorhinolaryngology-Head and Neck Surgery Research Group, Institute of Biomedical Research of A Coruña (INIBIC), Complexo Hospitalario Universitario de A Coruña (CHUAC), Universidade da Coruña (UDC), 15006 A Coruña, Spain
3. Health Sciences Programme, International Center for Doctorate (EIDUDC), Universidade da Coruña (UDC), 15001 A Coruña, Spain
4. Otorhinolaryngology—Head and Neck Surgery Department, Hospital Universitario Donostia—Biodonostia Research Institute, 20014 Donostia, Spain; chiesaestomba86@gmail.com
5. Otorhinolaryngology—Head and Neck Surgery Department, Hospital San Rafael (HSR), 15006 A Coruña, Spain
* Correspondence: miguel.mayo.yanez@sergas.es

Abstract: Background: Previous studies have assessed the capability of PRAAT for acoustic voice analysis in total laryngectomized (TL) patients, although this software was designed for acoustic analysis of laryngeal voice. Recently, we have witnessed the development of specialized acoustic analysis software, Tracheoesophageal Voice Analysis (TEVA). This study aims to compare the analysis with both programs in TL patients. **Methods:** Observational analytical study of 34 TL patients where a quantitative acoustic analysis was performed for stable phonation with vowels [a] and [i] as well as spectrographic characterization using the TEVA and PRAAT software. **Results:** The Voice Handicap Index (VHI-10) showed a mean score of 11.29 ± 11.16 points, categorized as a moderate handicap. TEVA analysis found lower values in the fundamental frequency vs. PRAAT ($p < 0.05$). A significant increase in shimmer values was observed with TEVA (>20%). No significant differences were found between spectrographic analysis with TEVA and PRAAT. **Conclusions:** Tracheoesophageal speech is an alaryngeal voice, characterized by a higher degree of irregularity and noise compared to laryngeal speech. Consequently, it necessitates a more tailored approach using objective assessment tools adapted to these distinct features, like TEVA, that are designed specifically for TL patients. This study provides statistical evidence supporting its reliability and suitability for the evaluation and tracking of tracheoesophageal speakers.

Keywords: larynx; tracheoesophageal puncture; speech; analysis; software; laryngectomy; rehabilitation; prosthesis

1. Introduction

The PRAAT software represents a prominent tool in contemporary objective acoustic analysis. Developed by Boersma and Weenik, this software enables the comprehensive analysis, synthesis, and manipulation of acoustic signals related to vocalization, achieved through the systematic adjustment of various parameters for the extraction of speech data and the evaluation of vocal quality [1]. PRAAT is a program designed especially for research in phonetics and to offer a tool to carry out general acoustic analysis of voice and speech as well as to use it for educational purposes.

Normally, the program is used under laryngeal speech conditions with rhythmic, periodic, and harmonic vocal fold movements.

The loss of vocal capacity in laryngectomized patients is a significant consequence of the total removal of the larynx, a critical structure for speech production. This surgical procedure compelled the laryngectomized patients to seek alternatives, such as tracheoesophageal speech (TES) or the use of voice prostheses (VP), to regain verbal communication that would lack the harmony and periodic vibration produced by the vocal folds [2]. The loss of natural voice is a complex emotional and functional transition for these patients, and vocal rehabilitation plays a crucial role in their adaptation to this new reality. The quality of voice in total laryngectomized (TL) patients relying on TES is intrinsically tied to the characteristics of the neo-glottis. Variability in the functioning of the neo-glottis and the vibration of the pharyngoesophageal tract following medical interventions, including surgery and radiation therapy (RT), results in substantial disparities in speech intelligibility and quality [3,4].

Previous studies have assessed the capability of PRAAT for acoustic voice analysis in TL patients. However, due to the subjective differences and phonatory physiology variances between patients with a larynx and those without, these findings appear to be less representative of vocal acoustics research [2,5]. For this reason, recent years have witnessed the development of specialized acoustic analysis software, such as Tracheoesophageal Voice Analysis (TEVA) [6]. This program was conceived to support the education, rehabilitation, and research endeavors of professionals working with TES and to benefit patients employing VP. The TEVA software is an integrated component within the phonetic analysis platform PRAAT, built upon the acoustic analysis framework outlined by Van As-Brooks, which categorizes voices based on phonation stability, duration, and the presence or absence of harmonics [3,7].

The difficulty of studying the speech of LT patients lies in the instability and irregularity of phonation, which is why precise and individualized calibrations and adjustments are required to obtain reliable results.

In acoustic signal typing, the voice characteristics are determined using acoustic analysis of speech. The typing is based on both visual inspection of plots of these analysis parameters and quantitative measures of a short (if possible, at least 2 s long) stretch of "stable" speech.

TEVA is a tool based on PRAAT software and designed for the specific analysis of patients with TES. Currently, there are not any studies comparing both analysis programs in laryngectomized patients. The aim of the study is to compare both acoustic analysis software in an attempt to find distinctions that will increase knowledge about transesophageal voice and thus improve education and rehabilitation for this type of patient.

2. Materials and Methods

2.1. Study Design

An observational analytical cohort study of TL patients recruited consecutively from the outpatient otorhinolaryngology clinics of a tertiary university hospital as they attended to routine follow-up from February 2019 to 2022. All patients were informed and invited to participate. The study was approved by the hospital's ethics committee (2022/094) and informed consent was obtained in all cases.

The objective of the study was to know if the results obtained with the TEVA program compared with PRAAT were more similar to what was initially expected. We would expect to find lower fundamental frequency values, as tracheoesophageal voices apparently subjectively seem to have. Also, with a higher frequency and amplitude variation component (jitter and shimmer). Apparently, at the beginning of the process, the differences in intensity should not be very striking between both programs.

2.2. Inclusion and Exclusion Criteria

The study exclusively involved voluntary participants who were users of Provox Vega® and met specific eligibility criteria.

The Provox Vega® prosthesis is a silicone device with a double flap that is placed on the tracheoesophageal wall. This prosthesis allows the passage of air from the trachea to the esophagus in a unidirectional way, so that the air vibrating in the pharyngoesophageal tract and the neopharynx generates the voice that is subsequently modulated and articulated in the oral cavity. Additionally, the valve prevents the passage of food or liquids from the esophagus to the trachea.

These criteria included being aged 18 or older, having undergone a total laryngectomy at least 3 months prior, having completed radiotherapy or chemotherapy (if applicable) at least 3 months ago, receiving treatment with proton-pump inhibitors, and having at least 3 months of experience using the Provox Vega®. Individuals were excluded from participation if they had medical conditions that prevented them from using the Provox system, had recurrent or metastatic diseases, had undergone a total or partial pharyngectomy, utilized alternative phonation methods instead of a voice prosthesis, experienced functional incapacity to independently maintain the voice prosthesis, or had impaired cognitive abilities. The presence or type of cervical dissection, as well as the type of tracheoesophageal puncture (primary or secondary), did not constitute an exclusion criterion.

The patients included had received phonatory rehabilitation from speech therapy. They had a pre-surgical evaluation, and later, after the intervention, they were evaluated even before discharge, normally 10 days after surgery. After discharge, the phonatory rehabilitation work continued in the speech therapy consultation.

In total, 47 patients were invited to participate; 6 patients who met the criteria refused to participate in the study because they did not want to participate in it. The main reason for not wanting to be included was the extension of the consultation by approximately 30–45 min to carry out the speech study.

Finally, 34 patients who fulfilled the criteria were included in the study.

At the time of the assessment, seven patients did not use the Provox System, which is the reason why they were excluded from the study. In all of these patients, a tracheoesophageal puncture (1st or 2nd) was performed, but due to complications related to it (mainly wide phonatory fistula with extrusions or ingestions of the prosthesis), it was finally decided to close the tracheoesophageal fistula, so at the time of assessment in consultation, it was not possible to include them in the study since the speech with the tracheoesophageal voice could not be recorded.

2.3. Collected Variables

Throughout the study, every patient received an anterograde voice prosthesis (VP) insertion, and their speech was evaluated while they manually occluded the stoma using a heat and moisture exchanger device. The assessment of the patients was carried out by both an otolaryngologist and a speech therapist. The following descriptive variables were recorded: age, months since surgery, complementary treatment with RT, primary or secondary tracheoesophageal puncture (TEP), number of VP (model), number of VP replacements, presence of pulmonary pathology or concomitant swallowing problems, and pharyngeal closure technique.

A perceptual analysis with the GRBAS scale (grade, roughness, breathiness, asthenia, strain) was carried out after reading a fragment of "Platero y Yo" (J.R. Jiménez) and the validated and adapted questionnaire Voice Handicap Index 10 (VHI-10) in Spanish [8].

The GRBAS was assessed on a 4-point scale (0 = normal, 1 = slight, 2 = moderate, 3 = extreme). The numbers included in the results are the total addition of the 5 variables included (GRBAS).

The included text is a fragment of "Platero y yo". It consists of 104 words with important phonetic richness and is widely used in subjective evaluations of the voice in the Spanish language.

The patient was recorded on 3 occasions, with the examiner selecting the best of the 3 attempts and evaluating the GRBAS scale at that time.

The assessment is carried out by two examiners independently, comparing one by one the results obtained for each item of GRBAS. If there are differences between the data recorded by each examiner, it is evaluated jointly to reach a common value according to the arguments of each one in a consensual way.

A subjective visual and acoustic adjustment was performed by viewing the spectrogram of the most stable segments of speech, lasting at least two seconds if possible. After this adjustment, the quantitative acoustic variables investigated were average sound pressure level (SPL) (dB), maximum SPL (dB), fundamental frequency (F0) Hz, jitter frequency disturbance, shimmer amplitude disturbance, and harmonic to noise ratio (HNR) for stable phonation of at least 2 s with vowels [a] and [i].

The variables were analyzed automatically with both of the software algorithms, and the numerical values were recorded for each of them.

The narrowband spectrographic characterization was developed according to spectrogram criteria [3].

The acoustic analysis was carried out using the NKI TE-Voice Analysis tool (TEVA) E5C4E4ADC5 2015-05-11T10:38:35Z software version and the PRAAT® 6.1.08 software version on a Hewlett-Packard computer (Intel® Core™ i5-4570SCPU 2.90Ghz) with an EliteDisplay® E231 monitor and Condenser® SF-666 microphone.

2.4. Recording Environment

All participants were recorded under the same conditions in a 4 × 3 m soundproof room with the Condenser® SF-666 microphone.

The microphone was calibrated with the PRAAT program, first performing phonation as soft as possible, with a whisper, and then performing phonation with a sustained vowel at a higher pitch, checking in the PRAAT sound recorder that the sound meter was not present at too high a threshold (red/yellow color). If it is yellow or red, the microphone was moved a little further away from the mouth to avoid a high component of noise [9]. The angle between the microphone and the mouth was around 45°, and the distance between them was 5–10 cm [9].

Finally, the SPL measurement was carried out using a mobile app (Niosh Sound Level Meter App). The mobile phone with the SPL app was placed about 30 cm in front of the mouth, and it is displayed to show how many dB the device measures, comparing with the result that was marked in the PRAAT of the same person performing a phonation with the phoneme [a] in the usual tone and, if possible, for a duration of 5 s. It was recorded in PRAAT and compared with the dB of the mobile app measurement. Adjusting the difference in dB obtained between both (adding or subtracting the dB that differs between the PRAAT and the SPL meter, taking the SPL meter as a more reliable reference).

Three attempts were made to record each phoneme [a] and [i], emitting a phonation for as long as possible in the usual conversational tone. The best of the 3 recordings was selected for each phoneme based on the existence or not and stability of a pitch curve, the dispersion of the formants, the noise, and the distribution of the pulses in the spectrogram. Visualizing these characteristics of regularity in the path of the sound wave, the 2 s of the recording that showed the most stable parameters, with less noise and dispersion of the sample, were identified, which were those that were included as a study sample to carry out the instrumental study.

Signal typing was categorized based on the visual characteristics observed in the narrowband spectrogram.

For TEVA, there are three options to adjust the pitch: a low and high pitch cutoff (300 and 600 Hz). We took a high-pitched cutoff (until 600 Hz). For PRAAT, we use a manual range of 30–600 Hz.

For the selection of vocal fragments for vocal analysis, the most stable parts were chosen, >2 s, with the largest component of visible, clear harmonics.

For the spectrographic analysis for both programs, the visualization of the narrow band spectrogram was carried out based on the Yanagihara classification [10].

- Type I: The regular harmonic components are mixed with the noise component, chiefly in the formant region of the vowels.
- Type II: The noise components in the second formants predominate over the harmonic components, and slight additional noise components appear in the high-frequency region above 3000 Hz.
- Type III: The second formants are totally replaced by noise components, and the additional noise components above 3000 Hz further intensify their energy and expand their range.
- Type IV: The second formants are replaced by noise components, and even the first formants of all vowels often lose their periodic components, which are supplemented by noise components. In addition, more intensified, high-frequency additional noise components are seen.

The detection of the formants was carried out one by one, and a manual adjustment of the phonatory intervals was made with greater stability and with more horizontal tracings in the spectrogram.

Above all, the difficulty was in cases in which the first formant was close to F0.

In TEVA, for example, a stable [a] sound will show a smooth spectrogram with many harmonics as horizontal lines. The more harmonics are clearly visible, the better the voice is.

2.5. Statistical Analysis

Statistical analysis was conducted using Stata 14.2 for Windows (StataCorp, LLC., College Station, TX, USA). Two-tailed statistical tests were employed, and a 95% confidence interval was utilized. Normality was assessed through the Kolmogorov–Smirnov test, while variances were examined using the Levene test. Quantitative variables were presented as mean ± standard deviation (SD) and median when applicable. Group mean comparisons were carried out using the Student's *t*-test, Mann–Whitney test, ANOVA, or Kruskal–Wallis test as appropriate. Qualitative variables were represented as frequency and percentage. Group differences were assessed through the chi-square test, Fisher's exact test, or their respective variants when suitable.

3. Results

3.1. Descriptive Analysis

A total of 34 patients were included (Table 1). All were men with a mean age of 63.41 ± 9.55 years (Table 2). With regard to the type of surgery performed, the most frequent intervention was TL with bilateral neck dissection in 21 patients (63.6%). The most frequent tumor locations were the glottis and supraglottic areas, with 20 patients affected (10 in each location, 30.3%, respectively), followed by the transglottic in 8 patients (24.2%). The pathological TNM in most cases was advanced stages T3–T4, with 30 patients (85.7%). The most commonly performed pharyngeal suture technique was a T-closure, to which a Tapia corset was added in 12 patients (35.30%), followed by a Hormaeche closure in 10 patients (29.4%). The remaining 12 patients (35.30%) were classified as others (including the association of the T-closure with other techniques, such as discontinuous closure, closure over a salivary tube, or a microvascular flap). More than half of the patients (n = 20, 58.8%) received adjunctive treatment with RT, with a mean of 54.62 Gy ± 4.43.

Table 1. Descriptive analysis.

Variables	Subgroups	N (%)
Surgery Type	TL [1] + BFND [2]	21 (63.6)
	TL + FLND [3] + RRND [4]	1 (3)
	TL + BFND + RFFF [5]	2 (6.1)
	TL + BFND	3 (9.1)
	TL + RLND [6] + FRND [7]	2 (6.1)
	TL + FLND	3 (9.1)
	TL + RRND	1 (3)
Tumor location	Transglottic	8 (24.2)
	Supraglottic	10 (30.3)
	Glottic	10 (30.3)
	Hypopharynx	5 (15.2)
pTNM	T4N1	2 (7.1)
	T3N1	2 (7.1)
	T4N0	3 (10.7)
	T2N0	4 (14.3)
	T3N2	10 (35.7)
	T3N0	6 (21.4)
	T4N2	1 (3.6)
TEP [8]	Primary	20 (58.8)
	Secondary	14 (41.2)
N. of voice prosthesis	8	17 (50)
	6	11 (32.4)
	4	5 (14.7)
	10	1 (2.9)
Radiotherapy treatment	Yes	20 (58.8)
	No	14 (41.2)
Pulmonary pathology	Yes	11 (32.4)
	No	23 (67.6)
Dysphagia	No	34 (100)
Pharyngeal closure	T + Tapia corset	12 (35.3)
	Hormaeche	12 (35.3)
	Others	10 (29.4)

[1] TL, total laryngectomy; [2] BFND, bilateral functional neck dissection; [3] FLND, functional left neck dissection; [4] RRND, radical right neck dissection; [5] RFFF, radial forearm free flap; [6] RLND, radical left neck dissection; [7] FRND, functional right neck dissection; [8] TEP, tracheoesophageal puncture.

Table 2. Descriptive analysis of continuous variables, subjective characterization of TES, and formants of [a] and [i] with PRAAT.

	Mean	Median	Standard Deviation	Min	Max
Age (years)	63.41	62.50	9.55	48.00	89.0
Number of VP [1] replacements	4.12	3.00	3.68	1.00	17.0
Gy [2] of RT [3] received	54.62	54.00	4.43	46.00	64.0
GRBAS [4]	7.35	7.50	3.36	1.00	14.0
VHI [5]	11.29	6.50	11.16	0.00	34.0
[a] Phonation time (s)	13.16	13.13	5.89	3.20	24.3
[a] 1° formant Frequency (F1)(Hz)	835.42	826.84	118.08	627.49	1059.1
[a] 2° formant Frequency (F2)(Hz)	1560.44	1553.92	209.94	1205.41	2272.2
[a] 3° formant Frequency (F3)(Hz)	2955.33	2948.03	242.54	2429.03	3477.7
[i] Phonation time (s)	12.11	11.15	5.84	2.89	25.6
[i] 1° formant Frequency (F1)(Hz)	472.86	388.39	210.93	283.26	1074.5
[i] 2° formant Frequency (F2)(Hz)	2450.03	2454.26	211.79	1838.55	2826.2
[i] 3° formant Frequency (F3)(Hz)	3112.98	3102.33	180.60	2865.25	3711.3

[1] VP, voice prosthesis; [2] Gy, gray; [3] RT, radiotherapy; [4] GRBAS scale (grade, roughness, breathiness, asthenia, strain), [5] Voice Handicap Index.

A primary TEP was performed in 20 patients (58.8%) and a secondary TEP in 14 patients (41.2%). In most cases of secondary TEP, a previous primary TEP was performed (71.42%).

The second intervention was due to local complications of the TEP or its closure. The number of the VP placed at the moment of study in most cases was Provox No. 8 (50%). The second most frequent was Provox No. 6 (32.35%).

3.2. Vocal Analysis

3.2.1. Subjective Analysis

The mean score of the GRBAS scale was 7.35 ± 3.35. Self-perception by the patients, evaluated with the Voice Handicap Index (VHI-10) test, showed a mean score of 11.29 ± 11.16 points, categorized as moderate handicap (Table 2).

3.2.2. Acoustic Analysis

The acoustic analysis comparing the TEVA and PRAAT programs for the phonemes [a] and [i] is summarized in Table 3. In all cases, differences were found in the acoustic analysis results between TEVA and PRAAT, except for Shimmer [a].

In the acoustic analysis of the [a] phoneme, the jitter analysis obtained an average of 2.09% with TEVA and 2.86% with PRAAT.

In the variation component of the amplitude studied with the shimmer of the [a] phoneme, the value is larger with the TEVA (mean 25.6%) compared to the PRAAT, which obtained a mean value of 15%.

The mean and maximum [a] frequencies have similar values, especially in the results of average intensity (TEVA 64.1 dB vs. PRAAT 63.9 dB). In the case of the maximum intensity, there was a greater difference (TEVA 74.8 dB vs. PRAAT 66.9 dB).

The mean fundamental frequency differs between both softwares, with the average in the analysis with TEVA being 105 Hz and with PRAAT being 275 Hz.

Finally, regarding [a] HNR, results with similar figures were obtained with both softwares (TEVA 3.36 dB vs. PRAAT 3.49 dB).

Table 3. Comparison of the results obtained in the instrumental analysis with the PRAAT and TEVA for the different variables (jitter, shimmer, mean and maximum intensity, fundamental frequency, and harmonic to noise ratio (HNR) obtained with the phonemes [a] and [i] with a microphone and mouth distance between 5 and 10 cm.

	TEVA [1]			PRAAT			p-Value
	Mean ± SD	Median	Range	Mean ± SD	Median	Range	
[a] Jitter (%)	2.09 ± 3.34	1.5	0.3–20	2.86 ± 2.61	1.75	0.34–9.19	<0.001
[a] Shimmer (%)	25.6 ± 12.8	21.3	8.70–57.3	15 ± 5.86	15.8	0.5–26.3	0.213
[a] Mean SPL (dB)	64.1 ± 6.22	64	50.6–78.5	63.9 ± 7.08	63.9	51–81	<0.001
[a] Maximum SPL (dB)	74.8 ± 10.1	73.1	54.8–91.4	66.9 ± 6.95	66.7	54.9–83.1	<0.001
[a] Fundamental frequency (F0) (Hz)	105 ± 41.7	96	49–215	275 ± 83	115	58.4–264	<0.001
[a] HNR [2] (dB)	3.36 ± 2.12	2.75	0.5–8	3.49 ± 2.36	3.13	0.07–7.99	<0.001
[i] Jitter (%)	1.57 ± 1.66	0.85	0.2–6.5	2.8 ± 2.54	1.82	0.29–11.1	<0.001
[i] Shimmer (%)	22.4 ± 12.4	17.9	4.1–52.2	14.9 ± 4.27	16	4.83–21.9	<0.001
[i] Mean intensity (dB)	63.3 ± 5.75	62.5	49.3–76.1	62 ± 6.24	61.7	48.4–74.8	<0.001
[i] Maximum intensity (dB)	66.9 ± 6.52	66.8	49.9–80.8	64.8 ± 5.9	64.5	51.1–76.4	<0.001
[i] Fundamental frequency (F0) (Hz)	109 ± 47.5	93	59–240	142 ± 117	90.3	54.8–635	<0.001
[i] HNR (dB)	5.46 ± 2.67	5.05	0.9–11.1	4.56 ± 2.47	4.2	1.39–10.9	<0.001

[1] TEVA, Tracheoesophageal Voice Analysis; [2] HNR, harmonic to noise ratio.

Regarding the acoustic analysis of the [i] phoneme, in this case, in the jitter value, there is a greater difference in the obtained result (TEVA 1.57% vs. PRAAT 2.8%).

The result of shimmer in the [i] phoneme, as occurred in the [a] analysis, is higher with the TEVA analysis, 22.4% vs. PRAAT 14.9%.

In the case of [i], the average and maximum intensities are much greater, even TEVA at 63.3 dB and 66.9 dB (mean and maximum, respectively) vs. PRAAT at 62 dB and 64.8 dB.

In relation to the fundamental frequency, statistically significant differences were also found (TEVA 109 Hz vs. PRAAT 142 Hz).

Finally, the [i] HNR was higher with TEVA at 5.46 dB vs. PRAAT at 4.56 dB.

Regarding the spectrographic analysis, no significant differences were found between both softwares, TEVA vs. PRAAT (Figure 1 and Table 4).

Table 4. Spectrogram analysis with TEVA and PRAAT (Yanagihara classification).

		Grade I N (%)	Grade II N (%)	Grade III N (%)	Grade IV N (%)	p-Value
[a]	TEVA	14 (41.2)	10 (29.4)	4 (11.8)	6 (17.6)	0.201
	PRAAT	15 (44.1)	15 (44.1)	3 (8.8)	1 (2.9)	
[i]	TEVA	8 (23.5)	15 (44.1)	8 (23.5)	3 (8.8)	0.414
	PRAAT	13 (38.2)	15 (44.1)	5 (14.7)	1 (2.9)	

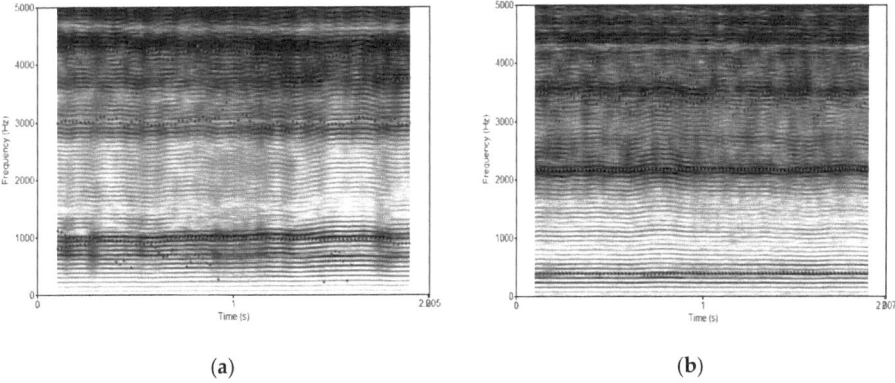

(a)   (b)

Figure 1. TEVA spectrographic analysis of [a] and [i]. Manually adjusted and selected sample in a sustained vowel of two-second duration. The stability and sharpness of the harmonics and formants are appreciated. (a) [a] Phoneme; (b) [i] phoneme.

4. Discussion

Acoustic signal typing and analysis is used in laryngeal voice and is often recorded with PRAAT software [11,12]. However, standard acoustic voice analyses are not always suitable to measure substitute voices because speech originating in the vibrating pharyngoesophageal segment, as TES, is known to contain more noise components and less regularity than laryngeal voice [2,13]. Therefore, the acoustic analysis of the tracheoesophageal voice continues to be a challenge today. Specific programs have been developed for TES [3,4]. This involved categorizing tracheoesophageal voices into four subtypes based on visual assessment of the acoustic content of narrow-band spectrograms supported by written guidelines [3,14,15].

Most of the recent studies demonstrate the superiority of the results obtained from instrumental and subjective acoustic analysis in patients using VP compared to other types of phonatory rehabilitation [16]. Recent reviews also demonstrated the best results in subjective questionnaires analyzing vocal quality, intelligibility, and quality of life [17].

Despite TEVA being a tool based on PRAAT, there are currently no studies comparing both analysis methods in laryngectomized patients. This study aims to conduct a comparative analysis of both objective acoustic analysis programs, with the objective of discerning any distinctions that may determine the suitability of one program over the other for the investigation of phonatory quality in TL patients.

In relation to the results obtained in our study in the VHI survey, an average of 11.29 was observed, classified as moderate handicap, but very close to a mild handicap value (less than 10 points) [18]. These results demonstrate the great satisfaction of patients with their speech rehabilitation method. The lower values in the fundamental frequency with the TEVA analysis are notable, considering that they are subjectively perceived as deep voices; therefore, these results are more in line with reality.

Regarding the speech stability values, the jitter evaluates the variation of the F0 between one cycle and the next [8,18,19]. The adaptation of the acoustic study to TES patients with TEVA demonstrates values closer to normalcy (<1%) for both phonemes [a] and [i] (2.09% and 1.57%, respectively) compared with the study with PRAAT (2.86% and 2.8%). Another equilibrium value is the shimmer parameter, which evaluates the variability of the amplitude from cycle to cycle and is inversely related to vocal intensity. For laryngeal voice (normal shimmer value <7%), the speech intensity during conversation is between 75 and 80 dB and depends on variables such as subglottal pressure, glottal closure, and respiratory capacity [18]. TL patients lose their laryngeal functions, and the airflow regulation needed for speech emission is worse. Furthermore, these patients, with a history of a smoking habit in most cases, usually have smaller lung capacities because of their respiratory pathology. For this reason, TL patients have intensity numbers lower than normal, considerably increasing shimmer values.

Despite the differences observed in our study in the formant analysis carried out with TEVA and PRAAT, no statistically significant differences were found, as were expected. It is worth noting the higher number of patients in III and IV grades for the [a] phoneme with TEVA (29.4%) than with PRAAT (11.7%). The same occurs for the phoneme [i] (TEVA n = 11; 32.3% vs. PRAAT n = 6; 17.6%). This fact can be explained because with TEVA, a more specific TES analysis is carried out, in which a less stable voice is identified and has fewer harmonic components than in the spectrographic analysis with PRAAT [3].

Tracheoesophageal speech (TES) seems to be more comparable to healthy speech, but it is necessary to go one step further to more precisely categorize this type of voice [2,7,11–14]. Therefore, analysis with a specific program for TES, such as TEVA, is more suitable for voices with VP since the adjustment of parameters for alaryngeal voices with a greater noise component is more accurate.

In the statistical analysis, significant results were observed in most of the variables. This means that the differences are not simply due to chance, and there are changes or differences between the two.

The difference between both programs that makes us think that TEVA is more specific and better adjusted to the characteristics of TES patients is that it categorizes the TES voices based on Van As-Brooks classification, keeping in mind the specific phonation stability, duration, and the presence or absence of harmonics in these kinds of voices.

On the other hand, PRAAT is a program designed for the analysis of laryngeal voices, with many of its algorithms focused on the fundamental frequency, which is much more irregular in patients with TES, so the analysis of these voices may be less adjusted to reality.

That is why, with exactly the same samples being studied, the TEVA software seems more adapted to the characteristics of laryngectomized patients who use TES. Furthermore, the results obtained with the TEVA are more similar to those expected initially, as we have commented before, especially in terms of fundamental frequency and amplitude variation.

The acoustic analysis was performed by individualizing each patient and adjusting the study to obtain the different variables in the most reliable way possible. For this reason, we believe that the values are as correct as possible.

5. Conclusions

In our study, the instrumental acoustic variables comparing the PRAAT and TEVA programs demonstrate with statistically significant evidence that the TEVA program could adjust more precisely and reliably to patients with alaryngeal voices who use TES. The differences observed between both types of software may be due to a better adjustment of the automatic parameters in the TEVA, and both may be complementary to categorize these types of voices in a more complete way. Furthermore, it would be interesting to expand the study sample, including patients of both genders, and try to improve the acoustic signal typing and objective vocal analysis of this type of patient.

Author Contributions: Conceptualization, A.K.-R., M.M.-Y. and F.V.-d.l.I.; methodology, A.K.-R., I.C.-V. and M.M.-Y.; software, A.K.-R. and M.M.-Y.; validation, C.M.C.-E., A.K.-R., I.C.-V. and M.M.-Y.; formal analysis, A.K.-R. and M.M.-Y.; investigation A.K.-R. and M.M.-Y.; resources, A.K.-R., I.C.-V. and M.M.-Y.; data curation, A.K.-R. and M.M.-Y.; writing—original draft preparation, A.K.-R.; writing—review and editing, C.M.C.-E., A.K.-R. and M.M.-Y.; visualization, A.K.-R. and M.M.-Y.; supervision, M.M.-Y.; project administration, A.K.-R. All authors have read and agreed to the published version of the manuscript.

Funding: The costs of the APC were covered by Fundación Profesor Nóvoa Santos (Hospital Teresa-Herrera, 1ª Planta. C/Xubias de Arriba, No. 84, 15006, A Coruña).

Institutional Review Board Statement: The study was conducted in accordance with the Declaration of Helsinki and approved by the Ethics Committee of Complexo Hospitalario Universitario de A Coruña (protocol code 2022/94, data of approval 25 April 2022) for studies involving humans.

Informed Consent Statement: Informed consent was obtained from all subjects involved in the study.

Data Availability Statement: The data presented in this study are available on request from the corresponding author due to privacy.

Conflicts of Interest: The authors declare no conflicts of interest.

References

1. Boersma, P.; Weenink, D. *PRAAT: Doing Phonetics by Computer*, (Version 5.3.51). 2007.
2. Klein-Rodríguez, A.; Cabo-Varela, I.; Vázquez-de la Iglesia, F. Acoustic Characterization of the Voice with a Tracheoesophageal Speech in Laryngectomized Patients. Similarities and Differences with the Laryngeal Voice. *J. Voice* **2020**, *37*, 144.e9–144.e14. [CrossRef] [PubMed]
3. van As-Brooks, C.J.; Koopmans-van Beinum, F.J.; Pols, L.C.; Hilgers, F.J. Acoustic Signal Typing for Evaluation of Voice Quality in Tracheoesophageal Speech. *J. Voice* **2006**, *20*, 355–368. [CrossRef] [PubMed]
4. Clapham, R.P.; van As-Brooks, C.J.; van Son, R.J.; Hilgers, F.J.; Brekel, M.W.v.D. The Relationship between Acoustic Signal Typing and Perceptual Evaluation of Tracheoesophageal Voice Quality for Sustained Vowels. *J. Voice* **2015**, *29*, 517.e23–517.e29. [CrossRef] [PubMed]
5. Cuenca, M.H.; Barrio, M.M. Acoustic Markers of Prosodic Boundaries in Spanish Spontaneous Alaryngeal Speech. *Clin. Linguist. Phon.* **2010**, *24*, 859–869. [CrossRef] [PubMed]
6. NKI TE-VOICE ANALYSIS Tool (EN). Available online: https://www.fon.hum.uva.nl/rob/NKI_TEVA/ (accessed on 26 May 2024).
7. van As, C.J. *Tracheoesophageal Speech. A Multidimensional Assessment of Voice Quality*; Budde-Elinkwijk Grafische Producties: Nieuwegein, The Netherlands, 2001; ISBN 978-90-90-15058-1.
8. Available online: https://www.atosmedical.es/productos/provox-vega (accessed on 26 May 2024).
9. Patel, R.R.; Awan, S.N.; Barkmeier-Kraemer, J.; Courey, M.; Deliyski, D.; Eadie, T.; Paul, D.; Švec, J.G.; Hillman, R. Recommended Protocols for Instrumental Assessment of Voice: American Speech-Language-Hearing Association Expert Panel to Develop a Protocol for Instrumental Assessment of Vocal Function. *Am. J. Speech-Lang. Pathol.* **2018**, *27*, 887–905. [CrossRef] [PubMed]
10. Yanagihara, N. Significance of harmonic changes and noise components in hoarseness. *J. Speech Hear. Res.* **1967**, *10*, 531–541. [CrossRef] [PubMed]
11. Núñez-Batalla, F.; Corte-Santos, P.; Señaris-González, B.; Llorente-Pendás, J.L.; Górriz-Gil, C.; Suárez-Nieto, C. Adaptation and validation to the Spanish of the Voice Handicap Index (VHI-30) and its shortened version (VHI-10). *Acta Otorrinolaringol. Esp.* **2007**, *58*, 386–392. [CrossRef] [PubMed]
12. Titze, I.R. *Workshop on Acoustic Voice Analysis: Summary Statement*; National Center for Voice and Speech: Iowa City, IA, USA, 1995.

13. Lechien, J.R.; Geneid, A. Consensus for Voice Quality Assessment in Clinical Practice: Guidelines of the European Laryngological Society and Union of the European Phoniatricians. *Eur. Arch. Otorhinolaryngol.* **2023**, *280*, 5459–5473. [CrossRef] [PubMed]
14. Moerman, M.; Martens, J.-P.; Dejonckere, P. Multidimensional Assessment of Strongly Irregular Voices Such as in Substitution Voicing and Spasmodic Dysphonia: A Compilation of Own Research. *Logop. Phoniatr. Vocol.* **2015**, *40*, 24–29. [CrossRef] [PubMed]
15. van Sluis, K.E.; van der Molen, L.; van Son, R.J.J.H.; Hilgers, F.J.M.; Bhairosing, P.A.; van den Brekel, M.W.M. Objective and Subjective Voice Outcomes after Total Laryngectomy: A Systematic Review. *Eur. Arch Otorhinolaryngol.* **2018**, *275*, 11–26. [CrossRef]
16. Hurren, A.; Miller, N. Voice Outcomes Post Total Laryngectomy. *Curr. Opin. Otolaryngol. Head Neck Surg.* **2017**, *25*, 205–210. [CrossRef] [PubMed]
17. Sirić, L.; Sos, D.; Rosso, M.; Stevanović, S. Objective Assessment of Tracheoesophageal and Esophageal Speech Using Acoustic Analysis of Voice. *Coll. Antropol.* **2012**, *36* (Suppl. S2), 111–114. [PubMed]
18. Maniaci, A.; Lechien, J.R.; Caruso, S.; Nocera, F.; Ferlito, S.; Iannella, G.; Grillo, C.M.; Magliulo, G.; Pace, A.; Vicini, C.; et al. Voice-Related Quality of Life After Total Laryngectomy: Systematic Review and Meta-Analysis. *J. Voice* **2021**, *38*, 539.e11–539.e19. [CrossRef]
19. Cobeta, I. Evaluación Clínica de la Fonación. Laboratorio de Voz. Suárez C, Gil-Carcedo LM. In *Tratado de Otorrinolaringología y Cirugía de Cabeza y Cuello*; Proyectos Médicos: Madrid, Spain, 2000.

Disclaimer/Publisher's Note: The statements, opinions and data contained in all publications are solely those of the individual author(s) and contributor(s) and not of MDPI and/or the editor(s). MDPI and/or the editor(s) disclaim responsibility for any injury to people or property resulting from any ideas, methods, instructions or products referred to in the content.

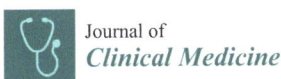

Article

It Sounds like It Feels: Preliminary Exploration of an Aeroacoustic Diagnostic Protocol for Singers

Calvin Peter Baker [1,2], Suzanne C. Purdy [1,*], Te Oti Rakena [2] and Stefano Bonnini [3]

[1] Speech Science, School of Psychology, University of Auckland, Auckland 1023, New Zealand; calvin.baker@auckland.ac.nz
[2] School of Music, University of Auckland, Auckland 1010, New Zealand; t.rakena@auckland.ac.nz
[3] Department of Economics & Management, University of Ferrara, 44121 Ferrara, Italy; bnnsfn@unife.it
* Correspondence: sc.purdy@auckland.ac.nz

Abstract: To date, no established protocol exists for measuring functional voice changes in singers with subclinical singing-voice complaints. Hence, these may go undiagnosed until they progress into greater severity. This exploratory study sought to (1) determine which scale items in the self-perceptual Evaluation of Ability to Sing Easily (EASE) are associated with instrumental voice measures, and (2) construct as proof-of-concept an instrumental index related to singers' perceptions of their vocal function and health status. Eighteen classical singers were acoustically recorded in a controlled environment singing an /a/ vowel using soft phonation. Aerodynamic data were collected during a softly sung /papapapapapapa/ task with the KayPENTAX Phonatory Aerodynamic System. Using multi and univariate linear regression techniques, CPPS, vibrato jitter, vibrato shimmer, and an efficiency ratio (SPL/P_{Sub}) were included in a significant model ($p < 0.001$) explaining 62.4% of variance in participants' composite scores of three scale items related to vocal fatigue. The instrumental index showed a significant association ($p = 0.001$) with the EASE vocal fatigue subscale overall. Findings illustrate that an aeroacoustic instrumental index may be useful for monitoring functional changes in the singing voice as part of a multidimensional diagnostic approach to preventative and rehabilitative voice healthcare for professional singing-voice users.

Keywords: functional diagnostics; preventative healthcare; self-perception; vocal fatigue; singing voice analysis

1. Introduction

The human voice is a versatile instrument that allows for the transmission of complex data including societal traditions, histories, codes, and emotions. Only small changes in voice production are needed to produce great shifts in intent and meaning. Professional singers rely on subtle and nuanced changes in voice function that require mobile, robust, and healthy vocal folds. Deterioration in voice production may significantly impact quality of life when a singer's voice is affected by organic (structural or neurological) or functional disorders [1–3]. Reputation in the artistic community and ability to earn a livelihood can also be negatively affected [4].

For voice researchers, clinicians, and pedagogues, singing-voice analysis presents unique challenges. Many of the widely used voice assessment techniques (e.g., local pitch and amplitude perturbation measures) rely on methods that may not be robust to singing-voice variables such as wide ranges in f_o, intensity, or vibrato characteristics (e.g., [5–9]). Additionally, traditional clinical voice analysis tasks (e.g., sustained vowels and reading passages at a comfortable pitch and intensity) do not incorporate the singing voice or consider singing-specific phenomena such as registration events or vibrato characteristics. While some may reason that speech samples are sufficient for all voice analyses, the analogous idea of analyzing task-specific movements of elite athletes without having them perform tasks relevant to their professional context is incongruous. If a singer presents with a singing-voice complaint, their singing voice should be analyzed.

Non-traumatic (i.e., not caused by a specific injury or event) clinical voice disorders (e.g., muscle tension dysphonia or nodules) are preceded by functional changes that increase risk of vocal injury [10,11]. Even without clear visual findings, maladaptive changes in vocal function result in inefficiencies and discomfort that are readily perceived by the trained voice user [12,13]. Therefore, determining biomarkers of early functional voice disorder is critical for preventative and habilitative healthcare for professional singing-voice users. Instruments that can measure functional changes in the singing voice related to singing-voice complaints may improve methods for monitoring vocal health through periods of hormonal or physiological change or periods of increased vocal demand (e.g., intense performance runs or leading up to performance exams). Patel et al. [14] recommend protocols for speech analysis but do not comment on the singing voice or the unique challenges related to singing voice analysis. To date no standardized protocol exists for quantitative singing-voice analysis in a clinical context, suggesting that these subclinical voice complaints must progress into greater severity before treatment is offered, i.e., when potential livelihood is impacted.

The Evaluation of Ability to Sing Easily (EASE) [15] was developed in acknowledgement of the unique voice complaints experienced by singers. The EASE is a self-rating scale consisting of three subscales that should be scored and interpreted separately: Vocal Fatigue (*VF*), Pathological Risk Indicators (*PRI*), and Voice Concerns (*VC*). The final instrument is a 22-item questionnaire using the four-point Likert-type responses *Not at all* (1); *Mildly* (2); *Moderately* (3); and *Extremely* (4). Appendix A provides a full list of the 22 items. Phyland (2014, unpublished data) reported good internal consistency for each subscale (Cronbach's α all > 0.8) and statistically significant correlations ($p < 0.001$) between each of the subscales. The EASE has shown promise in distinguishing between healthy and disordered singers and appears to be sensitive to subtle functional changes perceived by professional and semi-professional voice users [16–20]. The EASE is unique in that it was constructed to measure self-perceived vocal status without the assumption of voice disorder or injury [15,21], making it a particularly relevant tool for use with singers with subclinical voice complaints. While it has recently been recommended as part of a multidisciplinary approach when working with singers in the voice clinic [22], few studies have explored associations between EASE subscale items and instrumental voice measures.

1.1. Instrumental Analysis of the Singing Voice

Although there are many acoustic measures to choose from for speech-level analysis, fewer have proven efficacy for use with sung samples. Inverse filtering is a useful method for extracting voice-source information for both spoken and sung samples. The non-invasive nature of inverse filtering an acoustic signal allows singers to perform sung vocal tasks generally unencumbered. Inverse filters (or antiresonances) are used to counteract the vocal-tract transfer function, leaving only the estimated voice-source spectrum and the flow-glottogram (FLOGG). The normalized amplitude quotient (NAQ) is one parameter that can be calculated from the FLOGG and its first derivative [23,24]. It reflects the degree and quality of glottal closure related to phonation type, from breathy to pressed, and between singing styles [23,25–28]. The NAQ operates in the amplitude domain and hence is less affected by glottal event delineation [23,29]. As the NAQ infers glottal configuration related to phonation type, there may be an association between EASE subscale scores and NAQ values. One limitation is that the successful extraction of the FLOGG depends on accurate determination of the first two formants ($F_{1,2}$). Conveniently, the inverse filter module of *Sopran* [30] contains a real-time display of the FLOGG as the inverse filters are applied, allowing the user to adjust the frequencies to 'tune' the inverse filters to achieve a ripple-free closed phase in the FLOGG and a smooth source-spectrum tilt with no large dips surrounding the formants.

Relative average perturbation (RAP, %) and amplitude perturbation quotient 3 (APQ3, %) quantify pitch and amplitude perturbation in the glottal cycle, smoothed across three consecutive periods. They have been used successfully with singing voice samples [31,32] and are not widely affected by changes in f_o, intensity, or vibrato extent (VE) as are local jitter and shimmer (Baker et al., in review). An increase in EASE subscale scores may also be reflected in increased in RAP, APQ3, or both.

Smoothed cepstral peak prominence (CPPS) reflects the dB difference between the cepstral peak (most prominent rahmonic in the cepstrum), and a linear regression line at the same quefrency (ms). CPPS successfully discriminates between dysphonic and normophonic voices and has shown sensitivity to breathiness in normophonic speakers [33–37]. As CPPS is robust to factors such as environmental noise and microphone selection [38], it may be a useful clinical tool for tracking subtle changes in the singing voice. After controlling for the effects of f_o and intensity [7,39], a decrease in CPPS values may be associated with elevated EASE subscale scores.

The ubiquity of vibrato in the Western classical singing voice (WCSV) makes it a highly relevant candidate for singing-voice analysis in classically trained singers. Systematic contemporary commercial music (CCM) voice pedagogy is relatively young [40,41]. However, the present authors note growing consensus among practitioners that, while stylistic choices may influence vibrato characteristics, a well-balanced 'neutral' vocal production (i.e., not shaped by stylistic voice effects) that includes a stable and free vibrato should be a goal for CCM singers, from which artistry can be shaped. Stability in vibrato rate (VR) and VE is dependent on stable oscillatory mechanisms and fine intralaryngeal muscle coordination [42–44]. Morelli and colleagues [45] presented the *BioVoice* voice-analysis software that includes two measures for singing voice vibrato perturbation analysis: vibrato jitter and vibrato shimmer (hereafter V_{Jitt} and V_{Shim}). Like the well-known jitter and shimmer measures that measure frequency and amplitude perturbation in the acoustic waveform, V_{Jitt} and V_{Shim} quantify perturbation in the f_o vibrato waveform of a sung sample (for V_{Jitt} and V_{Shim} equations see [46]). Vibrato is a multidimensional phenomenon that includes cyclical muscular contractions producing a quasi-sinusoidal f_o oscillation. As such, inefficiencies in function or structural changes in the vocal folds are likely to result in decreased stability of VR and VE. Thus, the severity of singer-perceived voice complaints may increase with higher V_{Jitt} and V_{Shim}.

Aerodynamic measures provide complementary data to acoustic analyses that have clear physiological attributes. The Phonatory Aerodynamic System (PAS) [47] provides information on inferred subglottal pressure (P_{Sub}; cm H_2O, measured from intra-oral pressure during a /p/ occlusion), airflow during voicing (l/s), and sound-pressure-level (SPL [dB]). These data can be used to calculate various efficiency ratios. As described by Toles et al. [48], the SPL-to-P_{Sub} ratio decreases with incomplete adduction, perhaps due to functional or structural changes [49,50]. Thus, lower efficiency ratios may be associated with higher EASE subscale values. In this study, the ratio used will be referred to as Efficiency Ratio (ER), and is defined in Equation (1):

$$ER = \frac{SPL}{P_{Sub}} = \frac{dB}{cm\ H_2O} \quad (1)$$

While the measures explored here are not exhaustive, they offer complementary data on vocal function, can be successfully computed from sung samples, and can be easily implemented using existing tools in clinical and research contexts.

1.2. The Present Study

To date little research has been carried out exploring the links between instrumental voice measures and singers' perceptions of their own vocal function and health. These are needed to help determine biomarkers that indicate at-risk vocal function in professional singing-voice users with voice complaints and are critical for developing evidence-based preventative and rehabilitative healthcare approaches for singers.

The present exploratory study sought to (1) examine associations between selected acoustic and aerodynamic instrumental measures and the individual scale items of the EASE, and (2) to develop as proof-of-concept a multi-instrumental quantitative index of biomarkers that is sensitive to singers' self-perceived vocal function and health status. Instrumental measures were selected a priori based on their suitability for singing voice analysis and proven efficacy for tracking functional changes in voice behavior. We predicted that higher EASE item values would be associated with reduced vocal stability and efficiency as gauged through acoustic and aerodynamic voice measures.

2. Materials and Methods

2.1. Participants

A cross-sectional cohort of healthy cisgender male and female singers was recruited by a third party from the University of Auckland, School of Music Classical Voice Department. As the trans voice presents unique variations in function and may be structurally altered by hormonal or surgical intervention [51–54], only cisgender singers were included in this study. However, further specific research on non-binary and trans voice is needed. All singers were classically trained and had experience performing in solo, choral, and ensemble contexts. Data were collected between March and August 2022.

The singers were first asked to complete one online questionnaire which included the Singing-Voice Handicap Index-10 (SVHI-10) as a screening tool [55], and demographic data including self-reported ethnicity, stage of study, and total years of training. Participants were asked to disclose any previously diagnosed vocal injury or hearing loss and were seen by a laryngologist to assess vocal health and function. Female participants' recording sessions were scheduled to avoid the pre and perimenstrual period [56–58].

2.2. Acoustic and Aerodynamic Recordings

Each participant was first given five minutes alone in a sound-treated room to warm up their singing voice [59,60] and was asked to perform warmup tasks as if they were preparing for a solo performance. Following the warmup, participants were seated in the room with the researcher for recording. A headset omnidirectional condenser microphone (AKG HC 577L; AKG Acoustics, Vienna, Austria) positioned 7 cm adjacent (45°) to the right of the participant's mouth was used to capture the acoustic voice signal. The microphone was connected to a MacBook Pro running *PRAAT* v. 6.2.16 [61] via a pre-amplifier (MobilePre [MK II]; M-Audio, Rhode Island, USA). All recordings were captured at a 44.1 kHz sample rate. Participants were asked to sustain an /a/ vowel at any comfortable pitch and intensity, during which the C-weighted SPL was measured using an SPL-meter held adjacent to the microphone position. The SPL (L_{Ceq}) was announced by the researcher into the microphone to use later for dB SPL signal calibration before acoustic analyses [62].

Aerodynamic measurements were made using the PAS, a handheld device containing a transducer system that records airflow (through a mask), intra-oral pressure (through an intra-oral tube), and an acoustic signal. The microphone is fixed at a standard distance of approximately 15 cm from the mouth (5 cm preset position). Flow (l/s), pressure (cm H_2O), and SPL (dB) data were captured simultaneously in real time during the consonant-vowel (CV) train /papapapapapapa/.

2.3. Sung Tasks

Following warmup and calibration, participants were asked to sing a quiet /a/ vowel using their usual performance technique on C4 (261.63 Hz, low voice types) or C5 (523.25 Hz, high voice types). The starting f_o for each task was sounded on a digital keyboard before each attempt. Singers were asked to ensure the tone was sung as quietly as possible, whilst maintaining a solo-performance standard of volume, i.e., not a whisper. Soft (but not whispered) phonation requires a fine balance of P_{Sub} and glottal adduction [63–65], and therefore may be more useful in demonstrating vocal-fold related issues such as fatigue or oedema, which can be disguised by louder voicing, when the vocal-folds are more tightly adducted. High voice types were also asked to sing the same vowel on C4, which could be used later during inverse filtering as an approximate reference for F_1 and F_2 if necessary. After these tasks, participants completed the full EASE based on their voice production during the warmup and recording session only.

Following the acoustic recordings and completion of the EASE, participants were instructed how to use the PAS device. They were then asked to sing the CV train /papa-papapapapa/ on C4 (261.63 Hz, low voice types) or C5 (523.25 Hz, high voice types) in one breath as quietly as possible without whispering, in a similar manner to the acoustic recording. Raw data were visually inspected to ensure that the intra-oral pressure value returned to 0 cm H_2O during vowel phonation. The first and last utterances were discarded, and the averaged numerical data of the remaining five utterances were saved to a text file.

2.4. Acoustic Data Processing

Each participant's acoustic recording was saved in its entirety as a .wav file. Tasks were then separated and saved as individual files for analysis. The most stable medial five-second portion of the soft phonation sung task was used for acoustic analysis. Selections were made at the nearest zero-crossings and were checked for clipping, distortion, or extraneous noise aurally and through spectrographic review.

The trimmed acoustic signal was imported into *Sopran* [30] and calibrated with respect to SPL using the calibration tone collected at the time of recording [62]. The NAQ was obtained by first re-sampling the signal to 16 kHz, then inverse filtering the most stable one-second portion of the sung tone. As all singers performed an /a/ vowel, a reasonable estimate of the locations of F_1 and F_2 was possible based on a priori knowledge [66–68]. The inverse filters were tuned to obtain a waveform ideally with a ripple-free zero-flow phase in the FLOGG and a source-spectrum slope free from peaks or troughs surrounding formants [26,69,70]. If a zero-phase was not apparent (likely due to incomplete glottal closure), the inverse-filtered spectrum and negative peak of the flow derivative were used as guides for filter tuning [69,70]. If necessary, the C4 tone produced by the high voice type singers was used as a starting point for tuning formant frequencies. All data were checked for outliers and the process was repeated if a participant's NAQ values were well outside previously reported norms, i.e., 0.1–0.3 [23,25,29].

The CPPS was calculated in *PRAAT* v.6.2.16 [61] using the 'To PowerCepstrum' and 'Get CPPS' functions as described in earlier works [9,71,72]. All settings were kept as standard [61] apart from 'Peak search pitch range (Hz)' which was increased to 1000 Hz to ensure the f_o of all tasks were well accommodated [7]. The RAP and APQ3 were obtained in the 'voice report' function of *PRAAT* using standard settings. The freeware *BioVoice* [45] was used to calculate two measures of vibrato regularity for each signal: V_{Jitt} and V_{Shim}. Numerical results were saved in an *Excel* file after automatic analysis and then integrated into the combined data set.

2.5. Statistical Analyses

Data were statistically analyzed in *RStudio* v. 4.2.1 [73]. Box plots and histograms were used to explore the data and determine the presence of outliers. Multicollinearity was assessed using the variance inflation factor (VIF; Equation (2)), whereby each predictor variable was entered into a separate multiple linear regression model as the dependent variable and tested against the other predictors [74,75]. The VIF numerical threshold for variable inclusion was <5 [75].

$$\text{VIF} = \frac{1}{1 - R^2} \quad (2)$$

Multivariate regression and Pillai's trace with backward elimination were used to determine which instrumental measures (i.e., NAQ, RAP, APQ3, CPPS, V_{Jitt}, V_{Shim}, and ER) were associated with the individual EASE scale items. This approach allowed for the joint estimation of all coefficients and the evaluation of single effects in relation to all others. A composite score was then calculated from these scale items. Kendall's tau-b was used to determine the strength of association between the reduced-item scale and the *VF*, *PRI*, and *VC* subscales of the original EASE tool, respectively. To reduce the effect of possible Type-II errors arising from a small sample, the significance level was set at 0.10.

Predictor variables with a VIF < 5 were included in regression models [76], as well as gender, age, years of training, f_o, and SPL. Multiple linear regression was carried out using a backward elimination iterative method where predictor variables were systematically removed from the model using the largest *p*-value as criteria for exclusion in each iteration. The process was repeated until only predictor variables with *p*-values less than 0.10 were included [74,75]. Finally, multivariate normality was confirmed through non-significant skewness and kurtosis in the models' residuals and Mahalanobis' distances [77,78].

3. Results

Nineteen singers volunteered for participation (soprano [7], mezzo-soprano [1], alto [1], tenor [4], baritone [5], and bass [1]). The mean SVHI-10 score ($M = 10.89$; $SD = 5.28$) was higher than norms recorded by Sobol et al. [79], and one participant disclosed a history of diagnosed vocal injury. Their data was excluded from the ensuing analyses. The remaining 18 participants underwent visual inspection of the vocal folds by a laryngologist and were free of functional or organic voice disorder. Participants' mean age was 26.61 years ($SD = 8.94$, range = 19 to 59 years). Reported ethnicities included European (2), NZ European (9), Asian (3), Māori (3), and Pasifika (1). Mean years of lessons at a tertiary level was 9.94 ($SD = 7.67$, range = 1 to 37 years). Table 1 shows the descriptive statistics for included instrumental variables. In testing for multicollinearity, only RAP had a VIF greater than 5 and so was removed from ensuing analyses.

Table 1. Descriptive Statistics ($N = 18$) for All Included Instrumental Variables.

Measure	Min	Max	Mean	SD
NAQ ($[l/s]^2$)	0.131	0.301	0.209	0.042
RAP (%)	0.032	0.448	0.129	0.124
APQ3 (%)	0.204	1.83	0.727	0.418
CPPS (dB)	11.58	18.02	14.40	1.88
V_{Jitt} (%)	2.43	37.30	11.59	8.59
V_{Shim} %	11.40	47.95	27.27	11.55
ER (dB/cm H_2O)	7.78	15.90	10.74	2.34

Note. NAQ: Normalized Amplitude Quotient. RAP: Relative Average Perturbation. APQ3: Amplitude Perturbation Quotient 3. CPPS: Smoothed Cepstral Peak Prominence. V_{Jitt}: Vibrato Jitter. V_{Shim}: Vibrato Shimmer. ER: Efficiency Ratio.

Multivariate regression with backwards elimination revealed three scale items that were significantly associated ($p < 0.10$) with instrumental measures: Q1 'My voice is husky'; Q2 'My voice is dry/scratchy'; and Q11 'My top notes are breathy'. No age, gender, or training effects were found. The composite values for these three scale items are henceforth referred to as the EASE-3. The EASE-3 had a mean value of 5.17 (range = 3 to 8, $SD = 1.65$) out of a possible 12, where 3 indicates no difficulty at all and 12 indicates an extreme level of difficulty. Construct validity was tested against the original EASE *VF*, *PRI*, and *VC* subscales using Kendall's tau-b. A strong, statistically significant associations were seen between the *VF* subscales and the EASE-3 ($\tau = 0.742$, $p < 0.0001$). The *PRI* subscale was moderately associated with the EASE-3 ($\tau = 0.324$, $p = 0.089$). No correlation was found between the *VC* subscale and the EASE-3 ($\tau = 0.046$, $p > 0.10$).

Using Pillai's trace tests with backwards elimination, four significant coefficients' estimates were revealed (all $V > 0.55$, $p < 0.05$), corresponding to the explanatory variables CPPS, V_{Jitt}, V_{Shim}, ER. A univariate model including these measures showed a good fit for the EASE-3 data and was statistically significant, adjusted $R^2 = 0.624$, $p < 0.01$. Residual skewness and kurtosis for this model were non-significant ($p > 0.05$) and Mahalanobis' distance was below the critical D^2 value of 27.69 (12.88, $p < 0.01$). Signal SPL (dB), f_o, age, gender, and years of training showed no contribution in explaining variance, $p > 0.10$. The regression model for the EASE-3 is shown in Table 2. The regression equation is presented in Equation (3). Values derived from the model had a strong correlation with the original VF subscale ($\tau = 0.575$, $p = 0.001$), a moderate correlation with the PRI subscale $\tau = 0.295$, $p = 0.098$), and no correlation with the VC subscale ($\tau = 0.070$, $p > 0.10$).

$$\hat{y} = 14.0114 - 0.41753 * CPPS + 0.10822 * V_{Jitt} + 0.1164 * V_{Shim} - 0.6764 * ER \quad (3)$$

Table 2. Regression Model for the EASE-3.

	Estimate	Std. Error	T Value	Sig.
Intercept	14.0114	2.93662	4.771	<0.000 ***
CPPS (dB)	−0.41753	0.17085	−2.444	0.029 *
V_{Jitt} (%)	0.10822	0.03039	3.561	0.003 **
V_{Shim} (%)	0.1164	0.02927	3.977	0.002 **
ER (dB/cm H$_2$O)	−0.6764	0.14007	−4.829	<0.000 ***
Residual std. error: 1.014 on 13 df		Adjusted R^2 = 0.624		
F-statistic: 8.064 on 4 and 13 df		$p = 0.001696$ **		

Note. EASE-3: Evaluation of Ability to Sing Easily-3. CPPS: Smoothed cepstral peak prominence. V_{Jitt}: Vibrato jitter. V_{Shim}: Vibrato shimmer. ER: Efficiency ratio. Significance: *** $p < 0.001$, ** $p < 0.01$, * $p < 0.05$.

4. Discussion

Trained signers are sensitive to subtle changes in voice function that may not be apparent under visual examination. This does not mean, however, that these complaints should be taken lightly or dismissed; these subclinical functional changes may be precursors to developing functional or organic voice disorders such as muscle-tension dysphonia or space-occupying mass (e.g., nodules). To date, no established clinical protocols exist for working with the singing voice, and few studies have considered the suitability of traditional voice analysis techniques for singing voice analysis. This suggests that a singer's voice complaint must increase in severity (i.e., into dysphonia) before it is quantitatively measurable using clinical diagnostic instruments with speech samples. This is too late for the professional voice user who relies on optimal vocal function for livelihood. Furthermore, delay in diagnosis of subclinical functional disorders may lead to anxiety and loss of confidence and self-efficacy [80–83].

The EASE was developed to collect data on singers' self-perception of their vocal function and health at a single time point [15,21]. The EASE and its subscales have shown promise in distinguishing dysphonic from normophonic singers, and in measuring singers' perceptions of vocal function and health during periods of high vocal demand and in pre/postintervention studies [17,84,85]. We initially hypothesized that an increase in singers' EASE scores would be associated with increased values in acoustic measures, and decreased ER. Multiple linear regression with backwards elimination determined four instrumental predictors (CPPS, V_{Jitt}, V_{Shim}, and ER) that were significantly associated with three of the original 22 scale items: (1) My voice is husky, (2) My voice is dry/scratchy, and (3) My top notes are breathy. The significant association ($\tau = 0.742$, $p < 0.0001$) found between the combined EASE-3 score and the VF subscale of the original EASE supports that the EASE-3 primarily reflects biomarkers of vocal fatigue in the singing voice [15]. The significant relationship ($p = 0.001$) between the instrumental index and the original VF subscale in our data suggests that the development of a protocol and instrumental index for diagnosing and tracking vocal fatigue and effort-related symptoms in the singing voice is feasible. Given this association, we have termed the instrumental model constructed in this study the Aeroacoustic Singing Fatigue Index (ASFI).

4.1. Symptoms of Vocal Fatigue and the EASE-3

Hunter et al. [86] define vocal effort as the 'perceived exertion of a vocalist to a perceived communication scenario' (p. 516), and vocal fatigue as 'a quantifiable decline in function' (p. 516). Vocal effort is a commonly reported complaint for professional voice users in many sectors including performance, telemarketing/health, and education [4,13,87]. Reported symptoms of increased perceived vocal effort and measurable vocal fatigue include increased instability and breathiness, reduced agility and range, laryngeal discomfort, and increased phonation threshold pressures (PTP) [88–90]. The etiology of these symptoms is multifaceted and may arise (for example) from changes in vocal-fold viscosity, fatigue of intralaryngeal musculature and connective tissue, dehydration, or a combination of factors including these [91,92]. The nearly ubiquitous manifestation of vocal fatigue in functional, structural, and neurological dysphonia highlights its clinical significance [93]. There are clear connections between functional or organic pathologies and perceptual experiences of increased vocal effort. However, increased vocal effort and discomfort may also be present in the absence of visually identified pathology [94].

Vocal fatigue has an intuitive relationship with vocal demand and vocal demand response. Increased duration and intensity of vocal fold vibration during prolonged speech or singing incurs greater impact stress during vocal fold collision. Increased tissue viscosity in the vibrating portion of the vocal folds and reduced ability to mitigate the resulting increased friction (i.e., heat energy) have been proposed as contributing factors to vocal fatigue [91]. Despite these seemingly clear characteristics, few studies have found significant correlations between perceptions of vocal fatigue and instrumental voice measures; studies that have investigated this seem to present varied conclusions [87,95–97]. To the authors' knowledge, no research in this area has been carried out with a focus on the singing voice.

The items included in the EASE-3 have clear connections with known symptoms of vocal fatigue and functional disorder such as huskiness, dryness, scratchiness, and strain [98], some of which have also been included in the widely used Vocal Tract Discomfort Scale [12,99–101]. In the EASE-3 these sensations are reported in Q1 (My voice is husky) and Q2 (My voice is dry/scratchy). Breathiness is also part of the symptomology of vocal effort and fatigue [89] and is easily recognized by both singer and listener. Glottal sufficiency and its relation to breathiness is implied in scale item 11 (My top notes are breathy). For singers, the quality of high notes is particularly enlightening. Singing effectively at high frequencies requires fine coordination of aerodynamic and muscular function for optimal phonation that exposes the condition of the voice in a way that conversational speech may not. The third item in the EASE-3 (Q11 in the full EASE) relates directly to breathiness when singing high notes. Together, the EASE-3 is comprised of questions related to known traits of vocal fatigue and functional disorder and offer singer-specific contexts that are vital when analyzing the signing voice. We are not suggesting that the EASE-3 replace the original EASE VF subscale, however, in our data only these three questions offered psychometric data that could be related to quantitative aeroacoustic measures.

4.2. Perceptions of Singing Vocal Fatigue and Acoustic Measures

Acoustic voice measures offer instrumental (quantitative) and non-invasive insights into vocal function during phonation. However, few have been related to self-perceptual measures of vocal function and fatigue. The ASFI presented here includes CPPS, V_{Jitt}, and V_{Shim}, which, respectively, can be related to symptoms of vocal fatigue.

In our data, participants' CPPS values ranged from 11.58 to 18.02 dB ($M = 14.4$, $SD = 1.88$), which are within previously reported ranges for healthy speakers [39,102]. In previous research, Saeedi et al. [103] found associations between cepstral measures (CPP and CPPS) and elements of two different self-perceptual vocal health tools: the Vocal Tract Discomfort Scale (Persian) and the Non-Standard Hoarseness Self-Assessment. Their findings suggest that CPPS reflects some element of phonation that is directly perceivable by the speaker (or singer). Bhuta et al. [104] reported correlations between other noise-related measures (Noise-to-Harmonics Ratio [NHR], Voice Turbulence Index [VTI], and Soft Phonation Index [SPI]) and the perceptual Grade, Roughness, Breathiness, Aesthenia,

Strain (GRBAS) scale recorded from 37 dysphonic speakers. These associations between CPPS, breathiness, and perceptual voice analysis support the current findings.

The presence of breathiness in the voice is a readily-perceivable voice characteristic that classically trained singers typically work to eliminate [64,105]. CPPS offers insights into the presence of turbulent breath noise in the voice signal, and is strongly related to voice source behaviour. It may be that fatigue of vocal-fold adductor muscles or swelling of the vocal folds themselves contribute to incomplete glottal adduction or a non-simultaneous closing phase that increases noise components in the signal (i.e., reduces rahmonic distinguishability in the cepstrum). Although CPPS is affected by both f_o and SPL [7,9,39], no effect was seen in our data, likely owing to the controlled nature of the tasks in our protocol ('soft' singing on a prescribed frequency).

Vibrato perturbation was measured using the *BioVoice* V_{Jitt} and V_{Shim} parameters. In our study, V_{Jitt} values ranged from 2.43 to 37.3% ($M = 11.59$, $SD = 8.59$). V_{Shim} ranged from 11.4 to 47.95% ($M = 27.27$, $SD = 11.55$). These mean values are slightly higher than those reported in Manfredi et al. [46] but may result from task differences. In their study, singers were asked to perform a standardized melody in a comfortable key and volume from which one sustained tone was analyzed. In the present study singers sustained a quietly sung /a/ vowel on a prescribed f_o. Thus, lower P_{Sub} may have contributed to decreased vocal stability in our participants [106].

Vibrato is a significant feature of the WCSV and a common element in neutral CCM singing, the regularity and freedom of which is a mark of skilled and healthy singing voice production [63,64,107]. Several studies have identified regularity in VR and VE as important characteristics in perceptual rating tasks performed by both naïve and expert listeners. Ekholm et al. [108] found that a delay in vibrato onset was negatively associated with perceived vibrato appropriateness (rated by seven expert voice teachers). Anand et al. [109] found a relationship between f_o, VR and VE, and vibrato appropriateness as rated by four experts and five student judges. While this appropriateness was related to pedagogical and musico-aesthetic ideals, it is also of relevance to the present study. Small changes or instability in VR and VE evidently bear weight in perceptual judgement of vibrato, and these may have greater weight in self-assessment of singing function than smaller perturbations that are reflected in short-term perturbation measures (e.g., APQ3).

Although VE can be adjusted through training [43,44,110,111], no training effect was seen in our data, despite the large range of years of training in our participants. The use of the V_{Jitt} and V_{Shim} parameters somewhat reduces the potential confounding influence of training (where VR and VE can vary greatly across genres). Regardless of the VR or VE, if the vibrato is stable lower V_{Jitt} and V_{Shim} values should reflect such. It would be inappropriate for a clinician or researcher to request a singing participant to regulate their VR or VE for the sake of the voice analysis. Thus, vibrato-perturbation-related measures show great promise for singing voice analysis, allowing for application across genres and for intersubject and pre/posttreatment comparisons, ergo between singers with different vibrato rates and extents.

The relationships between V_{Jitt}, V_{Shim}, and voice condition, particularly vocal fatigue, is somewhat intuitive. As free vibrato originates in part through quasi-sinusoidal oscillatory contractions of the cricothyroid muscle (i.e., an oscillating f_o), muscle fatigue or vocal fold swelling may interfere with vibrato regularity. As a free vibrato involves a complex interaction between pressures, flows, resonances, and neuromuscular systems [43,112,113], measuring vibrato stability offers more detail about singing-voice function and condition than independent VR or VE values. It is possible that the same factors that contribute to huskiness or breathiness on high notes (e.g., reduced vocal fold adduction and motility through swelling or fatigue of adductory muscles) also affect vibrato stability.

4.3. Perceptions of Singing Voice Fatigue and the Efficiency Ratio

As singers are trained to proprioceptively evaluate their vocal function, small changes in their ability to perform specific vocal tasks (e.g., in efficiency) may be relevant contributors to their perception of vocal fatigue. Toles, Seidman, et al. [48] found the ER (SPL/P_{Sub}) to be sensitive pre/post excision of phonotraumatic lesions. They reported a mean ER of 9.25 (SD = 2.12) measured post-surgery during /papapapapa/ phonation at a comfortable pitch and volume. In the present study, participants' ER values ranged from 7.78 to 15.90 (M = 10.60, SD = 2.35). As classical singers are trained to optimize vocal efficiency, the ER maximum of 15.9 reached in our cohort is not surprising.

Titze [91] defined glottal efficiency as the ratio between aerodynamic input and acoustic output (p. 269). As unamplified voice production remains the norm in Western classical singing, finding maximum acoustic output with relatively minimal effort is key to maintaining sustainable and healthy (i.e., non-pressed) phonation. One potential limitation of P_{Sub}-based efficiency ratios is that, to a point, a high P_{Sub} and a well-adducted glottis will usually improve ER [63,114]. Thus, it may be difficult to distinguish between efficient (and sustainable) and hyperfunctional phonation solely based on ER. Further, f_o influences ER, as higher f_o are stronger in SPL owing to resonance-harmonics interactions and greater radiation efficiency [70,91,115,116]. Previous research has noted an increase in speakers' PTP after increased vocal demand [90,97,117], most likely owing to increased tissue viscosity, thickness of the vocal folds' colliding edge, and sub-optimal (i.e., too narrow or too wide) prephonatory glottal width [117–119]. Inadequate glottal adduction reduces acoustic power (i.e., ER), whereas high medial compression with P_{Sub} in the realm of pressed phonation would increase ER. A challenge then lies in identifying the line between practical (sustainable) singing-voice efficiency and potential hypertension represented in elevated ER values.

In our study, the use of soft phonation at a standardized f_o, and the inclusion of other voice-source-related acoustic measures may have somewhat mitigated this potential confounding influence: no dB or f_o effects were found. Soft phonation is used in the voice clinic (and studio) as an indication of not only behavioral adjustment, but also voice condition [120,121]. The ability to maintain adequate prephonatory glottal approximation for ease of oscillatory initiation as well as a relatively fast closing phase (i.e., improved power to output ratios), whilst simultaneously reducing intensity (dB) is a maneuver that requires fine muscle coordination challenging for the fatigued or otherwise dysfunctional singing voice [122,123]. The associations between ER and the scale items related to perceived huskiness (Q1) and breathiness (Q11) highlights this. The significant contribution of ER in the ASFI model offers support for the inclusion of aerodynamic measures (complementary to acoustic measures) in an instrumental index for diagnosing functional changes in singers with singing-voice complaints.

4.4. Limitations and Future Directions

To the authors' knowledge, this exploratory study represents the first attempt to explicitly examine relationships between the individual EASE scale items and instrumental aeroacoustic voice measures. The data presented illustrate how an instrumental index that relates to singers' nuanced perceptions of their singing-voice function can be constructed.

As the sample size in this study was small, it would be premature to widely generalize the findings. Future studies would benefit from larger cohorts of both normophonic and dysphonic singers. While useful for exploring possible associations in a novel field, we acknowledge that the use of stepwise regression with backward elimination may have excluded some relevant parameters. This statistical approach is widely used in contemporary research (e.g., [124–127]), and here provides some proof-of-concept supporting further validation research, which should utilize a wider range of analyses including permutation statistics, applied to larger datasets.

Some functional and perceptual changes in the singing voice may be traceable only intrasubject. For instance, given the wide range of norms within the human voice, one singer's baseline healthy measurements may be approaching dysphonic for another. It would be beneficial to compare intrasubject changes in the ASFI over time and after various levels of vocal demand. No instrumental measures were related to the *PRI* or *VC* subscales, and the ASFI showed only a moderate association with the *PRI* ($p < 0.10$). Further research with populations including disordered singers may clarify these relationships.

The use of the PAS with its mask may have somewhat altered the singing voice function of participants. Future research should explore less intrusive methods of collecting pressure data. More work is needed to determine which existing tools are suitable for use with the singing voice, and to develop robust, standardized singing-voice assessment protocols that can be implemented in clinical and pedagogical contexts. Although the instrumental measures explored in the present study represent a broad range across time, frequency, and aerodynamic domains, they are by no means exhaustive. Future research may benefit from exploring relationships between self-perception of singing voice function and health status and tools such as the voice range profile or non-linear analyses.

5. Conclusions

Subtle changes in singing-voice function are sensed by skilled voice users but are not always perceived aurally by a third party or readily identified using existing instrumental voice assessment techniques. Despite being a high-risk population, no standardized clinical protocol for singing voice analysis exists and little research has been carried out to determine the suitability of traditional clinical voice diagnosis approaches for use with the singing voice. Thus, singing-voice complaints presented by the professional voice user that indicate early signs of dysfunction may go undiagnosed until their severity progresses. This leaves a large gap in the care of professional singing-voice users who rely on optimal vocal function for livelihood. This exploratory study offers novel data illustrating associations between EASE scale items and instrumental aeroacoustic measures. Three of the 22 original items were correlated with instrumental voice measures, the composite score of which was significantly associated ($\tau = 0.742$, $p < 0.0001$) with the *VF* subscale. Multiple linear regression techniques indicated that CPPS, V_{Jitt}, V_{Shim}, and ER (measured during soft sung phonation) accounted for 62.4% of variation in the combined scores of the three scale items. This instrumental index was also significantly associated ($\tau = 0.575$, $p = 0.001$) with the original *VF* subscale. These instrumental measures show promise for singing voice analysis individually and as part of an instrumental index as illustrated here. Further development of diagnostic protocols for singers is needed for preventative and rehabilitative healthcare for professional singing-voice users.

Author Contributions: Conceptualization, C.P.B.; methodology, C.P.B., S.C.P. and T.O.R.; formal analysis, C.P.B. and S.B.; investigation, C.P.B. and S.C.P.; data curation, C.P.B.; writing—original draft preparation, C.P.B.; writing—review and editing, C.P.B., S.C.P., T.O.R. and S.B.; supervision, S.C.P. and T.O.R.; project administration, C.P.B. All authors have read and agreed to the published version of the manuscript.

Funding: This research received no external funding.

Institutional Review Board Statement: The study was conducted in accordance with the Declaration of Helsinki and approved by the University of Auckland Human Participants Ethics Committee (ref. 22159, 19 January 2022).

Informed Consent Statement: Informed consent was obtained from all participants.

Data Availability Statement: Participant recordings have not been made publicly available to protect confidentiality. Further inquiries can be directed to the corresponding author.

Acknowledgments: We gratefully acknowledge the singers who participated in this study.

Conflicts of Interest: The authors declare no conflict of interest.

Appendix A

Full list of items included in the Evaluation of Ability to Sing Easily, from Phyland et al., 2014 [15]. *VF*: Vocal fatigue. *PRI*: Pathological risk indicators. *VC*: Voice concerns.

1. My voice is husky (*VF*)
2. My voice is dry/scratchy (*VF*)
3. My voice cracks and breaks (*PRI*)
4. My throat muscles are feeling overworked (*VF*)
5. My voice is breathy (*PRI*)
6. My singing voice feels good (*VF*; reverse scored)
7. The onsets of my notes are delayed or breathy (*VF*)
8. My voice feels strained (*VF*)
9. I am worried about my voice (*VC*)
10. I am having difficulty with my breath for long phrases (*PRI*)
11. My top notes are breathy (*VF*)
12. My voice sounds rich and resonant (*VF*)
13. My voice is cutting out on some notes (*PRI*)
14. I am having difficulty singing softly (*PRI*)
15. My voice is tired (*VF*)
16. I am having difficulty changing registers (*PRI*)
17. I am having difficulty with my high notes (*PRI*)
18. Singing feels like hard work (*PRI*)
19. I am having difficulty projecting my voice (*PRI*)
20. I am concerned about my voice (*VC*)
21. My voice feels ready for performance if required (*VF*; reverse scored)
22. I am having difficulty sustaining long notes (*PRI*)

References

1. Hogikyan, N.D.; Sethuraman, G. Validation of an Instrument to Measure Voice-Related Quality of Life (V-RQOL). *J. Voice* **1999**, *13*, 557–569. [CrossRef]
2. Murry, T.; Medrado, R.; Hogikyan, N.D.; Aviv, J.E. The Relationship between Ratings of Voice Quality and Quality of Life Measures. *J. Voice* **2004**, *18*, 183–192. [CrossRef]
3. Krischke, S.; Weigelt, S.; Hoppe, U.; Köllner, V.; Klotz, M.; Eysholdt, U.; Rosanowski, F. Quality of Life in Dysphonic Patients. *J. Voice* **2005**, *19*, 132–137. [CrossRef]
4. Phyland, D.J.; Miles, A. Occupational Voice Is a Work in Progress: Active Risk Management, Habilitation and Rehabilitation. *Curr. Opin. Otolaryngol. Head Neck Surg.* **2019**, *27*, 439–447. [CrossRef]
5. Titze, I.R.; Horii, Y.; Scherer, R.C. Some Technical Considerations in Voice Perturbation Measurements. *J. Speech Hear. Res.* **1987**, *30*, 252–260. [CrossRef] [PubMed]
6. Dejonckere, P.H.; Giordano, A.; Schoentgen, J.; Fraj, S.; Bocchi, L.; Manfredi, C. To What Degree of Voice Perturbation Are Jitter Measurements Valid? A Novel Approach with Synthesized Vowels and Visuo-Perceptual Pattern Recognition. *Biomed. Signal Process. Control* **2012**, *7*, 37–42. [CrossRef]
7. Baker, C.P.; Sundberg, J.; Purdy, S.C.; Rakena, T.O.; Leão, S.H.d.S. CPPS and Voice-Source Parameters: Objective Analysis of the Singing Voice. *J. Voice* **2022**, in press. [CrossRef] [PubMed]
8. Brockmann, M.; Drinnan, M.J.; Storck, C.; Carding, P.N. Reliable Jitter and Shimmer Measurements in Voice Clinics: The Relevance of Vowel, Gender, Vocal Intensity, and Fundamental Frequency Effects in a Typical Clinical Task. *J. Voice* **2011**, *25*, 44–53. [CrossRef]
9. Sampaio, M.C.; Bohlender, J.E.; Brockmann-Bauser, M. Fundamental Frequency and Intensity Effects on Cepstral Measures in Vowels from Connected Speech of Speakers with Voice Disorders. *J. Voice* **2021**, *35*, 422–431. [CrossRef]
10. Kridgen, S.; Hillman, R.E.; Stadelman-Cohen, T.; Zeitels, S.; Burns, J.A.; Hron, T.; Krusemark, C.; Muise, J.; Van Stan, J.H. Patient-Reported Factors Associated with the Onset of Hyperfunctional Voice Disorders. *Ann. Otol. Rhinol. Laryngol.* **2021**, *130*, 389–394. [CrossRef] [PubMed]
11. Szkiełkowska, A.; Krasnodębska, P.; Mitas, A.; Bugdol, M.; Bugdol, M.; Romaniszyn-Kania, P.; Pollak, A. Electrophysiological Predictors of Hyperfunctional Dysphonia. *Acta Otolaryngol.* **2023**, *143*, 56–63. [CrossRef]
12. Mathieson, L.; Hirani, S.P.; Epstein, R.; Baken, R.J.; Wood, G.; Rubin, J.S. Laryngeal Manual Therapy: A Preliminary Study to Examine Its Treatment Effects in the Management of Muscle Tension Dysphonia. *J. Voice* **2009**, *23*, 353–366. [CrossRef] [PubMed]
13. Verdolini, K.; Ramig, L.O. Review: Occupational Risks for Voice Problems. *Logoped. Phoniatr. Vocol.* **2001**, *26*, 37–46. [CrossRef] [PubMed]

14. Patel, R.R.; Awan, S.N.; Barkmeier-Kraemer, J.; Coury, M.; Deliyski, D.; Eadie, T.; Paul, D.; Švec, J.G.; Hillman, R. Recommended Protocols for Instrumental Assessment of Voice: American Speech-Language-Hearing Association Expert Panel to Develop a Protocol for Instrumental Assessment of Vocal Function. *Am. J. Speech Lang. Pathol.* **2018**, *27*, 887–905. [CrossRef]
15. Phyland, D.J.; Pallant, J.F.; Thibeault, S.L.; Benninger, M.S.; Vallance, N.; Smith, J.A. Measuring Vocal Function in Professional Music Theater Singers: Construct Validation of the Evaluation of the Ability to Sing Easily (EASE). *Folia Phoniatr. Logop.* **2014**, *66*, 100–108. [CrossRef] [PubMed]
16. Devadas, U.; Vinod, D.; Maruthy, S. Immediate Effects of Straw Phonation in Water Exercises on Parameters of Vocal Loading in Carnatic Classical Singers. *J. Voice* **2020**, *37*, 142.e13–142.e22. [CrossRef] [PubMed]
17. Murphy Estes, C.; Chadwick, K.; Sadoughi, B.; Andreadis, K.; Sussman, S.; Sulica, L. Performers' Perceptions of Vocal Function during Oral Steroid Treatment of Vocal Fold Edema. *Laryngoscope* **2022**, *132*, 2434–2441. [CrossRef]
18. Zuim, A.F.; Stewart, C.F.; Titze, I.R. Vocal Dose and Vocal Demands in Contemporary Musical Theatre. *J. Voice* 2021, in press. [CrossRef]
19. Zuim, A.F.; Lloyd, A.T.; Gerhard, J.; Rosow, D.; Lundy, D. Associations of Education and Training with Perceived Singing Voice Function among Professional Singers. *J. Voice* **2021**, *35*, 500.e17–500.e24. [CrossRef]
20. Ragsdale, F.W.; Marchman, J.O.; Bretl, M.M.; Diaz, J.; Rosow, D.E.; Anis, M.; Zhang, H.; Landera, M.A.; Lloyd, A.T. Quantifying Subjective and Objective Measures of Singing after Different Warm-up Durations. *J. Voice* **2020**, *36*, 661–667. [CrossRef]
21. Phyland, D.J.; Pallant, J.F.; Benninger, M.S.; Thibeault, S.L.; Greenwood, K.M.; Smith, J.A.; Vallance, N. Development and Preliminary Validation of the EASE: A Tool to Measure Perceived Singing Voice Function. *J. Voice* **2013**, *27*, 454–462. [CrossRef]
22. Flock, L.; King, S.R.; Williams, J.; Finlay, E.; Smikle, H.; Benito, M.; Benton-Stace, F.; Brown, J.; Mann-Daraz, A.J.; Hart, L.; et al. Working Together to Find a Voice: Recommendations for Voice Healthcare Based on Expert-by-Experience and Practitioner Consensus. *J. Voice* 2023, in press. [CrossRef] [PubMed]
23. Alku, P.; Bäckström, T.; Vilkman, E. Normalized Amplitude Quotient for Parametrization of the Glottal Flow. *J. Acoust. Soc. Am.* **2002**, *112*, 701–710. [CrossRef] [PubMed]
24. Alku, P. Glottal Inverse Filtering Analysis of Human Voice Production—A Review of Estimation and Parameterization Methods of the Glottal Excitation and Their Applications. *Sādhanā* **2011**, *36*, 623–650. [CrossRef]
25. Björkner, E.; Sundberg, J.; Alku, P. Subglottal Pressure and Normalized Amplitude Quotient Variation in Classically Trained Baritone Singers. *Logoped. Phoniatr. Vocol.* **2006**, *31*, 157–165. [CrossRef]
26. Sundberg, J. Objective Characterization of Phonation Type Using Amplitude of Flow Glottogram Pulse and of Voice Source Fundamental. *J. Voice* **2022**, *36*, 4–14. [CrossRef]
27. Sundberg, J.; Thalén, M.; Alku, P.; Vilkman, E. Estimating Perceived Phonatory Pressedness in Singing from Flow Glottograms. *J. Voice* **2004**, *18*, 56–62. [CrossRef]
28. Sundberg, J.; Thalén, M. Respiratory and Acoustical Differences between Belt and Neutral Style of Singing. *J. Voice* **2015**, *29*, 418–425. [CrossRef]
29. Alku, P.; Airas, M.; Björkner, E.; Sundberg, J. An Amplitude Quotient Based Method to Analyze Changes in the Shape of the Glottal Pulse in the Regulation of Vocal Intensity. *J. Acoust. Soc. Am.* **2006**, *120*, 1052–1062. [CrossRef]
30. Granqvist, S. Sopran. Available online: www.tolvan.com (accessed on 20 June 2023).
31. Echternach, M.; Sundberg, J.; Zander, R.; Richter, B. Perturbation Measurements in Untrained Male Voices' Transitions from Modal to Falsetto Register. *J. Voice* **2011**, *25*, 663–669. [CrossRef]
32. Echternach, M.; Richter, B. Passaggio in the Professional Tenor Voice—Evaluation of Perturbation Measures. *J. Voice* **2012**, *26*, 440–446. [CrossRef] [PubMed]
33. Hillenbrand, J.; Houde, R.A. Acoustic Correlates of Breathy Vocal Quality: Dysphonic Voices and Continuous Speech. *J. Speech Lang. Hear. Res.* **1996**, *39*, 311–321. [CrossRef] [PubMed]
34. Hillenbrand, J.; Cleveland, R.A.; Erickson, R.L. Acoustic Correlates of Breathy Vocal Quality. *J. Speech Lang. Hear. Res.* **1994**, *37*, 769–779. [CrossRef]
35. Heman-Ackah, Y.D.; Heuer, R.J.; Michael, D.D.; Ostrowski, R.; Horman, M.; Baroody, M.M.; Hillenbrand, J.; Sataloff, R.T. Cepstral Peak Prominence: A More Reliable Measure of Dysphonia. *Ann. Hum. Biol.* **2003**, *112*, 324–333. [CrossRef]
36. Heman-Ackah, Y.D.; Michael, D.D.; Goding, G.S. The Relationship between Cepstral Peak Prominence and Selected Parameters of Dysphonia. *J. Voice* **2002**, *16*, 20–27. [CrossRef] [PubMed]
37. Sauder, C.; Bretl, M.; Eadie, T. Predicting Voice Disorder Status from Smoothed Measures of Cepstral Peak Prominence Using Praat and Analysis of Dysphonia in Speech and Voice (ADSV). *J. Voice* **2017**, *31*, 557–566. [CrossRef]
38. Bottalico, P.; Codino, J.; Cantor-Cutiva, L.C.; Marks, K.; Nudelman, C.J.; Skeffington, J.; Shrivastav, R.; Jackson-Menaldi, M.C.; Hunter, E.J.; Rubin, A.D. Reproducibility of Voice Parameters: The Effect of Room Acoustics and Microphones. *J. Voice* **2020**, *34*, 320–334. [CrossRef]
39. Brockmann-Bauser, M.; Van Stan, J.H.; Sampaio, M.C.; Bohlender, J.E.; Hillman, R.E.; Mehta, D.D. Effects of Vocal Intensity and Fundamental Frequency on Cepstral Peak Prominence in Patients with Voice Disorders and Vocally Healthy Controls. *J. Voice* **2021**, *35*, 411–417. [CrossRef]
40. Weekly, E.M.; LoVetri, J.L. Follow-up Contemporary Commercial Music (CCM) Survey: Who's Teaching What in Nonclassical Music. *J. Voice* **2009**, *23*, 367–375. [CrossRef]

41. Chandler, K. Teaching Popular Music Styles. In *Teaching Singing in the 21 Century. Landscapes: The Arts, Aesthetics, and Education*; Harrison, S.D., O'Bryan, J., Eds.; Springer: Dordrecht, The Netherlands, 2014; Volume 14, pp. 35–51.
42. Sangiorgi, T.; Manfredi, C.; Bruscaglioni, P. Objective Analysis of the Singing Voice as a Training Aid. *Logoped. Phoniatr. Vocol.* **2009**, *30*, 136–146. [CrossRef]
43. Titze, I.R.; Story, B.; Smith, M.; Long, R. A Reflex Resonance Model of Vocal Vibrato. *J. Acoust. Soc. Am.* **2002**, *111*, 2272. [CrossRef] [PubMed]
44. Sundberg, J. Acoustic and Psychoacoustic Aspects of Vocal Vibrato. *STL-QPSR* **1994**, *35*, 45–68.
45. Morelli, M.S.; Orlandi, S.; Manfredi, C. BioVoice: A Multipurpose Tool for Voice Analysis. *Biomed. Signal Process. Control* **2021**, *64*, 102302. [CrossRef]
46. Manfredi, C.; Barbagallo, D.; Baracca, G.; Orlandi, S.; Bandini, A.; Dejonckere, P.H. Automatic Assessment of Acoustic Parameters of the Singing Voice: Application to Professional Western Operatic and Jazz Singers. *J. Voice* **2015**, *29*, 517.e1–517.e9. [CrossRef] [PubMed]
47. Stemple, J.; Weinrich, B.; Brehm, S.B. *Phonatory Aerodynamic System: A Clinical Manual*; KayPENTAX Corp.: Lincoln Park, NJ, USA, 2008; Available online: https://www.pentaxmedical.com/pentax/en/99/1/Phonatory-Aerodynamic-System-PAS-Model-6600 (accessed on 20 June 2023).
48. Toles, L.E.; Seidman, A.Y.; Hillman, R.E.; Mehta, D.D. Clinical Utility of the Ratio of Sound Pressure Level to Subglottal Pressure in Patients Surgically Treated for Phonotraumatic Vocal Fold Lesions. *J. Speech Lang. Hear. Res.* **2022**, *65*, 2778–2788. [CrossRef]
49. Grillo, E.U.; Verdolini, K. Evidence for Distinguishing Pressed, Normal, Resonant, and Breathy Voice Qualities by Laryngeal Resistance and Vocal Efficiency in Vocally Trained Subjects. *J. Voice* **2008**, *22*, 542–546. [CrossRef]
50. Baken, R.J.; Orlikoff, R.F. *Clinical Measurement of Speech and Voice*, 2nd ed.; Singular Publishing Group: San Diego, CA, USA, 2000.
51. Oates, J.M.; Dacakis, G. Speech Pathology Considerations in the Management of Transsexualism—A Review. *Int. J. Lang. Commun. Disord.* **1983**, *18*, 139–151. [CrossRef]
52. Dahl, K.L.; Mahler, L.A. Acoustic Features of Transfeminine Voices and Perceptions of Voice Femininity. *J. Voice* **2020**, *34*, 961.e19–961.e26. [CrossRef]
53. Gelfer, M.P.; Schofield, K.J. Comparison of Acoustic and Perceptual Measures of Voice in Male-to-Female Transsexuals Perceived as Female versus Those Perceived as Male. *J. Voice* **2000**, *14*, 22–33. [CrossRef]
54. Romano, T. The Singing Voice during the First Two Years of Testosterone Therapy: Working with the Trans or Gender Queer Voice. Ph.D. Thesis, University of Colorado, Boulder, CO, USA, 2018.
55. Cohen, S.M.; Statham, M.; Rosen, C.A.; Zullo, T. Development and Validation of the Singing Voice Handicap-10. *Laryngoscope* **2009**, *119*, 1864–1869. [CrossRef]
56. Lã, F.M.B.; Sundberg, J.; Howard, D.M.; Sa-Couto, P.; Freitas, A. Effects of the Menstrual Cycle and Oral Contraception on Singers' Pitch Control. *J. Speech Lang. Hear. Res.* **2012**, *55*, 247–361. [CrossRef]
57. Abitbol, J.; Abitbol, P.; Abitbol, B. Sex Hormones and the Female Voice. *J. Voice* **1999**, *13*, 424–446. [CrossRef] [PubMed]
58. Abitbol, J.; de Brux, J.; Millot, G.; Masson, M.-F.; Mimoun, O.L.; Pau, H.; Abitbol, B. Does a Hormonal Vocal Cord Cycle Exist in Women? Study of Vocal Premenstrual Syndrome in Voice Performers by Videostroboscopy-Glottography and Cytology on 38 Women. *J. Voice* **1989**, *3*, 157–162. [CrossRef]
59. Pomfret, B. Vocalizing Vocalises. *J. Sing.* **2012**, *69*, 61–66.
60. Gish, A.; Kunduk, M.; Sims, L.; McWhorter, A.J. Vocal Warm-up Practices and Perceptions in Vocalists: A Pilot Survey. *J. Voice* **2012**, *26*, e1–e10. [CrossRef] [PubMed]
61. Boersma, P.; Weenink, D. Praat: Doing Phonetics by Computer [Computer Program]. Version 6.2.16. 2023. Available online: http://www.praat.org/ (accessed on 19 August 2022).
62. Švec, J.G.; Granqvist, S. Tutorial and Guidelines on Measurement of Sound Pressure Level in Voice and Speech. *J. Speech Lang. Hear. Res.* **2018**, *61*, 441–461. [CrossRef] [PubMed]
63. Sundberg, J. *The Science of the Singing Voice*; Northern Illinoise University Press: DeKalb, IL, USA, 1987.
64. Miller, R. *The Structure of Singing: System and Art in Vocal Technique*; Schirmer: Boston, MA, USA, 1996.
65. Miller, D.G.; Schutte, H.K.; Doing, D. Soft Phonation in the Male Singing Voice. *J. Voice* **2001**, *15*, 483–491. [CrossRef] [PubMed]
66. Hillenbrand, J.; Getty, L.A.; Clark, M.J.; Wheeler, K. Acoustic Characteristics of American English Vowels. *J. Acoust. Soc. Am.* **1995**, *97*, 3099–3111. [CrossRef]
67. Kent, R.D.; Vorperian, H.K. Static Measurements of Vowel Formant Frequencies and Bandwidths: A Review. *J. Commun. Disord.* **2018**, *74*, 74–97. [CrossRef]
68. Kent, R.D. Vocal Tract Acoustics. *J. Voice* **1993**, *7*, 97–117. [CrossRef]
69. Fant, G.; Liljencrants, J.; Lin, Q. A Four-Parameter Model of Glottal Flow. *STL-QPSR* **1985**, *26*, 1–13.
70. Stevens, K.N. *Acoustic Phonetics*; MIT Press: Cambridge, MA, USA, 2000.
71. Maryn, Y.; Weenink, D. Objective Dysphonia Measures in the Program PRAAT: Smoothed Cepstral Peak Prominence and Acoustic Voice Quality Index. *J. Voice* **2015**, *29*, 35–43. [CrossRef] [PubMed]
72. Watts, C.R.; Awan, S.N.; Maryn, Y. A Comparison of Cepstral Peak Prominence Measures from Two Acoustic Analysis Programs. *J. Voice* **2017**, *31*, 387.e1–387.e10. [CrossRef]
73. R Core Team. *R: A Language Environment for Statistical Computing*; R Foundation for Statistical Computing: Vienna, Austria, 2022.

74. Vu, D.H.; Muttaqi, K.M.; Agalgaonkar, A.P. A Variance Inflation Factor and Backward Elimination Based Robust Regression Model for Forecasting Monthly Electricity Demand Using Climatic Variables. *Appl. Energy* **2015**, *140*, 385–394. [CrossRef]
75. Sheather, S. *A Modern Approach to Regression with R*; Springer: New York, NY, USA, 2009.
76. James, G.; Witten, D.; Hastie, T.; Tibshirani, R. *An Introduction to Statistical Learning*; Springer: New York, NY, USA, 2013; Volume 103, ISBN 978-1-4614-7137-0.
77. Mahalanobis, P.C. Reprint of: Mahalanobis, P.C. (1936) "On the Generalised Distance in Statistics". *Sankhya A* **2018**, *80*, 1–7. [CrossRef]
78. Khattree, R.; Naik, D.N. *Applied Multivariate Statistics with SAS®Software*, 2nd ed.; SAS Institude Inc.: Cary, NC, USA, 1999.
79. Sobol, M.; Sielska-Badurek, E.M.; Rzepakowska, A.; Osuch-Wójcikiewicz, E. Normative Values of SVHI-10. Systematic Meta-Analysis. *J. Voice* **2019**, *34*, 808.e25–808.e28. [CrossRef] [PubMed]
80. Misono, S.; Peterson, C.B.; Meredith, L.; Banks, K.; Bandyopadhyay, D.; Yueh, B.; Frazier, P.A. Psychosocial Distress in Patients Presenting with Voice Concerns. *J. Voice* **2014**, *28*, 753–761. [CrossRef]
81. Rosen, D.C.; Heuer, R.J.; Sasso, D.A.; Sataloff, R.T. Psychological Aspects of Voice Disorders. In *Clinical Assessment of Voice*; Sataloff, R.T., Ed.; Plural Publishing, Inc.: San Diego, CA, USA, 2017; pp. 303–333.
82. Li-Jessen, N.Y.K.; Jones, C. Keeping Injured Voices Hush-Hush: Why Professional Singers and Actors Often Don't Seek Treatment for Vocal Illness. Available online: https://theconversation.com/keeping-injured-voices-hush-hush-why-professional-singers-and-actors-often-dont-seek-treatment-for-vocal-illness-183330 (accessed on 8 June 2023).
83. Huston, C. Speaking Out about Vocal Injuries on Broadway. Available online: https://www.broadwaynews.com/speaking-out-about-vocal-injuries-on-broadway (accessed on 8 June 2023).
84. Randolph, G.W.; Sritharan, N.; Song, P.; Franco, R.; Kamani, D.; Woodson, G. Thyroidectomy in the Professional Singer-Neural Monitored Surgical Outcomes. *Thyroid* **2015**, *25*, 665–671. [CrossRef]
85. Vella, B.; Brown, L.; Phyland, D.J. Amateur Music Theatre Singers' Perceptions of Their Current Singing Voice Function. *J. Voice* **2021**, *35*, 589–596. [CrossRef]
86. Hunter, E.J.; Cantor-Cutiva, L.C.; van Leer, E.; van Mersbergen, M.; Nanjundeswaran, C.D.; Bottalico, P.; Sandage, M.J.; Whitling, S. Toward a Consensus Description of Vocal Effort, Vocal Load, Vocal Loading, and Vocal Fatigue. *J. Speech Lang. Hear. Res.* **2020**, *63*, 509–532. [CrossRef]
87. Lehto, L.; Laaksonen, L.; Vilkman, E.; Alku, P. Occupational Voice Complaints and Objective Acoustic Measurements—Do They Correlate? *Logoped. Phoniatr. Vocol.* **2006**, *31*, 147–152. [CrossRef]
88. Aronson, A.E.; Bless, D.M. *Clinical Voice Disorders*, 4th ed.; Thieme Medical Publishers, Inc.: New York, NY, USA, 2009.
89. Nanjundeswaran, C.; Shembel, A.C. Laying the Groundwork to Study the Heterogeneous Nature of Vocal Fatigue. *J. Voice* **2022**, in press. [CrossRef] [PubMed]
90. Enflo, L.; Sundberg, J.; McAllister, A. Collision and Phonation Threshold Pressures before and after Loud, Prolonged Vocalization in Trained and Untrained Voices. *J. Voice* **2013**, *27*, 527–530. [CrossRef] [PubMed]
91. Titze, I.R. *Principles of Voice Production*; National Center for Voice and Speech: Iowa City, IA, USA, 2000.
92. Shembel, A.C.; Nanjundeswaran, C. Potential Biophysiological Mechanisms Underlying Vocal Demands and Vocal Fatigue. *J. Voice* **2022**, in press. [CrossRef]
93. Verdolini, K.; Rosen, C.A.; Branski, R.C. (Eds.) *Classification Manual for Voice Disorders-I*, 1st ed.; Psychology Press: New York, NY, USA, 2014; ISBN 9781135600204.
94. Solomon, N.P. Vocal Fatigue and Its Relation to Vocal Hyperfunction. *Int. J. Speech Lang. Pathol.* **2008**, *10*, 254–266. [CrossRef] [PubMed]
95. Eustace, C.S.; Stemple, J.C.; Lee, L. Objective Measures of Voice Production in Patients Complaining of Laryngeal Fatigue. *J. Voice* **1996**, *10*, 146–154. [CrossRef]
96. Laukkanen, A.-M.; Ilomäki, I.; Leppänen, K.; Vilkman, E. Acoustic Measures and Self-Reports of Vocal Fatigue by Female Teachers. *J. Voice* **2008**, *22*, 283–289. [CrossRef]
97. Chang, A.; Karnell, M.P. Perceived Phonatory Effort and Phonation Threshold Pressure across a Prolonged Voice Loading Task: A Study of Vocal Fatigue. *J. Voice* **2004**, *18*, 454–466. [CrossRef] [PubMed]
98. Wingate, J.M.; Brown, W.S.; Shrivastav, R.; Davenport, P.; Sapienza, C.M. Treatment Outcomes for Professional Voice Users. *J. Voice* **2007**, *21*, 433–449. [CrossRef]
99. De Oliveira Lemos, I.; Picanço Marchand, D.L.; Oliveira Cunha, E.; Alves Silvério, K.C.; Cassol, M. What Are the Symptoms That Characterize the Clinical Condition of Vocal Fatigue? A Scoping Review and Meta-Analysis. *J. Voice* **2023**, in press. [CrossRef]
100. Lukaschyk, J.; Abel, J.; Brockmann-Bauser, M.; Keilmann, A.; Braun, A.; Rohlfs, A.-K. Cross-Validation and Normative Values for the German Vocal Tract Discomfort Scale. *J. Speech Lang. Hear. Res.* **2021**, *64*, 1855–1868. [CrossRef]
101. Lopes, L.W.; Cabral, G.F.; Figueiredo de Almeida, A.A. Vocal Tract Discomfort Symptoms in Patients with Different Voice Disorders. *J. Voice* **2015**, *29*, 317–323. [CrossRef] [PubMed]
102. Batthyany, C.; Maryn, Y.; Trauwaen, I.; Caelenberghe, E.; van Dinther, J.; Zarowski, A.; Wuyts, F. A Case of Specificity: How Does the Acoustic Voice Quality Index Perform in Normophonic Subjects? *Appl. Sci.* **2019**, *9*, 2527. [CrossRef]
103. Saeedi, S.; Aghajanzadeh, M.; Khoddami, S.M.; Dabirmoghaddam, P.; Jalaie, S. Relationship of Cepstral Analysis with Voice Self-Assessments in Dysphonic and Normal Speakers. *Eur. Arch. Oto-Rhino-Laryngol.* **2022**, *280*, 1803–1813. [CrossRef] [PubMed]

104. Bhuta, T.; Patrick, L.; Garnett, J.D. Perceptual Evaluation of Voice Quality and Its Correlation with Acoustic Measurements. *J. Voice* **2004**, *18*, 299–304. [CrossRef]
105. Miller, R. *Solutions for Singers: Tools for Performers and Teachers*; Oxford University Press, Inc.: New York, NY, USA, 2004.
106. Brockmann-Bauser, M.; Bohlender, J.E.; Mehta, D.D. Acoustic Perturbation Measures Improve with Increasing Vocal Intensity in Individuals with and without Voice Disorders. *J. Voice* **2018**, *32*, 162–168. [CrossRef]
107. Stark, J. *Bel Canto: A History of Vocal Pedagogy*; University of Toronto Press Incorporated: Toronto, ON, Canada, 2008.
108. Ekholm, E.; Papagiannis, G.C.; Chagnon, F.P. Relating Objective Measurements to Expert Evaluation of Voice Quality in Western Classical Singing: Critical Perceptual Parameters. *J. Voice* **1998**, *12*, 182–196. [CrossRef]
109. Anand, S.; Wingate, J.M.; Smith, B.; Shrivastav, R. Acoustic Parameters Critical for an Appropriate Vibrato. *J. Voice* **2012**, *26*, 820.e19–820.e25. [CrossRef]
110. Lester-Smith, R.A.; Kim, J.H.; Hilger, A.; Chan, C.-L.; Larson, C.R. Auditory-Motor Control of Fundamental Frequency in Vibrato. *J. Voice* **2021**, *37*, 296.e9–296.e19. [CrossRef]
111. Ramig, L.A.; Shipp, T. Comparative Measures of Vocal Tremor and Vocal Vibrato. *J. Voice* **1987**, *1*, 162–167. [CrossRef]
112. Shipp, T.; Doherty, E.T.; Haglund, S. Physiologic Factors in Vocal Vibrato Production. *J. Voice* **1990**, *4*, 300–304. [CrossRef]
113. Large, J.; Iwata, S. Aerodynamic Study of Vibrato and Voluntary 'Straight Tone' Pairs in Singing. *Folia Phoniatr. Logop.* **1971**, *23*, 50–65. [CrossRef]
114. Titze, I.R. Regulation of Vocal Power and Efficiency by Subglottal Pressure and Glottal Width. In *Vocal Fold Physiology: Voice Production, Mechanisms and Functions*; Fujimura, O., Ed.; Raven Press: New York, NY, USA, 1988; Volume 2, pp. 227–238.
115. Gramming, P.; Sundberg, J. Spectrum Factors Relevant to Phonetogram Measurement. *J. Acoust. Soc. Am.* **1988**, *83*, 2352–2360. [CrossRef] [PubMed]
116. Titze, I.R. Acoustic Interpretation of the Voice Range Profile (Phonetogram). *J. Speech Lang. Hear. Res.* **1992**, *35*, 21–34. [CrossRef] [PubMed]
117. Xue, C.; Kang, J.; Hedberg, C.; Zhang, Y.; Jiang, J.J. Dynamically Monitoring Vocal Fatigue and Recovery Using Aerodynamic, Acoustic, and Subjective Self-Rating Measurements. *J. Voice* **2019**, *33*, 809.e11–809.e18. [CrossRef] [PubMed]
118. Titze, I.R.; Schmidt, S.S.; Titze, M.R. Phonation Threshold Pressure in a Physical Model of the Vocal Fold Mucosa. *J. Acoust. Soc. Am.* **1995**, *97*, 3080–3084. [CrossRef]
119. Titze, I.R. The Physics of Small-Amplitude Oscillation of the Vocal Folds. *J. Acoust. Soc. Am.* **1988**, *83*, 1538–1552. [CrossRef]
120. Rousell, N.C.; Lobdell, M. The Clinical Utility of the Soft Phonation Index. *Clin. Linguist. Phon.* **2006**, *20*, 181–186. [CrossRef]
121. Mathew, M.M.; Bhat, J.S. Soft Phonation Index—A Sensitive Parameter? *Indian J. Otolaryngol. Head Neck Surg.* **2009**, *61*, 127–130. [CrossRef]
122. Herbst, C.T.; Hess, M.; Müller, F.; Švec, J.G.; Sundberg, J. Glottal Adduction and Subglottal Pressure in Singing. *J. Voice* **2015**, *29*, 391–402. [CrossRef]
123. Titze, I.R. Unsolved Mysteries about Vocal Fatigue and Recovery. *J. Sing.* **2009**, *65*, 449–450.
124. Lee, S.J.; Park, Y.M.; Lim, J.-Y. Comprehensive Index of Vocal Fatigue (CIVF): Development and Clinical Validation. *J. Voice* **2023**, in press. [CrossRef] [PubMed]
125. Lisowska, A.; Dubatówka, M.; Chlabicz, M.; Jamiołkowski, J.; Kondraciuk, M.; Szyszkowska, A.; Knapp, M.; Szpakowicz, A.; Łukasiewicz, A.; Kamiński, K. Disparities in the Prevalence and Risk Factors for Carotid and Lower Extremities Atherosclerosis in a General Population—Bialystok PLUS Study. *J. Clin. Med.* **2023**, *12*, 2627. [CrossRef] [PubMed]
126. Schweer, J.T.; Neumann, P.-A.; Doebler, P.; Doebler, A.; Pascher, A.; Mennigen, R.; Rijcken, E. Crohn's Disease as a Possible Risk Factor for Failed Healing in Ileocolic Anastomoses. *J. Clin. Med.* **2023**, *12*, 2805. [CrossRef] [PubMed]
127. Cha, D.S.; Moshirfar, M.; Herron, M.S.; Santos, J.M.; Hoopes, P.C. Prediction of Posterior-to-Anterior Corneal Curvature Radii Ratio in Myopic Patients after LASIK, SMILE, and PRK Using Multivariate Regression Analysis. *J. Clin. Med.* **2023**, *12*, 4536. [CrossRef] [PubMed]

Disclaimer/Publisher's Note: The statements, opinions and data contained in all publications are solely those of the individual author(s) and contributor(s) and not of MDPI and/or the editor(s). MDPI and/or the editor(s) disclaim responsibility for any injury to people or property resulting from any ideas, methods, instructions or products referred to in the content.

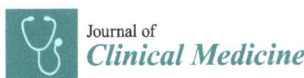

Article

Comparative Evaluation of High-Speed Videoendoscopy and Laryngovideostroboscopy for Functional Laryngeal Assessment in Clinical Practice

Joanna Hoffman, Magda Barańska *, Ewa Niebudek-Bogusz † and Wioletta Pietruszewska †

Department of Otolaryngology, Head and Neck Oncology, Medical University of Lodz, 90-153 Lodz, Poland; ewa.niebudek-bogusz@umed.lodz.pl (E.N.-B.); wioletta.pietruszewska@umed.lodz.pl (W.P.)
* Correspondence: magda.a.baranska@gmail.com
† These authors contributed equally to this work.

Abstract: Advancements in dynamic laryngeal imaging, particularly high-speed videoendoscopy (HSV), have addressed several limitations of laryngovideostroboscopy (LVS). This study aimed to compare the success rates of LVS and HSV in generating recordings suitable for objective functional assessment of vocal fold movements. **Methods:** This study included 200 patients with voice disorders (123 with benign glottal lesions, 56 with malignant lesions, and 21 with functional voice disorders) and 47 normophonic individuals. All participants underwent LVS followed by HSV. Kymographic analysis was performed to evaluate phonatory parameters, including amplitude, symmetry, and glottal dynamics. The success of both methods in generating analyzable kymograms was assessed, and statistical comparisons were made using the chi-square test (significance level set at $p < 0.05$). **Results:** The failure rate for LVS was significantly higher (43.32%) compared to HSV. HSV successfully generated kymograms in 68.22% of cases where LVS failed. The primary factors contributing to LVS failure included synchronization issues, inadequate recording brightness, unstable phonation, and hidden glottal opening. Failure rates related to structural obstacles were similar between the two methods. HSV demonstrated superior kymogram feasibility across all subgroups, with the highest success observed in cases of organic glottal pathologies (30.73%). A significant advantage of HSV was observed for both benign and malignant glottal lesions, especially in cases of asynchronous vocal fold oscillations. **Conclusions.** By overcoming the inherent limitations of LVS, HSV provides a more reliable and objective assessment of phonatory function. Its ability to generate suitable kymograms with greater precision makes HSV a valuable tool for routine clinical diagnostics, enabling the accurate identification of subtle laryngeal pathologies and enhancing diagnostic accuracy.

Keywords: high-speed videoendoscopy (HSV); laryngovideostroboscopy (LVS); kymographic analysis; phonatory function; vocal fold oscillations; voice disorders; benign glottal lesions; malignant glottal lesions

1. Introduction

The assessment of voice function necessitates a comprehensive array of diagnostic tools, encompassing perceptual voice evaluation, subjective patient assessments, acoustic measurements, and laryngostroboscopic examination [1]. Each modality provides unique insights into vocal function, reflecting the complexity of voice diagnostics. Among these, the accurate visualization of vocal fold vibrations remains pivotal for diagnosing and managing laryngeal disorders [1–3]. Of the available visualization techniques, laryngovideostroboscopy (LVS) and high-speed videoendoscopy (HSV) are particularly valuable for evaluating the dynamic function of the glottis.

Laryngovideostroboscopy is the standard imaging technique for assessing phonatory movements of the vocal folds and remains widely used in clinical practice [1]. This method relies on digital video recordings that reconstruct vocal fold movement over multiple phonation cycles. However, LVS does not provide real-time visualization of vocal fold function. Instead, it generates an averaged representation of the phonation cycle by combining sequential frames from multiple cycles, capturing minor variations that may occur. As such, LVS is most effective when vocal fold vibrations are regular and synchronous and when stable phonation samples of sufficient duration can be recorded [4,5].

A stroboscopic visual-perceptual assessment via LVS is recommended for analyzing various aspects of vocal fold function, including vibratory amplitude, mucosal wave propagation, phase symmetry, vertical positioning, and glottal closure patterns. However, as noted by the European Laryngological Society, the interpretation of LVS findings can be affected by observer bias, potentially compromising objectivity [1]. The use of blinded evaluations or panel-based ratings, particularly in post-surgical follow-ups, may improve their reliability, though such practices are challenging to implement in routine clinical settings. The American Speech–Language–Hearing Association also underscores the importance of integrating quantitative measures into vocal fold assessments to enhance diagnostic precision as technological advancements progress [6].

High-speed videoendoscopy (HSV) addresses many limitations inherent in LVS by providing real-time imaging of vocal fold vibrations. This technology captures detailed and reliable data on vocal fold dynamics, enabling the assessment of both synchronous and asynchronous phonatory patterns [7–9]. HSV operates at frame rates higher than 2000 frames per second, offering high-resolution visualization of vocal fold oscillations. Unlike LVS, which captures approximately 10 phonatory cycles over a 10 s interval, HSV achieves comparable detail within just one-tenth of a second [5,10–13].

This capability allows HSV to analyze vocal fold function even in challenging cases, such as dysphonic voices, irregular glottal movements, or short phonation times, which are often inadequately captured by LVS. Furthermore, HSV recordings generate high-quality kinematic images that enable more accurate kymograms—graphical representations of vocal fold movement over time and space [14–19]. Kymography derived from HSV is widely regarded as one of the most effective methods for objectively assessing the temporal aspects of phonatory function [10].

While kymographic analysis can also be applied to LVS recordings (termed strobovideokymography), this process is labor-intensive and depends on the availability of high-quality stroboscopic images [4,5]. HSV offers a significant advantage in this regard due to its ability to produce kymographic data from brief recording sessions, thereby expanding the range of patients who can undergo this type of analysis [11].

This study aims to compare the success rates of obtaining LVS and HSV recordings suitable for objective evaluation in routine clinical practice. The analysis focuses on identifying the causes of examination failure across the entire study cohort, stratified by patient categories including normophonic individuals, as well as those with functional, benign, and malignant vocal fold lesions.

2. Materials and Methods

2.1. Study Group

This study included 247 patients from the Department of Otolaryngology, Head and Neck Oncology at the Medical University of Lodz and its affiliated outpatient clinic, evaluated from 2020 to 2023 for various laryngeal lesions. The mean age of the total group was 58.6 years (median 62, range 21–90). A control group was established, comprising 47 normophonic subjects with no history of dysphonia and no organic or functional abnormalities of the larynx. The study group consisted of 200 patients with voice disorders, including 123 with benign glottal lesions, 56 with malignant lesions, and 21 with functional voice disorders. All patients with organic lesions underwent laser microsurgery, confirming the initial diagnosis histopathologically. The inclusion criteria for the study group encompassed the following: age $\geq$ 18 years, the ability to perform HSV and LVS tests without structural barriers (e.g., hypopharyngeal or epiglottic tumors obstructing the glottis), and patient cooperation. After each examination, attempts were made to generate kymograms. Detailed group characteristics are shown in Table 1.

Table 1. Characteristics of the study group.

Variables	Benign Lesions	Malignant Lesions	Functional Disorders	Control Group
n	123	56	21	47
median age	57	70	59	50
males/females	35/88	46/10	7/14	13/34

This study received approval from the Ethical Committee of the Medical University of Lodz (no. RNN/96/20/KE, dated 8 April 2020), and written informed consent was obtained from all participants.

2.2. Methods of Examination

All patients first underwent an otolaryngological examination, including a comprehensive interview regarding voice-related issues. Each subject then underwent a baseline endoscopic examination of the larynx under white light, followed by a strobe light examination (LVS) using the same endoscope. Laryngovideostroboscopy was performed using a rigid 90° endoscope (Olympus WA96105A, Olympus Medical Systems, Tokyo, Japan). In select cases where rigid endoscopy was not feasible due to anatomical constraints or patient discomfort, a flexible endoscope (Olympus ENF-VH2, Olympus Medical Systems, Tokyo, Japan) was used. Digital imaging was recorded with an Olympus Visera Elite OTV-S190 camera (Olympus Medical Systems, Tokyo, Japan) paired with a xenon light source and an Olympus CLL-S1 (Olympus Medical Systems, Tokyo, Japan) strobe lamp. Following LVS, subjects were examined with an HSV camera. HSV images were recorded using the Advanced Larynx Imager System (ALIS) [20] equipped with laser diode lighting (ALIS Lum-MF1, Diagnova Technologies, Wroclaw, Poland) and a high-speed camera (ALIS Cam HS-1, Diagnova Technologies, Wroclaw, Poland) connected to a rigid oval endoscope (Fiegert–Endotech ϕ12.4/7.2, Tuttlingen, Germany) with a light guide using a 4.8 mm fiber optic cable.

High-speed videoendoscopy (HSV) was performed using a color high-speed camera with a frame rate of 4000 frames per second (fps) and a pixel resolution of 512 × 512. This configuration allowed for high temporal and spatial resolution, facilitating the precise analysis of vocal fold vibrations. For laryngovideostroboscopy (LVS), images were captured at a rate of one stroboscopic cycle per second, ensuring that periodic vocal fold vibrations were effectively reconstructed, with a pixel resolution of 480 × 400. The stroboscopic system used an LED light source synchronized with the patient's fundamental frequency to achieve optimal imaging conditions. Regarding the duration of analyzed sequences, LVS recordings required a minimum phonation time of 10 s to ensure the capture of sufficient vibration cycles for meaningful analysis. In contrast, HSV recordings were completed within 0.06–0.08 s, corresponding to 10–20 phonation cycles (depending on the fundamental frequency), thereby enabling the real-time visualization of vocal fold oscillations in a much shorter time frame.

Among the 200 subjects with dysphonia, 178 with hypertrophic glottal pathologies underwent laser microsurgery, and final diagnoses were based on histopathological examination of tissue specimens. The classification of benign lesions adhered to the WHO 2017 dysplasia grading, while all malignant lesions were confirmed as squamous cell carcinoma. The study design was applied to both the control and study groups (Figure 1).

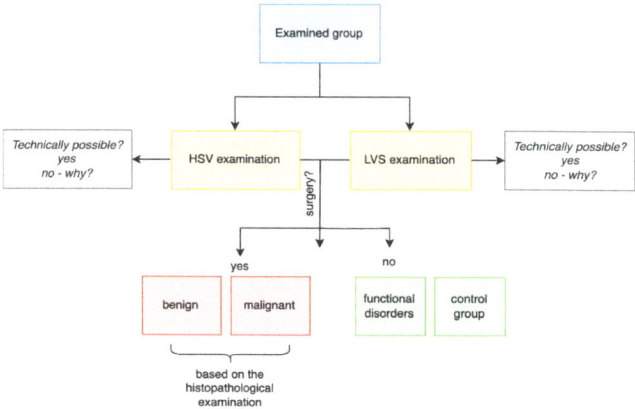

Figure 1. Sequential steps of the study protocol.

Figure 1 illustrates the sequential steps of the study protocol, outlining the diagnostic workflow applied to all participants. The process commenced with an initial otolaryngological examination, including a comprehensive medical interview to assess voice-related symptoms. Following the baseline assessment, each participant underwent laryngovideostroboscopy (LVS) as the first imaging modality, which was subsequently followed by high-speed videoendoscopy (HSV).

The examination sequence was standardized for all subjects to ensure consistency and minimize potential biases. The LVS examination involved recording vocal fold vibrations using strobe light synchronization, whereas the HSV examination captured high-frame-rate recordings to assess real-time vocal fold dynamics. After data acquisition, kymographic analysis was performed on both LVS and HSV recordings to evaluate phonatory parameters, such as vibratory amplitude, symmetry, and glottal closure.

Additionally, the protocol included specific criteria for determining successful kymogram generation, focusing on the quality of the extracted images and their suitability for objective assessment. The study protocol also accounted for potential challenges, such as insufficient phonation stability or anatomical obstructions, which were systematically documented and analyzed.

2.2.1. Differences Between LVS and HSV Recordings

LVS synchronizes strobe light with the patient's voice frequency to produce an apparent slow-motion image of vocal fold vibrations. However, this is achieved by capturing frames from different phonation cycles, often from widely separated points in the cycle.

(Figure 2—adapted and modified based on the illustration from Deliyski (2010) to provide a clearer representation of HSV functionality within the context of our study. The original source has been accordingly cited to acknowledge the contribution [16].) As a result, LVS imaging requires regular vibration periodicity to produce accurate results. This dependence makes LVS unsuitable for assessing irregular vocal fold vibrations or short, stable phonation cycles in patients with severe dysphonia, where the glottal image may appear blurred, resembling static light endoscopy. Additionally, the recorded sample must be long enough to yield a reliable image. These limitations were observed in patients where LVS could not be conducted due to unstable phonation. Similar challenges are noted in the literature [21].

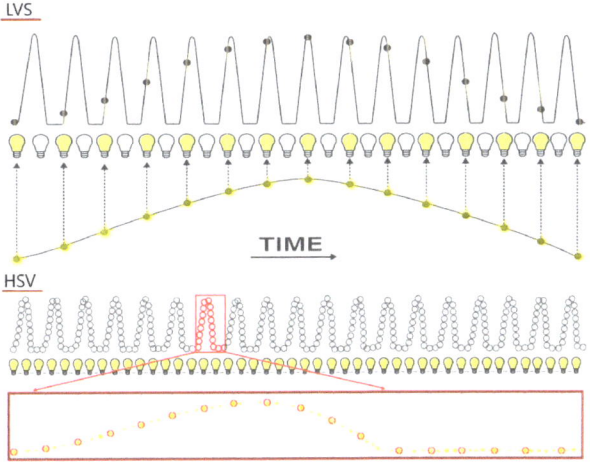

Figure 2. Schematic illustration of the creation of a videostroboscopic and high-speed video recording, adapted and modified based on the illustration from Deliyski (2010) [16].

High-speed videoendoscopy (HSV) overcomes these limitations by recording the actual vibrations of the vocal folds at a speed of several thousand frames per second, enabling the detailed visualization of successive phonation cycles. HSV thus facilitates the analysis of vibratory cyclicity over extended periods in asynchronous voices, where strobe light synchronization is ineffective. This method is applicable for both irregular glottal function and severe vocal fold pathology, where patients may not sustain a stable phonation for long periods. While LVS typically requires capturing 10 cycles over a 10 s period for a fundamental frequency of 100 Hz, the duration may vary depending on the strobe unit settings, which can range from 0.5 to 1.5 cycles per second. In contrast, HSV records the same data within a fraction of a second, independent of cycle synchronization settings. These recordings provide a robust basis for generating a kymographic analysis of successive phonatory cycles (Figure 3).

2.2.2. Kymographic Analysis

Following image acquisition, LVS and HSV recordings were subjected to detailed kymographic analysis using DiagNova Technologies software version 1.3 [20]. Kymographic section plots were generated at three levels along the entire vertical axis of the vocal folds (posterior, middle, and anterior) for both LVS and HSV recordings (Figures 3(A1–A3) and 4(A1–A3)). A sample analysis for a normophonic subject based on LVS is shown in Figure 3.

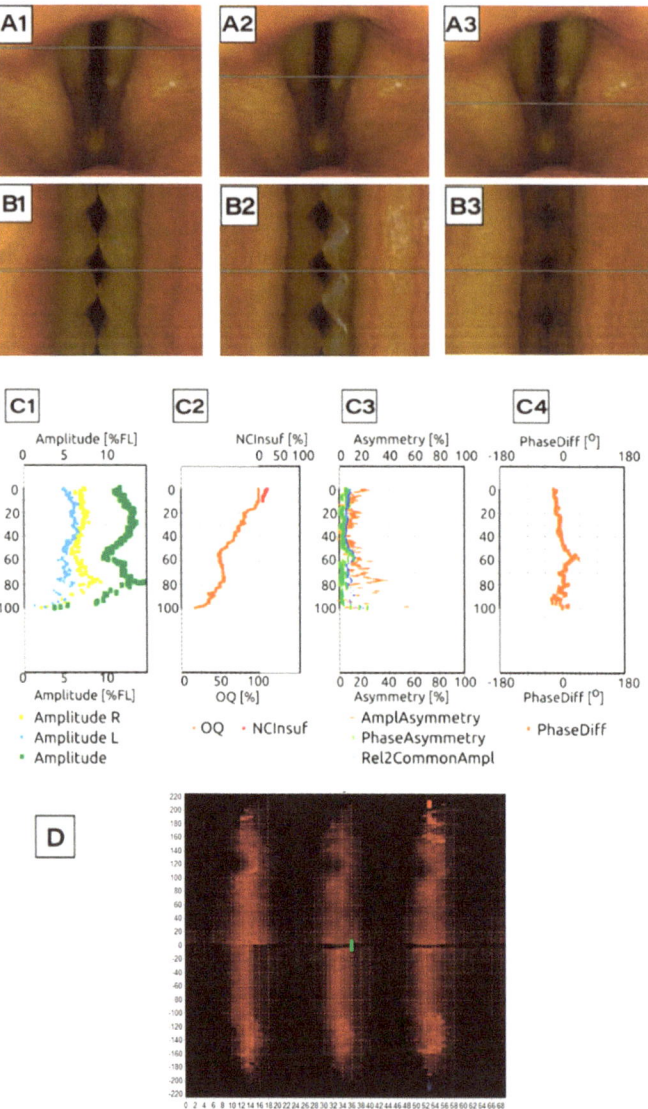

Figure 3. Analysis of data generated on the basis of an LVS record for Subject 1 (normophonic patient, 40 years old woman with 3 cycles of vocal folds movement); (**A1–A3**) image of the glottis with the reference line along the course of the vocal folds marked with a gray line, for which a videokymogram was obtained at the posterior, middle, and anterior sections, respectively; (**B1–B3**) videokymograms generated at the marked sections: the posterior, middle, and anterior parts of the glottis, respectively; (**C1**) graphs showing (y-axis presents the glottal axis) the amplitude movement of the vocal folds: blue—right vocal fold, yellow—left vocal fold, and green resultant of the movement of both vocal folds; (**C2**) graph showing the degree of glottal closure: orange line—value of Open Quotient alongside the longitudinal axis of the glottis and red line—non-Closure Quotient determining the insufficiency of the glottis; (**C3**) asymmetry rate; (**C4**) phase difference; (**D**) phonovibrogram: a diagram presenting the movement of the vocal folds in time in relation to the center of the glottis; the center of the diagram indicates the anterior part of the glottis; the upper part describes the movement of the left vocal fold, while the lower part describes the movement of the right vocal fold.

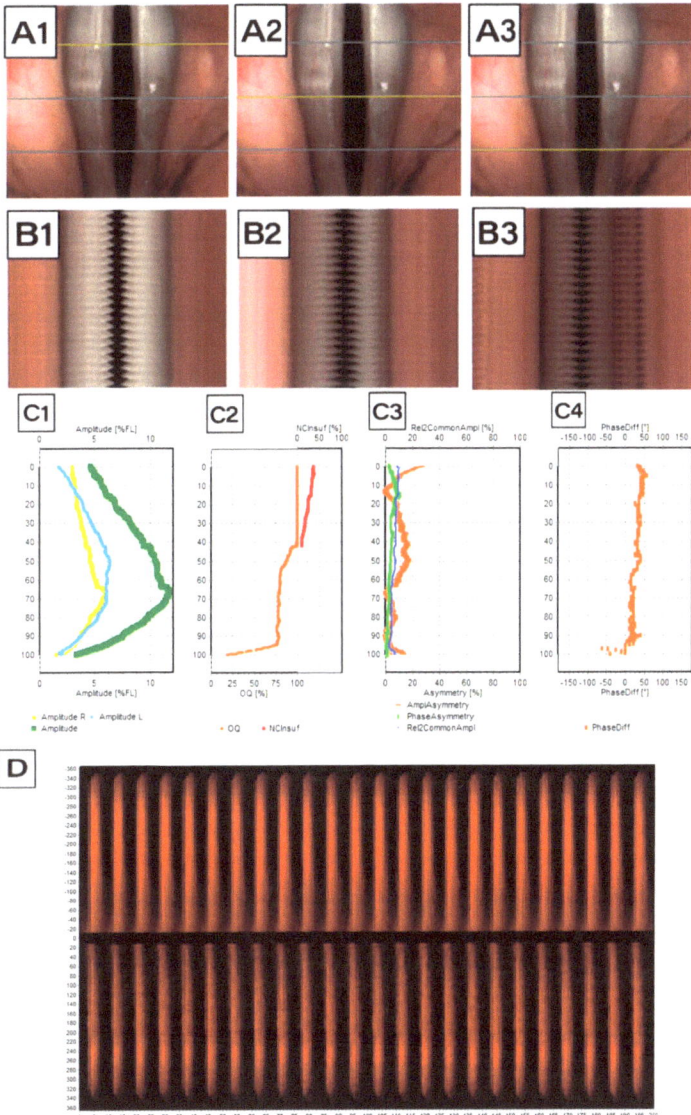

Figure 4. Analysis of data generated on the basis of an HSV record for Subject 1 (normophonic patient, 40 years old woman; 21 cycles of vocal folds movement): (**A1**–**A3**) image of the glottis with the cross-section along the course of the vocal folds marked with a gray line, for which a videokymogram was obtained at the posterior, middle, and anterior sections, respectively; (**B1**–**B3**) videokymograms generated at the marked sections: the posterior, middle, and anterior parts of the glottis, respectively; (**C1**) graphs showing (y-axis presents the glottal axis) the amplitude movement of the vocal folds: blue—right vocal fold, yellow—left vocal fold, and green resultant of the movement of both vocal folds; (**C2**) graph showing the degree of glottal closure: orange line—value of Open Quotient alongside the longitudinal axis of the glottis and red line—non-Closure Quotient determining the insufficiency of the glottis; (**C3**) asymmetry rate; (**C4**) phase difference; (**D**) phonovibrogram: a diagram presenting the movement of the vocal folds in time in relation to the center of the glottis; the center of the diagram indicates the anterior part of the glottis; the upper part describes the movement of the left vocal fold, while the lower part describes the movement of the right vocal fold.

Each LVS sample, after semi-automatic image stabilization, required manual preparation by an ENT specialist or phoniatrician. This process involved outlining the vocal fold edges and glottal area and adjusting individual frames as necessary. Following this, the software generated a kymographic cross-section at 1/3, 2/3, and 3/3 of the glottal length (Figure 3(B1–B3)), which was subsequently digitally equalized for brightness due to fluctuations in strobe light intensity. At least three full recording cycles were necessary to generate an LVS-based kymographic analysis, but often, more cycles were required. This limitation affects the reliability of the results from strobovideokymography.

The usability of a kymogram was determined based on the clear visualization of vocal fold oscillations without artifacts that could impair quantitative analysis. A kymogram was considered usable if it allowed for the extraction of phonatory parameters, such as amplitude, symmetry, and glottal closure, with sufficient clarity and accuracy to support objective functional assessment. In contrast, unsuccessful kymogram generation was defined as cases where visualization was obscured due to factors such as excessive movement artifacts, hidden glottal opening, or synchronization issues that prevented accurate analysis.

Kymograms derived from HSV recordings are simpler and faster to produce. Unlike LVS, which requires multiple cycles, HSV allows for kymogram generation even with short phonation times. Additionally, HSV kymograms directly correspond to the selected phonation cycles, providing more precise data on actual vocal fold movements at specific glottal levels during each cycle phase (Figure 4(B1–B3)). Due to the shorter recording time required for HSV (0.06–0.08 s of phonation), glottal axis correction was not necessary. The stabilized view in HSV recordings ensured a stable position of the glottis, reducing the risk of human error and enhancing kymogram quality and accuracy.

Phonovibrograms, which graphically represent vocal fold movement, were also generated based on both LVS and HSV recordings (Figures 3D and 4D). Phonovibrograms effectively consolidate data on vocal fold oscillations in a color-coded map over a specified time interval [22]. The X-axis represents time, while the Y-axis represents points along the vocal fold edge. In the map, red intensity indicates the degree of vocal fold opening (the momentary distance between the vocal fold edge and the glottis axis), while black denotes that the distance equals zero and the vocal fold is aligned to the glottal axis center. A comparison of LVS-based and HSV-based phonovibrograms shows that HSV provides a clearer, more detailed visualization of vocal fold oscillations.

2.2.3. Statistical Analysis

A comprehensive statistical analysis was performed to evaluate the effectiveness of LVS and HSV in generating analyzable kymograms. Descriptive statistics were calculated for all measured parameters, and categorical variables were compared using the chi-square test to determine statistical significance. A p-value of <0.05 was considered statistically significant. All statistical analyses were conducted using GraphPad Prism software version 9.3.1. The statistical methodology ensured robust comparisons between the two imaging modalities, enabling the accurate assessment of their diagnostic capabilities.

3. Results

In this study, it was possible to generate kymographic records for 205 patients (82.99% of the total) using HSV, compared to 140 patients (56.68%) using LVS (Figure 5), and a statistically significant difference favoring HSV ($p < 0.001$) was found.

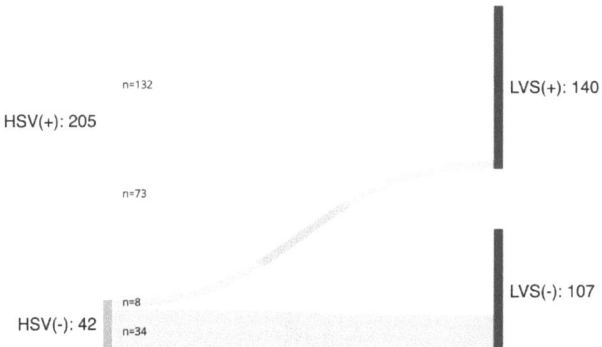

Figure 5. Groups of patients qualified for the study: HSV(+)—successful HSV examination; HSV(−) unsuccessful HSV examination; LVS(+)—successful LVS examination; LVS(−)—unsuccessful LVS examination.

Only eight patients (3.24%) had kymograms generated solely using LVS without concomitant HSV results. In all these cases, anatomical or structural obstacles, such as a prominent epiglottal pedicle or a flat epiglottis obscuring the anterior vocal folds, impeded HSV imaging due to the limitations of rigid optics. This challenge was mitigated in LVS by using flexible optics.

However, both LVS and HSV examinations failed to produce kymograms suitable for analysis in 34 patients (13.77%). We analyze and discuss the reasons for the difficulties encountered with HSV and LVS testing (Figures 6 and 7).

3.1. Observed Issues

3.1.1. Challenges with Adequate Glottal Opening and Vocal Fold Visualization (Figure 7A)

Generating a kymogram requires a clear visualization of the glottal area to define the medial edges of the vocal folds. Hidden glottal opening was observed in both LVS and HSV recordings. In the LVS group, this limitation prevented kymogram generation in 42 patients (42/205; 20.48%), whereas it impacted only 18 patients in the HSV group (18/229; 8.61%), and a statistically significant difference ($p < 0.001$) was found. This issue was especially prevalent among patients with large lesions. Additionally, visualizing the entire vocal fold structure, including the lower edge, was challenging in some cases. While both LVS and HSV theoretically provide similar laryngeal views, clinical experience and technical factors suggest that the HSV system more frequently allows for clear visualization of the lower vocal fold edge. This advantage is likely due to HSV's ability to capture phonation at lower fundamental frequencies with higher temporal and spatial resolution, reducing the impact of vibratory irregularities that may blur the stroboscopic image.

3.1.2. Structural Obstacles Hindering Glottis Visualization (Figure 7B–D)

Structural abnormalities or variations in the supraglottal region, such as a pedunculated epiglottis obstructing the anterior glottal part, a flat epiglottis, or intrinsic pathologies like vocal fold tumors, impeded glottal visualization. This issue divided patients into two subgroups: The first included those with anatomical variations like an omega-shaped epiglottis or an epiglottal pedicle covering the anterior commissure, obstructing the glottis (Figure 7(B1,B2)). The second subgroup (Figure 7(C1,C2)) included patients whose glottal visualization was hindered by extensive pathologies like large glottal tumors (Figure 7(D1,D2)).

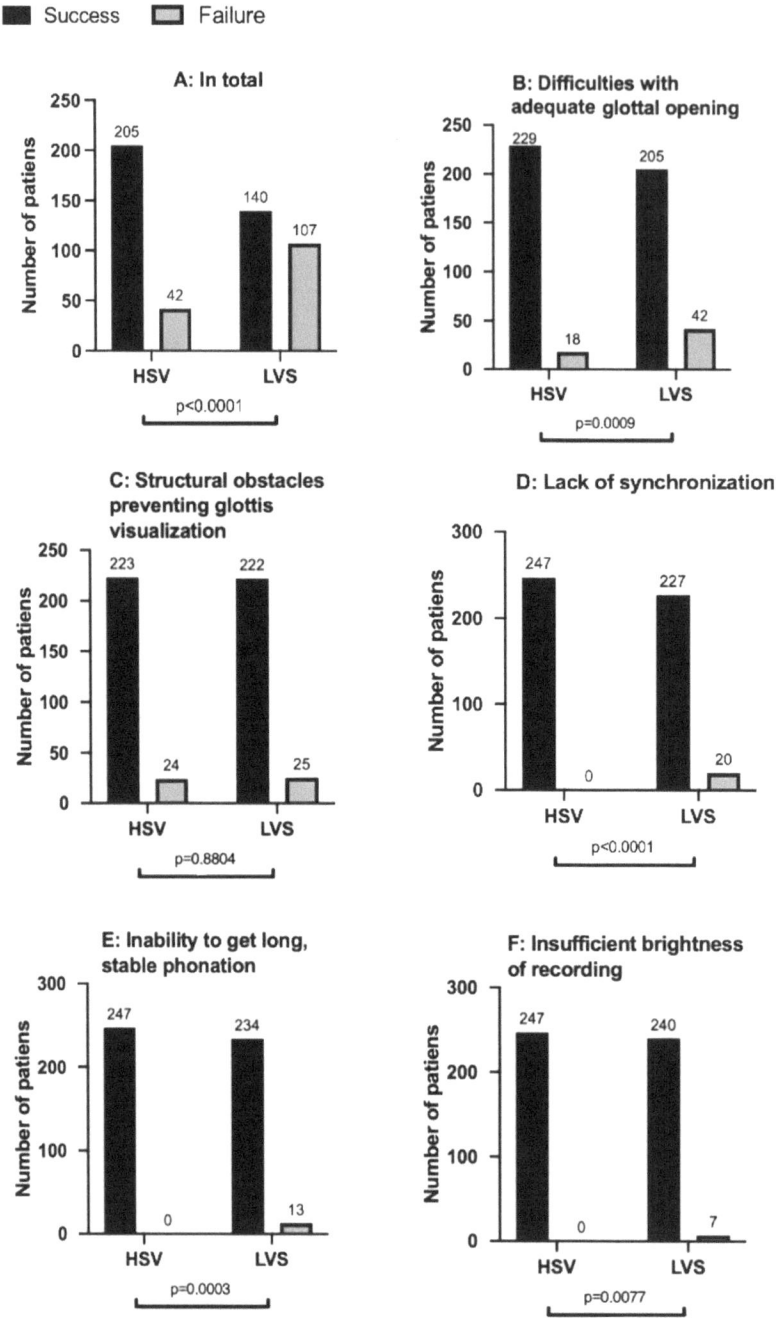

Figure 6. Difficulties with kymographic analysis in the HSV and LVS groups (total group n = 247): (**A**) for the whole study group and (**B**–**F**) for the following difficulties described in Section 3.1.

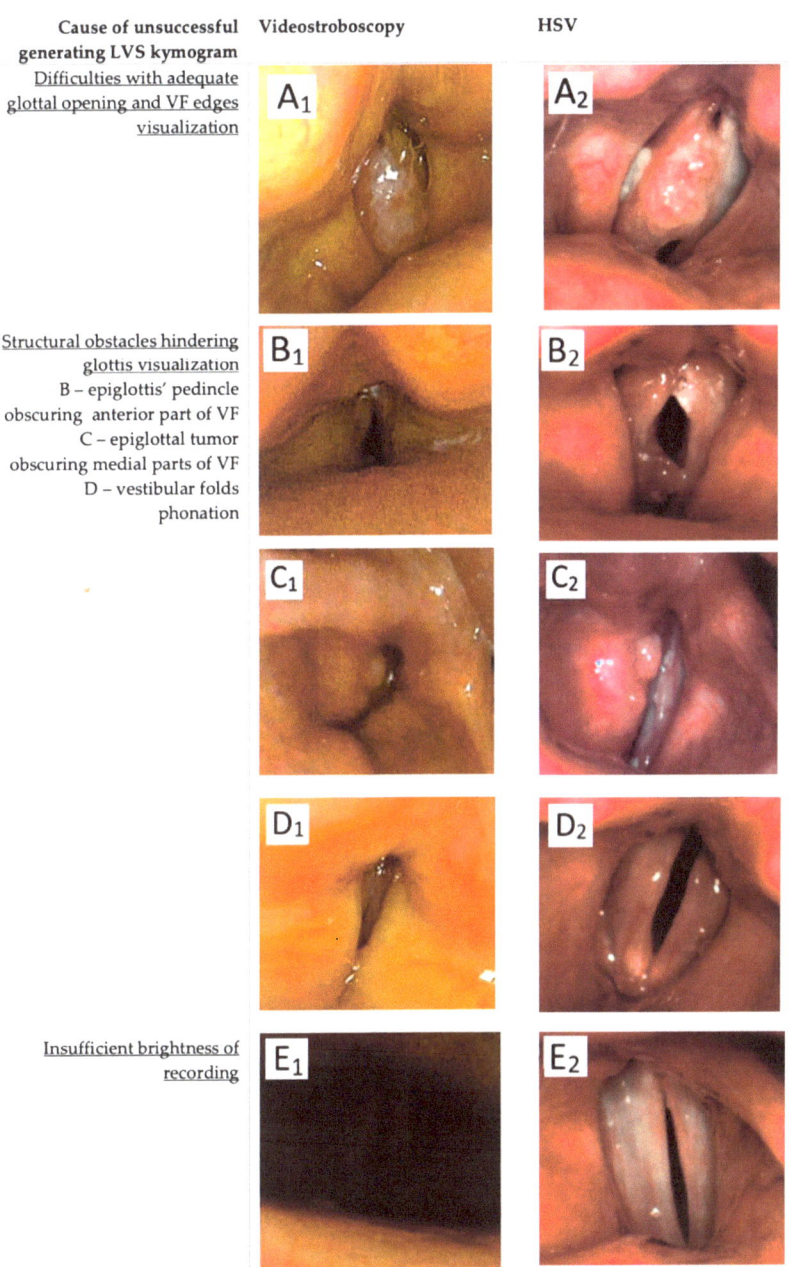

Figure 7. Images of patients' larynx in whom generating LVS-based kymogram was insufficient to generate kymograms (**A1,B1,C1,D1,E1**) compared with images from successful HSV-based kymography (**A2,B2,C2,D2,E2**). Subject (**A**): a male patient with carcinoma planoepitheliale G-3 in the right vocal fold; Subject (**B**): a male patient with a fibrovascular polyp in the right vocal fold; Subject (**C**): a male patient with epiglottal carcinoma planoepitheliale G-2; Subject (**D**): a female patient with functional voice disorders; Subject (**E**): a male patient with vocal fold inflammation and incomplete glottal closure, resulting in too short stable phonation to obtain an LVS recording. The causes of unsuccessful LVS-based kymogram creation are described in the table. VF—vocal folds.

Vestibular fold phonation was more common in LVS recordings (Figure 7(D1)), observed even in cases where flexible optics were used for improved visualization, whereas HSV was more affected by rigid optics, particularly in cases of a drooping or omega-shaped epiglottis. Furthermore, extensive proliferative lesions, such as carcinomas that obscured both vocal folds, limited the use of both LVS and HSV in clinical practice due to the inability to generate reliable kymograms for these cases.

3.1.3. Lack of Light Synchronization (Figure 6D)

The synchronization of strobe light with the patient's vocal frequency is essential for LVS. In 20 patients (8.1% of the total), this was the primary reason for failed LVS kymograms. However, this issue was not present in HSV recordings visualizing the actual motion of the vocal folds, thus eliminating the need for light synchronization.

3.1.4. Inability to Sustain Long, Stable Phonation (Figure 6E)

This issue affected only LVS recordings. Generating high-quality LVS images requires at least 10 s of stable phonation, which some patients with extensive lesions could not maintain. This hindered the ability to assess mucosal wave movement and identify asymmetries. In the LVS group, this problem impacted 13 patients (5.26%).

In Figure 6, "long phonation" is defined as the ability of the patient to sustain a stable phonatory sound for at least 10 s. The "Lack of synchronization" refers to the inability of the strobe light to properly align with the vocal fold vibration frequency, leading to inconsistent or blurred images. These factors were rated by two experienced otolaryngologists and phoniatricians (EN-B and WP) based on the criteria of the instrumental assessment of the voice, ensuring consistency and reliability in the assessment [6].

3.1.5. Insufficient Recording Brightness (Figure 6F)

This issue was not encountered in HSV recordings due to the laser illumination for sufficient laryngeal brightness [23]. However, in the LVS group, insufficient brightness affected seven patients (2.83%).

3.1.6. Summary of Observed Issues

To summarize the evaluation of the unsuccessful generation of LVS kymograms in comparison to HSV-based kymograms (Figure 6), the total failure rate was significantly higher ($p < 0.001$) and resulted in a failure rate of 43.32% (failure of LVS recordings—107/247). The significant difference was observed for the following reasons: hidden glottal opening: $p = 0.009$ (LVS 42/247 vs. HSV 18/247), lack of synchronization: $p < 0.001$ (20/247 vs. 0/247), insufficiently long phonation: $p = 0.0003$ (13/247 vs. 0/247), and insufficient brightness of recordings: $p = 0.0077$ (7/247 vs. 0/247). No significant differences were found for structural obstacles obscuring the glottis $p = 0.8804$ (25/247 vs. 24/247). In our analysis, we categorized visualization challenges into two distinct groups:

1. Hidden glottal opening: This category includes cases where the vocal folds failed to sufficiently open to allow for effective kymographic analysis. This issue primarily arose in patients with functional dysphonia or glottic pathologies that restricted the natural opening of the vocal folds during phonation;
2. Structural Hindrances in Glottal Visualization: this category encompasses cases where visualization was obstructed by anatomical structures such as an omega-shaped epiglottis, a large epiglottic petiole, or supraglottic hyperfunction, leading to incomplete or distorted views of the glottis.

For HSV, the main obstacles were structural hindrances in glottal visualization (24/223; 9.72%) and hidden glottal opening (18/229; 7.28%). HSV exhibited a success rate of 83.00%, a 26.31% higher success rate than LVS. Notably, HSV significantly outperformed LVS in most of the observed challenges (Figure 6).

3.2. Analysis of Cases with Inconclusive Kymograms Using Only One Technique

In cases where initial kymogram generation was unsuccessful with both HSV and LVS, we further explored whether optimized HSV and LVS settings and improved patient cooperation could allow for successful kymogram acquisition, especially in patients where one method had already proven inadequate. Among the 107 patients for whom LVS kymograms were not feasible, reliable kymograms were obtained in 73 patients (68.22%) through HSV. However, in 34 cases, neither HSV nor LVS produced a kymogram.

In eight cases where HSV kymograms could not be generated, LVS was successful. In six of these cases, structural obstacles, such as a prominent epiglottis, obstructed HSV visualization, and in the remaining two, hyperfunctional phonation enabled sufficient opening of the glottis.

3.3. Comparison of Kymogram Feasibility by Lesion Type

HSV demonstrated a notable advantage in generating kymograms, particularly in patients with organic glottal pathologies. In normophonic patients, HSV yielded additional (in comparison to LSV) kymograms in four out of forty-seven patients (8.51%), while in those with benign lesions, 32 additional kymograms were obtained (26.02%). For patients with malignant lesions, HSV generated additional kymograms in 23 cases (41.07%). A significant difference ($p < 0.0001$) was observed for both benign and malignant hypertrophic masses of the glottis. For patients with functional voice disorders, HSV generated six additional kymograms (28.57%) compared to LVS ($p = 0.006$). The success rate difference across all examined groups is presented in Figure 8.

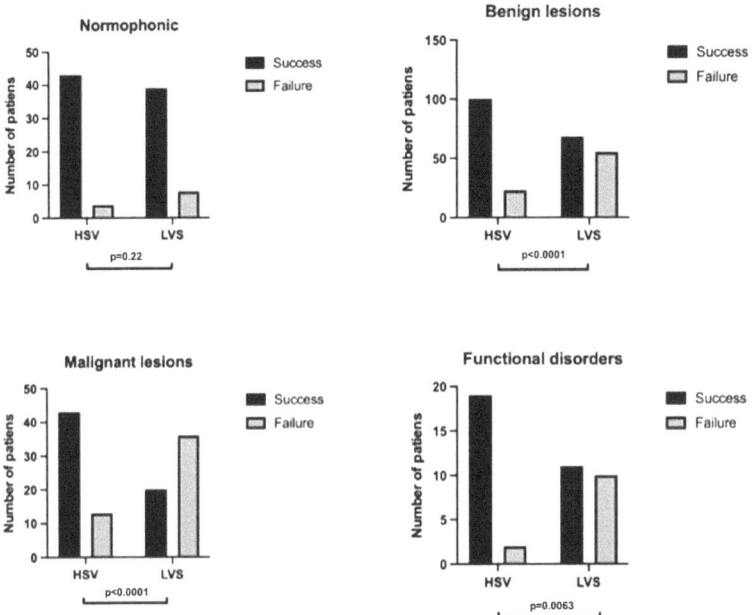

Figure 8. Feasibility of obtaining the kymograms from LVS recordings in comparison to HSV in the patients' groups divided by diagnosis.

In all patient groups with organic lesions, the HSV method resulted in a 30.73% higher rate of kymogram generation. Notably, failure causes such as insufficient light, synchronization issues, and insufficient phonation cycles did not occur in HSV recordings.

Among patients with carcinoma, hidden glottal opening was a common cause of failure in LVS compared to HSV (Figure 7(A1,A2)), with a difference in occurrence of 29% in carcinoma cases. Moreover, kymograms generated by HSV (Figure 9) provided superior temporal resolution, enhanced visualization of asynchronous vibrations, and greater structural detail compared to LVS kymograms (Figure 10), which rely on periodic phonation cycles and may obscure irregularities. The parameters presented in Figures 3, 4, 9 and 10 were computed using a dedicated kymographic analysis software, which applies semi-automated edge detection algorithms to track vocal fold movement along pre-defined glottal axes. The amplitude, symmetry, and phase differences were calculated based on pixel intensity changes over time, allowing for an objective assessment of vocal fold vibrations. Each computed value represents an average over multiple phonatory cycles to improve measurement accuracy.

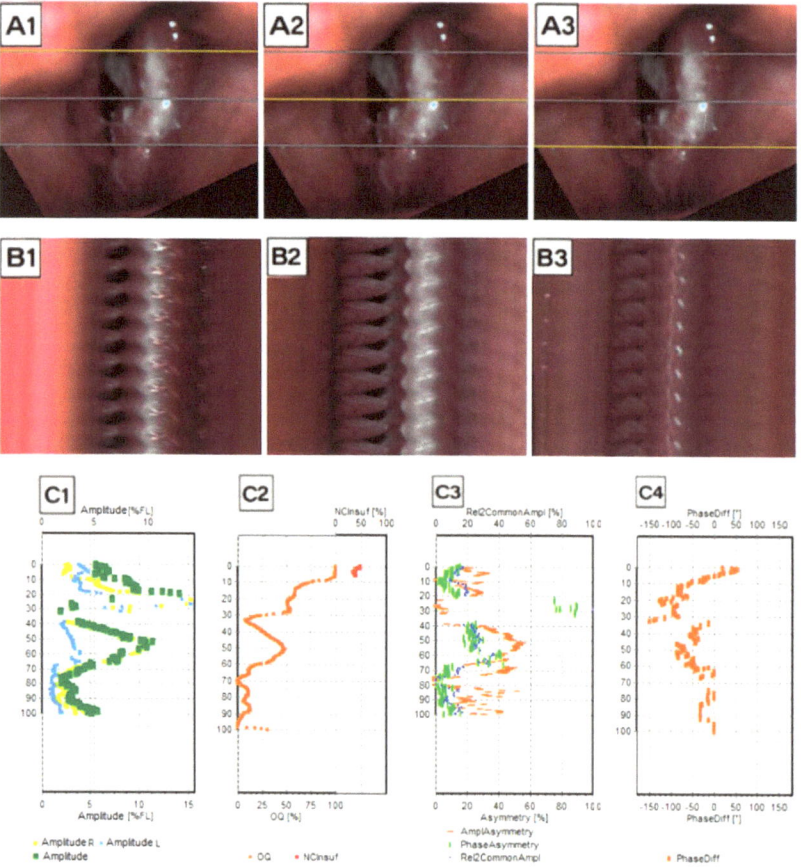

Figure 9. *Cont.*

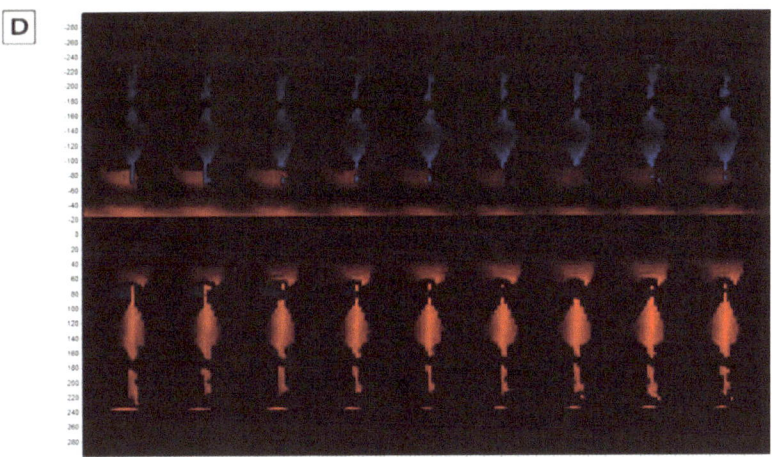

Figure 9. Analysis of data generated on the basis of HSV record for Subject 3: Patient with malignant lesion (61 years old man with cancer of the left vocal fold). Representative kymographic analysis derived from HSV recordings with 9 cycles of vocal fold movement. For a detailed description of the analysis process, please refer to the caption of Figures 3 and 4.

The phonovibrograms displayed in these figures provide a comprehensive visualization of vocal fold oscillation patterns over time. They are two-dimensional spatiotemporal representations of changes in the glottal area during phonation; the horizontal axis is time, and the vertical axis represents the length along the glottis. They represent the numeric value of the width of the space between the vocal folds (glottal gap). Darker color indicates decreased amplitude of vocal fold oscillations and increased glottal gap. They consolidate multiple vocal fold oscillation parameters into a single graphical representation, highlighting temporal variations in amplitude and phase relationships. This enables clinicians to visualize asymmetries, irregular vibrations, and insufficient glottal closure.

The last phase of our analysis compared the feasibility of generating kymograms from LVS and HSV recordings in patients with unilateral and bilateral lesions. The data showed a significant difference in kymogram generation success rates between HSV and LVS for both lesion types. Specifically, HSV achieved a 30% higher success rate than LVS, with HSV generating 115 successful recordings compared to 72 for LVS in unilateral lesions and 26 compared to 14 for bilateral lesions. These differences were statistically significant: $p < 0.00001$ for the unilateral lesions and $p = 0.0058$ for the bilateral lesions.

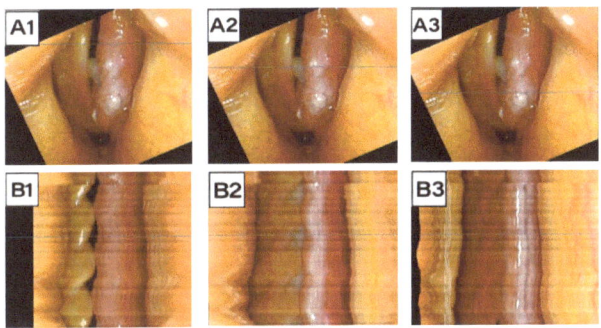

Figure 10. *Cont.*

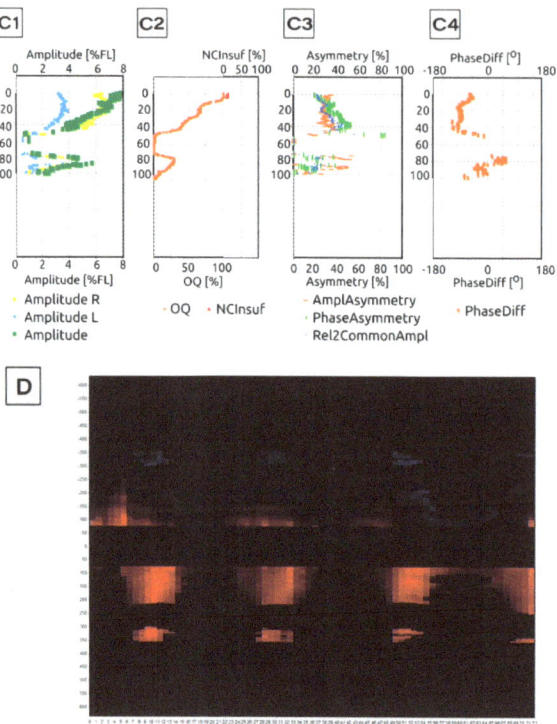

Figure 10. Analysis of data generated on the basis of HSV record for Subject 3: Patient with malignant lesion (61 years old man with cancer of the left vocal fold). Representative kymographic analysis derived from LVS recordings with 3 cycles of vocal fold movement. For a detailed description of the analysis process, please refer to the caption of Figures 3 and 4.

4. Discussion

High-speed videolaryngoscopy has become a valuable tool for visualizing vocal fold vibrations, providing an objective assessment and precise structural and functional evaluation of the glottis, and it is crucial for diagnosing various glottic pathologies [10]. Initially used for functional voice disorders, HSV is now increasingly applied to organic glottic lesions [24,25]. Unlike laryngovideostroboscopy (LVS), HSV captures real vocal fold vibrations at thousands of frames per second, enabling the analysis of vibration patterns in asynchronous voices and severe pathologies where strobe synchronization fails [2,5].

This study aimed to assess the effectiveness of generating kymograms for quantifying vocal fold oscillations using LVS and HSV recordings. A total of 247 subjects underwent both stroboscopy and HSV as part of standard diagnostic protocols, providing data for analysis. To our knowledge, this is the largest study assessing glottic pathologies in both methods. Of these, 179 presented with hypertrophic glottic masses, including 123 benign and 56 malignant lesions. The findings confirmed HSV as a valuable method for assessing organic glottic lesions, providing a higher rate of successful kymogram generation compared to LVS, which may aid in the evaluation of vocal fold oscillations. Consistent with previous studies, HSV outperformed LVS in generating kymograms, delivering faster, higher-quality results that address LVS's inherent limitations [13,26]. HSV-based kymograms allow for more objective evaluations of phonatory vibrations and quantitative parameter analysis, aiding less experienced clinicians in the preoperative diagnosis of glottic hypertrophic masses.

The existing literature highlights the subjective nature of vocal fold vibration assessments in both LVS and HSV examinations that are often influenced by clinician experience. Fujiki et al. explored subjective laryngeal ratings from LVS and HSV by categorizing raters by experience levels (over or under five years) [11]. They found high inter-rater reliability for amplitude, mucosal wave, and non-vibrating portions but noted challenges in assessing phase symmetry and periodicity [11]. In 9% of LVS and 6% of HSV exams, clinicians failed to identify at least one parameter. Similarly, Poburka et al. noted that inter-judge reliability ranged from 0.57 to 0.96 for LVS and from 0.81 to 0.94 for HSV in their assessment of mucosal wave and non-vibrating portions [8]. Efforts to improve objectivity in LVS and HSV assessments, such as through visuoperceptual variables, have been explored [27].

While previous studies have compared LVS and HSV, our research uniquely focuses on the specific challenges and success rates in generating analyzable kymograms across different patient groups, including normophonic individuals and those with functional, benign, and malignant vocal fold lesions. Additionally, our study provides a detailed analysis of the reasons behind LVS failure and the extent to which HSV can overcome these challenges [5,8,9].

For years, our department has used kymographic analysis to evaluate glottal phonatory function, transitioning from LVS- to HSV-based methods [23,28]. Advanced HSV techniques provide objective metrics for vocal fold amplitude, symmetry, and periodicity. Consistent with literature data, HSV-generated kymograms are faster and easier to produce than those derived from LVS [5,29].

Research demonstrates that high-speed videoendoscopy (HSV) significantly outperformed low-speed videoendoscopy (LVS) in generating kymograms. The observed better outcomes for unilateral lesions may be attributed to greater asynchrony in vocal fold vibrations, which HSV captures effectively through kymographic analysis.

In the functional dysphonia group, HSV also showed a significantly higher success rate than LVS; however, no significant difference was observed in the normophonic control group. Nevertheless, in clinical practice, obtaining high-quality recordings in patients with voice pathologies is prioritized, where HSV seems particularly advantageous [30].

Our results are consistent with prior studies suggesting the utility of HSV in diagnosing organic dysphonia [8,31]. Asymmetric hypertrophic glottal masses can often cause asynchronous vocal fold vibrations, which HSV can precisely capture, facilitating the detailed analysis of affected versus unaffected folds [12,32]. In this research, for benign glottic lesions, HSV achieved a 26% higher kymogram success rate than LVS, and for malignant lesions, this advantage rose to 41%. These differences were highly significant and support HSV's advantage in morphological insights into vocal fold oscillations compared to stroboscopy [10,21]. Additionally, HSV-based kymograms provided accurate measurements of parameters such as amplitude, glottic dynamics, asymmetry, phase difference, and periodicity of vibrations. Figures 9 and 10 highlight the improved quality of HSV kymograms compared to LVS. Consistent with the findings by Powell et al., HSV's higher frame rate and resolution facilitated the assessment of laryngeal pliability [24]. Yamauchi et al. further noted HSV's ability to identify non-vibrating areas in infiltrative malignant lesions, such as invasive carcinoma [32].

Our study compared factors affecting kymogram generation with LVS and HSV. Hidden glottal opening (due to prolonged closing phases) was a notable challenge, affecting 7.3% of HSV recordings versus 17% for LVS ($p = 0.0009$). This difference likely arises from LVS sampling incomplete glottal cycles, which is unlike HSV, which captures full cycles, enabling precise measurements of medial vocal fold edge distances. Previous studies confirm that HSV provides a more accurate representation of laryngeal vibrations than LVS [13,21,24]. The limitations of both methods are detailed in Table 2.

Improved lighting in HSV using laser illumination enhanced kymogram quality by increasing the brightness. According to manufacturer specifications and clinical observations, laser illumination did not significantly raise the endoscope's temperature; however, the potential for localized heating and its effects on the tongue root and vocal tract tissues should be considered when using high-intensity light sources. In our study, HSV captured full-color images, which improved visibility compared to the specific LVS system used, where images were often darker due to the limitations of the LED strobe lamp. However, it is important to note that some LVS systems with higher-intensity strobe lamps can provide bright and well-illuminated images, potentially mitigating this issue. Although some authors suggest that grayscale is beneficial for HSV recordings, others identify insufficient brightness as a common limitation in color HSV recordings [8,9,11].

Another limitation of LVS is its reliance on light synchronization, particularly in moderate or severe dysphonia cases where an unstable voice signal can disrupt synchronization, producing asynchronous sequences that are challenging to interpret. This limitation affected 8.1% of our LVS recordings and was a significant barrier to kymogram generation compared to HSV ($p < 0.001$ for synchronization issues; $p = 0.0003$ for unstable phonation). Prior studies report a 17–63% failure rate for LVS in similar cases [21,38]. HSV, by contrast, proved superior for assessing glottic malignant lesions and cases of asynchronicity, aligning with recommendations for its use in complex pathologies [24].

Table 2. Comparison of limitations of the HSV and LVS techniques based on our experience and the literature cited in the discussion.

TECHNICAL AND EQUIPMENT LIMITATIONS	
HSV	- expensive equipment limits accessibility. - large datasets require specialized software. - optics can discomfort patients and restrict anatomical visualization.
LVS	- limited resolution and brightness reduce detail visibility. (however, the resolution and brightness of LVS recordings in our study were limited by the specific system used, which may not reflect the capabilities of newer high-resolution LVS systems available on the market.) - sometimes, images fail to reflect irregular vibrations, preventing the examination.
COMPARISON	HSV provides high-quality, real-time vibratory tracking but entails higher costs and demanding data management. LVS is more accessible and uses flexible scopes but lacks resolution and precision for detailed assessments.
LIGHTING AND IMAGING SYNCHRONIZATION	
HSV	- HSV requires specialized lighting for optimal imaging, though newer systems are improving illumination technology.
LVS	- LVS requires stable phonation for strobe synchronization, as it struggles with strobe synchronization in cases of asynchronic voices or severe dysphonia, reducing interpretable images.
COMPARISON	HSV delivers superior imaging, aided by advanced lighting, while LVS often inhibits the examination in severe dysphonic patients lacking stable vocal patterns.

Table 2. Cont.

DEPENDENCE ON STABLE PHONATION	
HSV	- our HSV examination was limited to rigid optics; however, various studies have demonstrated the feasibility of flexible high-speed videoendoscopy [23,31,33–37].
LVS	- LVS needs around 10 s of stable phonation, which poses a challenge for patients with severe voice disorders.
COMPARISON	LVS relies on stable phonation, which is necessary for light synchronization, limiting its use in severe dysphonia, while HSV effectively captures all irregular vibrations in real time without requiring synchronization.
STRUCTURAL AND ANATOMICAL CHALLENGES	
HSV	- challenges in visualizing the glottis with anatomical variations (e.g., prominent epiglottis) which disturbs kymogram generation; this is related to the use of rigid optics in our HSV system. - while HSV provides high-resolution imaging, large lesions that cover the glottis may still prevent a full assessment.
LVS	- lower resolution and frame averaging hinder the assessment of intricate lesions or non-vibrating areas. - flexible scopes improve comfort but struggle with large masses and reduce resolution in complex cases.
COMPARISON	Our HSV system offers clearer imaging but is restricted by rigid scopes, while LVS provides less detail but gains flexibility with adaptable scopes.
DATA INTERPRETATION AND OBJECTIVITY	
HSV	- HSV result interpretation from the software requires expertise.
LVS	- LVS assessments rely on subjective interpretation, causing inconsistencies, especially for phase symmetry and periodicity. - Quantitative analysis in LVS is time-consuming, delaying real-time diagnostic feedback.
COMPARISON	HSV offers greater accuracy but requires costly equipment and advanced expertise. LVS is prone to subjective interpretation and observer variability, especially for less experienced users, and objective analysis is time-consuming.

Our findings provide several new insights into the feasibility and accuracy of HSV compared to LVS for kymographic analysis. We confirmed previous studies indicating the superior ability of HSV in capturing detailed vibratory patterns and overcoming synchronization limitations inherent to LVS. However, our study extends existing knowledge by offering a comprehensive analysis of failure rates and success factors in a larger patient cohort, particularly in cases of organic glottal lesions.

In contrast to earlier research, our results highlight the specific challenges associated with LVS, such as its dependency on phonation stability and lighting conditions, which have not been thoroughly quantified before; however, some technical aspects, like lightning conditions, should not be generalized across all HSV and LVS systems available on the market today. Our findings align with those by Patel et al. (2008) and Poburka et al. (2017) but provide new evidence regarding the practical implications of these limitations in clinical practice [8,21].

In the future perspective, artificial intelligence (AI), which has shown significant potential in the recognition of both functional and non-functional glottic pathologies, may be further investigated in HSV or LVS to help differentiate laryngeal lesions. Studies have demonstrated that machine learning algorithms, combined with imaging modalities such as narrow-band imaging (NBI) and white light imaging (WLI), can enhance the early detection and classification of glottic lesions, including benign and malignant conditions [39,40]. Additionally, AI models utilizing voice signals, demographics, and structured medical records have been developed to differentiate glottic neoplasms from benign voice disorders, offering a non-invasive diagnostic approach with promising accuracy [41].

Overall, our study supports and expands upon the existing literature, reinforcing the advantages of HSV while providing new data on its applicability across different clinical scenarios. Future research should focus on optimizing HSV protocols to further improve diagnostic accuracy and efficiency in voice disorder assessments.

5. Conclusions

This study highlights the comparative effectiveness of high-speed videolaryngoscopy (HSV) and laryngovideostroboscopy (LVS) in generating kymograms and objectively assessing vocal fold function in patients with voice disorders. HSV demonstrated a significantly higher kymogram generation success rate (83% vs. 57% for LVS), particularly in cases of patients with asynchronous vocal fold oscillations associated with both organic and functional pathologies, with statistically significant differences across all patient groups, including those with benign and malignant glottic lesions. By overcoming LVS limitations through high frame rates and real-time imaging, HSV enables detailed assessments even in severe dysphonia or extensive glottic lesions. Its ability to provide precise quantitative parameters such as amplitude, asymmetry, and glottal closure underlines HSV's potential as a routine diagnostic tool, offering improved diagnostic accuracy and outcomes in specialized laryngeal assessments.

Future research could aim to improve HSV accessibility and develop automated data analysis tools to facilitate its clinical integration. Hybrid approaches combining HSV's detailed accuracy with the practicality of LVS, as explored in our department's previous work, may further optimize laryngeal imaging practices. Broader adoption of HSV could significantly enhance the quality and precision of voice disorder diagnostics, ultimately leading to better therapeutic outcomes for patients.

Author Contributions: Conceptualization, J.H., E.N.-B., and W.P.; methodology, W.P and E.N.-B.; validation, W.P and E.N.-B.; formal analysis, J.H.; investigation, W.P., E.N.-B., J.H., and M.B.; data curation, J.H. and W.P.; writing—original draft preparation, J.H., W.P., M.B., and E.N.-B.; writing—review and editing, J.H., W.P., M.B., and E.N.-B.; visualization, J.H. and M.B.; supervision, W.P. and E.N.-B.; project administration, W.P. All authors have read and agreed to the published version of the manuscript.

Funding: This research received no external funding.

Institutional Review Board Statement: The study was conducted in accordance with the Declaration of Helsinki and approved by the Ethics Committee of Medical University of Lodz no. RNN/96/20/KE, date of approval 8 April 2020, for studies involving humans.

Informed Consent Statement: Informed consent was obtained from all subjects involved in the study.

Data Availability Statement: The data presented in this study are available upon request from the corresponding author due to restrictions regarding patients' privacy.

Conflicts of Interest: The authors declare no conflicts of interest.

References

1. Dejonckere, P.H.; Bradley, P.; Clemente, P.; Cornut, G.; Crevier-Buchman, L.; Friedrich, G.; Van De Heyning, P.; Remacle, M.; Woisard, V. A Basic Protocol for Functional Assessment of Voice Pathology, Especially for Investigating the Efficacy of (Phonosurgical) Treatments and Evaluating New Assessment Techniques: Guideline Elaborated by the Committee on Phoniatrics of the European Laryngological Society (ELS). *Eur. Arch. Oto-Rhino-Laryngol.* **2001**, *258*, 77–82. [CrossRef]
2. Eysholdt, U. Laryngoscopy, Stroboscopy, High-Speed Video and Phonovibrogram. In *Phoniatrics I Fundamentals–Voice Disorders–Disorders of Language and Hearing Development*; Springer: Berlin/Heidelberg, Germany, 2020; pp. 364–376.

3. Prufer, N.; Woo, P.; Altman, K.W. Pulse Dye and Other Laser Treatments for Vocal Scar. *Curr. Opin. Otolaryngol. Head Neck Surg.* **2010**, *18*, 492–497. [CrossRef] [PubMed]
4. Sielska-Badurek, E.M.; Jędra, K.; Sobol, M.; Niemczyk, K.; Osuch-Wójcikiewicz, E. Laryngeal Stroboscopy-Normative Values for Amplitude, Open Quotient, Asymmetry and Phase Difference in Young Adults. *Clin. Otolaryngol.* **2019**, *44*, 158–165. [CrossRef] [PubMed]
5. Woo, P. Objective Measures of Laryngeal Imaging: What Have We Learned since Dr. Paul Moore. *J. Voice* **2014**, *28*, 69–81. [CrossRef]
6. Patel, R.R.; Awan, S.N.; Barkmeier-Kraemer, J.; Courey, M.; Deliyski, D.; Eadie, T.; Paul, D.; Švec, J.G.; Hillman, R. Recommended Protocols for Instrumental Assessment of Voice: American Speech-Language-Hearing Association Expert Panel to Develop a Protocol for Instrumental Assessment of Vocal Function. *Am. J. Speech Lang. Pathol.* **2018**, *27*, 887–905. [CrossRef]
7. Doellinger, M.; Lohscheller, J.; McWhorter, A.; Kunduk, M. Variability of Normal Vocal Fold Dynamics for Different Vocal Loading in One Healthy Subject Investigated by Phonovibrograms. *J. Voice* **2009**, *23*, 175–181. [CrossRef]
8. Poburka, B.J.; Patel, R.R.; Bless, D.M. Voice-Vibratory Assessment With Laryngeal Imaging (VALI) Form: Reliability of Rating Stroboscopy and High-Speed Videoendoscopy. *J. Voice* **2017**, *31*, 513.e1–513.e14. [CrossRef]
9. Zacharias, S.R.C.; Deliyski, D.D.; Gerlach, T.T. Utility of Laryngeal High-Speed Videoendoscopy in Clinical Voice Assessment. *J. Voice* **2018**, *32*, 216–220. [CrossRef]
10. Powell, M.E.; Deliyski, D.D.; Zeitels, S.M.; Burns, J.A.; Hillman, R.E.; Gerlach, T.T.; Mehta, D.D. Efficacy of Videostroboscopy and High-Speed Videoendoscopy to Obtain Functional Outcomes From Perioperative Ratings in Patients with Vocal Fold Mass Lesions. *J. Voice* **2020**, *34*, 769–782. [CrossRef]
11. Fujiki, R.B.; Croegaert-Koch, C.K.; Thibeault, S.L. Videostroboscopy Versus High-Speed Videoendoscopy: Factors Influencing Ratings of Laryngeal Oscillation. *J. Speech Lang. Hear. Res.* **2023**, *66*, 1496–1510. [CrossRef]
12. Kaluza, J.; Niebudek-Bogusz, E.; Malinowski, J.; Strumillo, P.; Pietruszewska, W. Assessment of Vocal Fold Stiffness by Means of High-Speed Videolaryngoscopy with Laryngotopography in Prediction of Early Glottic Malignancy: Preliminary Report. *Cancers* **2022**, *14*, 4697. [CrossRef] [PubMed]
13. Kist, A.M.; Dürr, S.; Schützenberger, A.; Döllinger, M. OpenHSV: An Open Platform for Laryngeal High-Speed Videoendoscopy. *Sci. Rep.* **2021**, *11*, 13760. [CrossRef]
14. Tigges, M.; Wittenberg, T.; Mergell, P.; Eysholdt, U. Imaging of Vocal Fold Vibration by Digital Multi-Plane Kymography. *Comput. Med. Imaging Graph.* **1999**, *23*, 323–330. [CrossRef]
15. Švec, J.G.; Schutte, H.K. Videokymography: High-Speed Line Scanning of Vocal Fold Vibration. *J. Voice* **1996**, *10*, 201–205. [CrossRef] [PubMed]
16. Deliyski, D. *Laryngeal Evaluation: Indirect Laryngoscopy to High-Speed Digital Imaging*; Kendall, K.A., Leonard, R.J., Eds.; Thieme: New York, NY, USA, 2010; ISBN 9781604062724.
17. Woo, P. Objective Measures of Stroboscopy and High-Speed Video. *Adv. Otorhinolaryngol.* **2020**, *85*, 25–44. [CrossRef] [PubMed]
18. Hertegård, S. What Have We Learned about Laryngeal Physiology from High-Speed Digital Videoendoscopy? *Curr. Opin. Otolaryngol. Head Neck Surg.* **2005**, *13*, 152–156. [CrossRef]
19. Švec, J.G.; Schutte, H.K. Kymographic Imaging of Laryngeal Vibrations. *Curr. Opin. Otolaryngol. Head Neck Surg.* **2012**, *20*, 458–465. [CrossRef]
20. Racino, A.; Just, M.; Tyc, M.; DiagNova I Resources. Medical Video Recording. *Part V: High-Speed Camera in Practice*. Available online: https://diagnova.eu/pages/resources/video_recording_V_hsv_2.html (accessed on 1 May 2021).
21. Patel, R.; Dailey, S.; Bless, D. Comparison of High-Speed Digital Imaging with Stroboscopy for Laryngeal Imaging of Glottal Disorders. *Ann. Otol. Rhinol. Laryngol.* **2008**, *117*, 413–424. [CrossRef]
22. Lohscheller, J.; Eysholdt, U. Phonovibrogram Visualization of Entire Vocal Fold Dynamics. *Laryngoscope* **2008**, *118*, 753–758. [CrossRef]
23. Pietruszewska, W.; Just, M.; Morawska, J.; Malinowski, J.; Hoffman, J.; Racino, A.; Barańska, M.; Kowalczyk, M.; Niebudek-Bogusz, E. Comparative Analysis of High-Speed Videolaryngoscopy Images and Sound Data Simultaneously Acquired from Rigid and Flexible Laryngoscope: A Pilot Study. *Sci. Rep.* **2021**, *11*, 20480. [CrossRef]
24. Powell, M.E.; Deliyski, D.D.; Hillman, R.E.; Zeitels, S.M.; Burns, J.A.; Mehta, D.D. Comparison of Videostroboscopy to Stroboscopy Derived from High-Speed Videoendoscopy for Evaluating Patients with Vocal Fold Mass Lesions. *Am. J. Speech Lang. Pathol.* **2016**, *25*, 576–589. [CrossRef]
25. Yamauchi, A.; Imagawa, H.; Yokonishi, H.; Sakakibara, K.I.; Tayama, N. Multivariate Analysis of Vocal Fold Vibrations on Various Voice Disorders Using High-Speed Digital Imaging. *Appl. Sci.* **2021**, *11*, 6284. [CrossRef]
26. Shinghal, T.; Low, A.; Russell, L.; Propst, E.J.; Eskander, A.; Campisi, P. High-Speed Video or Video Stroboscopy in Adolescents: Which Sheds More Light? *Otolaryngol. Head Neck Surg.* **2014**, *151*, 1041–1045. [CrossRef] [PubMed]
27. Brunings, J.W.; Vanbelle, S.; Akkermans, A.; Heemskerk, N.M.M.; Kremer, B.; Stokroos, R.J.; Baijens, L.W.J. Observer Agreement for Measurements in Videolaryngostroboscopy. *J. Voice* **2018**, *32*, 756–762. [CrossRef]

28. Malinowski, J.; Pietruszewska, W.; Kowalczyk, M.; Niebudek-Boguz, E. Value of High-Speed Videoendoscopy as an Auxiliary Tool in Differentiation of Benign and Malignant Unilateral Vocal Lesions. *J. Cancer Res. Clin. Oncol.* **2024**, *150*, 10. [CrossRef]
29. Kang, D.H.; Wang, S.G.; Park, H.J.; Lee, J.C.; Jeon, G.R.; Choi, I.S.; Kim, S.J.; Shin, B.J. Real-Time Simultaneous DKG and 2D DKG Using High-Speed Digital Camera. *J. Voice* **2017**, *31*, 247.e1–247.e7. [CrossRef] [PubMed]
30. Panchami, B.; Kumar, S.P.; Phadke, K.V. Visualization and Analysis of Vocal Fold Dynamics in Various Voice Disorders. *J. Voice* **2024**. [CrossRef] [PubMed]
31. Lohscheller, J.; Švec, J.G.; Döllinger, M. Vocal Fold Vibration Amplitude, Open Quotient, Speed Quotient and Their Variability along Glottal Length: Kymographic Data from Normal Subjects. *Logoped. Phoniatr. Vocol.* **2013**, *38*, 182–192. [CrossRef]
32. Yamauchi, A.; Yokonishi, H.; Imagawa, H.; Sakakibara, K.I.; Nito, T.; Tayama, N.; Yamasoba, T. Quantitative Analysis of Digital Videokymography: A Preliminary Study on Age- and Gender-Related Difference of Vocal Fold Vibration in Normal Speakers. *J. Voice* **2015**, *29*, 109–119. [CrossRef]
33. Woo, P. Simultaneous High-Speed Video Laryngoscopy and Acoustic Aerodynamic Recordings during Vocal Onset of Variable Sound Pressure Level: A Preliminary Study. *Bioengineering* **2024**, *11*, 334. [CrossRef]
34. Echternach, M.; Burk, F.; Köberlein, M.; Döllinger, M.; Burdumy, M.; Richter, B.; Titze, I.R.; Elemans, C.P.H.; Herbst, C.T. Biomechanics of Sound Production in High-Pitched Classical Singing. *Sci. Rep.* **2024**, *14*, 13132. [CrossRef] [PubMed]
35. Woo, P.; Baxter, P. Flexible Fiber-Optic High-Speed Imaging of Vocal Fold Vibration: A Preliminary Report. *J. Voice* **2017**, *31*, 175–181. [CrossRef] [PubMed]
36. Naghibolhosseini, M.; Deliyski, D.D.; Zacharias, S.R.C.; de Alarcon, A.; Orlikoff, R.F. Temporal Segmentation for Laryngeal High-Speed Videoendoscopy in Connected Speech. *J. Voice* **2018**, *32*, 256.e1–256.e12. [CrossRef]
37. Petermann, S.; Döllinger, M.; Kniesburges, S.; Ziethe, A. Analysis Method for the Neurological and Physiological Processes Underlying the Pitch-Shift Reflex. *Acta Acust. United Acust.* **2016**, *102*, 284–297. [CrossRef]
38. Woo, P.; Colton, R.; Casper, J.; Brewer, D. Diagnostic Value of Stroboscopic Examination in Hoarse Patients. *J. Voice* **1991**, *5*, 231–238. [CrossRef]
39. Tie, C.W.; Li, D.Y.; Zhu, J.Q.; Wang, M.L.; Wang, J.H.; Chen, B.H.; Li, Y.; Zhang, S.; Liu, L.; Guo, L.; et al. Multi-Instance Learning for Vocal Fold Leukoplakia Diagnosis Using White Light and Narrow-Band Imaging: A Multicenter Study. *Laryngoscope* **2024**, *134*, 4321–4328. [CrossRef]
40. Li, Y.; Gu, W.; Yue, H.; Lei, G.; Guo, W.; Wen, Y.; Tang, H.; Luo, X.; Tu, W.; Ye, J.; et al. Real-Time Detection of Laryngopharyngeal Cancer Using an Artificial Intelligence-Assisted System with Multimodal Data. *J. Transl. Med.* **2023**, *21*, 698. [CrossRef]
41. Wang, C.T.; Chen, T.M.; Lee, N.T.; Fang, S.H. AI Detection of Glottic Neoplasm Using Voice Signals, Demographics, and Structured Medical Records. *Laryngoscope* **2024**, *134*, 4585–4592. [CrossRef]

Disclaimer/Publisher's Note: The statements, opinions and data contained in all publications are solely those of the individual author(s) and contributor(s) and not of MDPI and/or the editor(s). MDPI and/or the editor(s) disclaim responsibility for any injury to people or property resulting from any ideas, methods, instructions or products referred to in the content.

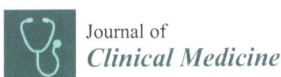

Article

Determining the Mouth-to-Microphone Distance in Rigid Laryngoscopy: A Simple Solution Based on the Newly Measured Values of the Depth of Endoscope Insertion into the Mouth

Dominika Valášková [1], Jitka Vydrová [2] and Jan G. Švec [1,2,*]

[1] Voice Research Lab, Department of Experimental Physics, Faculty of Sciences, Palacký University, 779 00 Olomouc, Czech Republic; dominika.valaskova01@upol.cz
[2] Voice and Hearing Centre Prague, Medical Healthcom, Ltd., 110 00 Prague, Czech Republic
* Correspondence: jan.svec@upol.cz

Abstract: Mouth-to-microphone (MTM) distance is important when measuring the sound of voice. However, determining the MTM distance for laryngoscope-mounted microphones during laryngoscopic examinations is cumbersome. We introduce a novel solution for such cases, using the depth of insertion of the laryngoscope into the mouth D_I as a reference distance. We measured the average insertion depth, D_I, in 60 adult women and 60 adult men for rigid laryngoscopes with 70° and 90° view. We found the D_I for the 70°/90° laryngoscope to be 9.7 ± 0.9/9.4 ± 0.6 cm in men, 8.9 ± 0.9/8.7 ± 0.7 cm in women, and 9.3 ± 0.9/9.0 ± 0.7 cm in all adults. Using these values, we show that, for microphones fixed at 15–40 cm from the tip of the laryngoscope, the final MTM distances are between 5 and 35 cm from the lips, and the standard uncertainties of these distances are between 16% and 2.5%. Our solution allows laryngologists and laryngoscope manufacturers to set and estimate the MTM distance for any rigid laryngeal endoscope with a microphone attached with reasonable accuracy, avoiding the need to measure this distance in vivo in routine practice.

Keywords: rigid laryngoscopy; oral cavity length; mouth-to-microphone distance; voice recording

1. Introduction

Laryngeal endoscopy (laryngoscopy) is the basic tool for the clinical examination of the voice. State-of-the-art laryngoscopy utilizes rigid and flexible laryngeal endoscopes (laryngoscopes) that are inserted into the mouth or nose, respectively, in order to visualize the larynx and the vocal folds (Figure 1). Here, we focus on the rigid endoscopes that allow for different types of endoscopic video cameras to be attached to capture laryngeal motion during phonation. Three basic laryngeal endoscopic techniques are used in laryngology for this purpose: laryngeal stroboscopy, high-speed videoendoscopy, and videokymography [1–5]. These methods visualize the larynx by using the same laryngoscopic approach but utilize three different types of video cameras, providing different types of laryngeal videos. All mentioned techniques aim at observing the vocal fold vibrations, revealing possible abnormalities of the vocal fold function.

Modern laryngoscopic devices capture the sound by a small microphone attached directly to the laryngoscope or to a camera head to relate the vocal fold abnormalities to the produced vocal sound. The captured sound is used to determine basic vocal characteristics, e.g., the vocal fold vibrational frequency (f_o) and sound pressure level (SPL), which can be displayed on a monitor [6]. This is relevant because the laryngeal adjustment and vocal fold behavior change with the f_o and SPL.

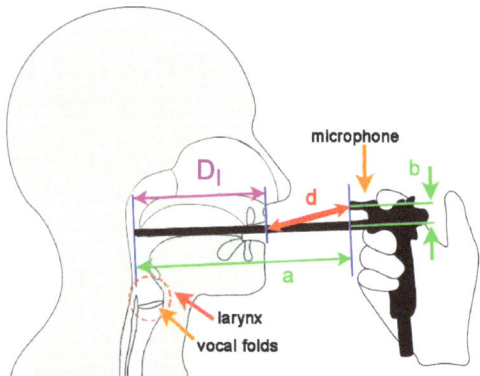

Figure 1. Insertion of a rigid laryngeal endoscope (laryngoscope) into the mouth to observe the larynx and the vocal folds during voice production in clinical voice examination. A small microphone attached to the laryngoscope captures the produced voice. The mouth-to-microphone (MTM) distance, d, influences the properties of the captured sound. This distance depends on the position of the microphone with respect to the tip of the laryngoscope (parameters a and b) and the depth of insertion of the laryngoscope into the mouth, D_I.

In order to interpret the recorded sound correctly, it is important to know the distance of the microphone from the mouth [7,8]. Wendler recommended setting this distance to 15 cm during laryngoscopy [9]; however, this recommendation has not been universally adopted. When the microphone is attached to the laryngoscope, or to the camera head mounted on the laryngoscope, the mouth-to-microphone (MTM) distance, d, cannot be set directly, because it depends on the depth of insertion of the laryngoscope into the mouth D_I (Figure 1). Therefore, to determine the MTM distance, d, we need to measure it directly during the laryngoscopic procedure. This measurement normally requires three people to be involved (the examiner performing the laryngoscopy, the examiner performing the distance measurement, and the subject undergoing the rigid laryngoscopy). Such a measurement is doable but cumbersome and time-consuming to perform in clinical practice for every examined client.

In this paper, we introduce an alternative method of determining the MTM distance for microphones attached to rigid laryngoscopes or to camera heads mounted on rigid laryngoscopes. Our method is based on knowledge of one key parameter—the depth of insertion of the laryngoscope into the mouth, D_I. As shown in Figure 1, the MTM distance, d, can be determined by subtracting the D_I value from the microphone position with respect to the tip of the laryngoscope. If the laryngoscope insertion depth, D_I, is reasonably similar across adult males and across adult females, the MTM distance does not have to be measured for each patient but can rather be universally specified for each laryngoscope, using a simple formula. However, to the best of our knowledge, so far, there is no reliable information on how deep the endoscope is placed into the mouth when performing rigid laryngoscopy and how the variability changes across subjects. Therefore, the first aim of this study is to determine the average insertion depth and its variation in adults for two common types of rigid laryngoscopes used in clinical practice—those with angles of view of 70 and 90 degrees [10,11]. Our specific questions and hypotheses related to the measurements of the laryngoscope insertion depth, D_I, were as follows:

1. Is the insertion depth different between male and female patients? We hypothesized the insertion depth to be larger in males, due to their longer vocal tract.
2. Is the insertion depth different for the laryngoscopes with a 70° and 90° view? We hypothesized the insertion depth to be larger in the 70° laryngoscope type since its tip is expected to be placed lower in the oropharynx, closer to the larynx.

The second aim of this study is to formulate empirical rules for determining the universal laryngoscopic MTM distance, d, in adults for the 70° and 90° rigid laryngoscopes with an attached microphone. To determine the possible difference in the MTM distance, d, estimated by the rules from its real value, the standard uncertainty is specified for adult males, adult females, and for all adults from the measured variability of the laryngoscope insertion depth, D_I, across subjects.

2. Materials and Methods

This is a cross-sectional study of 120 adult subjects. Three rigid laryngoscopes with 90° and 70° angles of view were used for the study. The measurements were performed from side photographs of the subjects taken during laryngoscopy. The length of the laryngoscope tube visible outside the mouth, z (Figure 2), was subtracted from the known full length of the laryngoscope, l, to derive the laryngoscope insertion depth, D_I. The details of the materials and methods are given below.

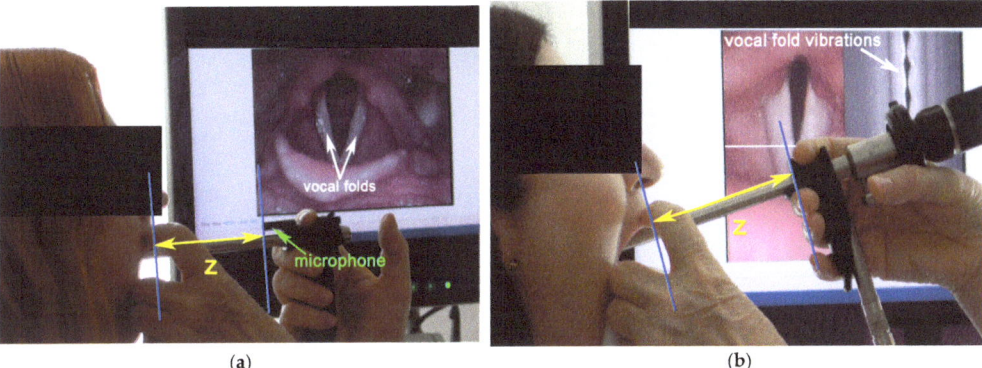

Figure 2. Side images obtained during (**a**) laryngeal stroboscopy (90° laryngoscope with an embedded microphone, L90S) and (**b**) videokymography (70° laryngoscope, L70K). The outside distance, z, was measured to derive the laryngoscope insertion depth into the mouth. Notice the monitor in the background showing the laryngeal images with the vocal folds—these were used for checking the correct placement of the laryngoscope in the mouth.

2.1. Subjects

One hundred twenty human adults (sixty male, age 50 ± 18, age range 19–91; sixty female, age 45 ± 18, age range 18–89) served as subjects for our study. The subjects were prospectively recruited from patients visiting a laryngologist at the clinical institute to which the second and last author belong. They were White Czech patients, except for one Hispanic patient. They visited the clinic for an outpatient laryngeal examination for various voice disorders or prevention purposes. The specific laryngeal diagnoses were of no significance for this study; we were interested only in measuring the depth of laryngoscope insertion into the mouth during the examinations. None of the subjects had the laryngeal skeleton deformed due to an accident or removed due to cancer. Only those subjects in which the laryngeal exam could be successfully completed and who gave their consent to the examination were included in the study. The patients with an obstructed view or no view of the vocal folds during phonation were excluded.

2.2. Examination Procedures and Division of the Subjects into Groups

The subjects were photographed from the side while undergoing a routine laryngoscopic examination procedure. All the subjects gave their consent for the photography. The Ethics Board of the clinical institute that the second and last authors belong to approved of the consent form and the study. Apart from taking the photographs, no special investigations were performed for the purpose of this study. The patients were seated comfortably in the examination chair and instructed to sustain a phonation of vowel /e/ or syllable /he/ at a comfortable pitch and loudness. Both the insertion of rigid laryngoscopes and the examination process were performed by a laryngologist with 30 years of clinical experience.

In the beginning, each participant underwent a laryngeal stroboscopic examination. This was performed using a 90° view laryngoscope (further labeled L90S), which is commonly used in Europe. The participants were then divided into three equally sized groups, each containing 40 subjects (20 females and 20 males). The division was based on the need for an additional laryngeal videokymographic examination, which was performed to obtain more accurate information on vocal fold vibrations, thus allowing for a more detailed diagnosis when needed. Group 1 underwent laryngeal videokymographic examination using the 70°-view laryngoscope (L70K). Group 2 underwent laryngeal videokymographic examination using the 90°-view laryngoscope (L90K). The division of the subjects into Groups 1 and 2 was random. Subjects from Group 3 were not indicated for any additional laryngeal examination procedure. The distribution of the subjects into the groups is summarized in Table 1. The ANOVA test revealed no statistically significant difference in age among the subgroups (ANOVA: $p_{age\text{-females}} = 0.397$; $p_{age\text{-males}} = 0.590$).

Table 1. The division of the patients into three groups according to used laryngoscope types (L70K, L90K, and L90S). No statistically significant differences in age were found among the groups. SD = standard deviation.

Group	Number of Males (M), Females (F)	Type of Used Laryngoscope	Age (Mean ± SD)
1	20 M 20 F	L70K + L90S	M 53 ± 17 F 42 ± 20
2	20 M 20 F	L90K + L90S	M 47 ± 17 F 50 ± 18
3	20 M 20 F	L90S	M 50 ± 17 F 44 ± 15

2.3. Examination Equipment

For the stroboscopic examination, we used the endoscopic system Xion EndoSTROB together with a L90S laryngoscope. This was a 90° rigid endoscope containing an integrated camera and microphone (Xion zoom laryngoscope type 130 310 629, Ø 10 mm, with handle and integrated light guide cable). For the subsequent VKG examination, we used the 2nd-generation videokymographic camera (Cymo 2156) and the 300 W endoscopic xenon light source (FX 300 A, Fentex Medical, Neuhausen ob Eck, Germany). The camera was alternately attached to one of two different rigid laryngoscopes for the VKG examinations. For Group 1, we used the L70K laryngoscope, i.e., the 70° Xion zoom laryngoscope (type 130 3210 527, Ø 10 mm). For Group 2, we used the L90K laryngoscope, i.e., the 90° Xion zoom laryngoscope (type 130 310 529, Ø 10 mm). The laryngoscopes were attached to the VKG camera head, using a C-mount objective adapter (R. Wolf, Knittlingen, Germany, type 8523.272, 27 mm focal length). The only reason for using the two different laryngoscopes for videokymography was the interest in finding whether there is a difference in the depth of laryngoscope insertion into the mouth between the 70° and 90° laryngoscope types since these two laryngoscope types are commonly used at different laryngology departments around the world [10,11].

Photographs were taken from the client's side, using the Nikon D3100 camera with a 4608 × 3072 pixel resolution. The photographic view was focused on the client's head and included the hand of the examiner holding the laryngoscope inserted into the mouth. A computer monitor displaying the laryngoscopic view was intentionally placed in the background (Figure 2) and was utilized to check whether the laryngoscope was fully inserted into the mouth, providing the full view of the vocal folds (Figure 2a). In the photographs taken during the VKG examination, the display monitor had to show the VKG line being placed perpendicularly to the glottis, as well as visible vocal fold vibrations in the videokymograms (Figure 2b). Multiple photographs were taken during every single examination. In total, 962 photographs (464 photos of 60 females; 498 photos of 60 males) were taken. For each subject, the age was noted.

2.4. Calibration Measurements—Laryngoscope Lengths

Multiple photographs of the rigid laryngoscopes used for this study were taken for reference purposes to find the length of the tubes of the used laryngoscopes. In total, 20 photos were taken (L70K: 8 photos; L90K: 7 photos; L90S: 5 photos) and used for calibration measurements of the lengths. The laryngoscopes were laid on a white background next to the ruler, giving clearly visible marks of lengths (Figure 3). The ruler was used to calibrate the photograph measurements in millimeters. The length of the tube, l, and the reference part, r, was determined from the photographs, as well as the distances a and b defining the microphone's position with respect to the tip of the laryngoscope, and the distance c of the center of the objective lens from the tip of the laryngoscope (Table 2). The calibration and the measurements were performed using the freeware program ImageJ.

Table 2. Sizes of laryngoscopes used for laryngeal examination, the microphone positions with respect to the tip of the laryngoscope, and the distance of the center of the objective lens from the tip of the laryngoscope. VKG = videokymography.

Laryngoscope Code	Type of Examination	Angle (°)	Length of Tube, l (cm)	Reference Length, r (cm)	Microphone Distance, a (cm)	Microphone Distance, b (cm)	Lens to Tip Distance, c (cm)
L70K	VKG	70	18.64 ± 0.08	4.44 ± 0.02	30.52 ± 0.05	2.67 ± 0.06	0.46 ± 0.01
L90K	VKG	90	19.09 ± 0.06	4.31 ± 0.08	30.26 ± 0.04	2.67 ± 0.06	0.61 ± 0.01
L90S	Stroboscopy	90	17.27 ± 0.06	7.26 ± 0.05	17.27 ± 0.06	1.08 ± 0.03	0.30 ± 0.01

2.5. Measurements of the Depth of Laryngoscope Insertion into the Mouth

In order to find out the depth of the laryngoscope insertion into the mouth, we measured the length of the tube remaining outside the mouth during laryngoscopy from the photographic images (Figure 2, distance z). To find this distance in centimeters, we used the known size of the reference part, r, of each laryngoscope (Table 2 and Figure 3). The end of the mouth was determined by drawing a line touching the upper lip that was perpendicular to the laryngoscopic tube for each patient (solid blue line touching lips, Figure 2). The depth of the laryngoscope insertion into the mouth, D_I (Table 3), was obtained by subtracting the measured outside length, z, from the known total length, l, of the laryngoscope tube (Table 2).

The statistical analysis was performed using the programs MS Excel and Statistica. The one-sample Kolmogorov–Smirnov test (K-S test) was used for the results from each laryngoscope to find whether the data were normally distributed. To compare the different groups (sex or laryngoscope type), we first performed the test of equality of variances: the F-test with the null hypothesis of two groups having the same variances. The F-test was a prerequisite for the choice of the subsequent two-sample t-test with equality or inequality variances and paired two-sample t-test for means. To determine significance, we used α values of 0.05, 0.01, and 0.001. To counteract the problem of multiple comparisons during the K-S test and t-tests, we used the Holm method [12]. For the Holm method, we sorted all p-values from the lowest to highest ($p_1, p_2 \ldots p_i \ldots p_K$) and defined corrected alpha levels as follows:

$$\alpha^* = \frac{\alpha}{K - i + 1} \quad (1)$$

where K is the number of p-values, and i is the order of p_i-values. Every p-value had a different α^* value to be compared with. A more detailed explanation of the measuring steps can be found in [13,14].

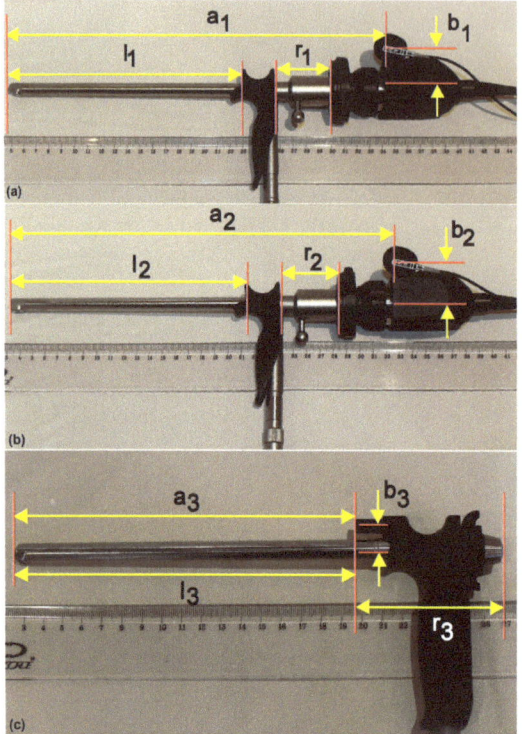

Figure 3. Examples of calibration photographs of the three rigid laryngoscopes used in this study: (**a**) L70K, (**b**) L90K, and (**c**) L90S. The lengths of the tubes, l_1, l_2, l_3, and of the reference parts, r_1, r_2, r_3, as well as the horizontal and vertical positions of the microphone from the tip of the laryngoscope (distances a_1, a_2, a_3, and b_1, b_2, b_3, respectively), were determined for the three laryngoscopes, respectively, using these photographs. The results are listed in Table 2. In (**a**,**b**), the microphone is fixed to the VKG camera head and covered by a protective acoustic foam; the location of the microphone inside the foam is indicated by the drawing. In (**c**), the microphone is embedded directly in the laryngoscope L90S.

Table 3. The measured laryngoscope insertion depths for the three different laryngoscopes (L70K, L90K, and L90S) and for L90S pooled with L90K. The measurement results are listed as mean values and standard deviations (this holds for the other tables too). The results of the statistical tests for female–male differences are shown at the bottom of the table. Levels of significance were highlighted as p-value < 0.01 (**), and <0.001 (***).

		L70K		L90K		L90S		L90K + L90S	
	Sex	n	Insertion Depth, D_I (cm)	n	Insertion Depth, D_I (cm)	n	Insertion Depth, D_I (cm)	n	Insertion Depth, D_I (cm)
Insertion Depth	Females (F)	20	8.91 ± 0.86	20	8.84 ± 0.68	60	8.63 ± 0.63	80	8.68 ± 0.65
	Males (M)	20	9.70 ± 0.90	20	9.47 ± 0.63	60	9.39 ± 0.65	80	9.41 ± 0.64
	Adults (F + M)	40	9.31 ± 0.90	40	9.15 ± 0.72	120	9.01 ± 0.74	160	9.05 ± 0.74
F-test (p-value)	Females vs. Males	20/20	0.44	20/20	0.38	60/60	0.42	80/80	0.47
t-test (p-value)	Females vs. Males	20/20	0.009 **	20/20	0.005 **	60/60	<0.001 ***	80/80	<0.001 ***

3. Results

Figure 4 shows the average insertion depth in females and males, as well as in all adults (i.e., females pooled with males), measured for the three different types of rigid laryngoscopes, L70K, L90K, and L90S. The numerical results are provided in Table 3. The K-S test proved that all data were normally distributed (K-S test: $\alpha^*_{0.05} = 0.006$–0.05, $p = 0.06$–0.6 for the nine subgroups displayed in Figure 4).

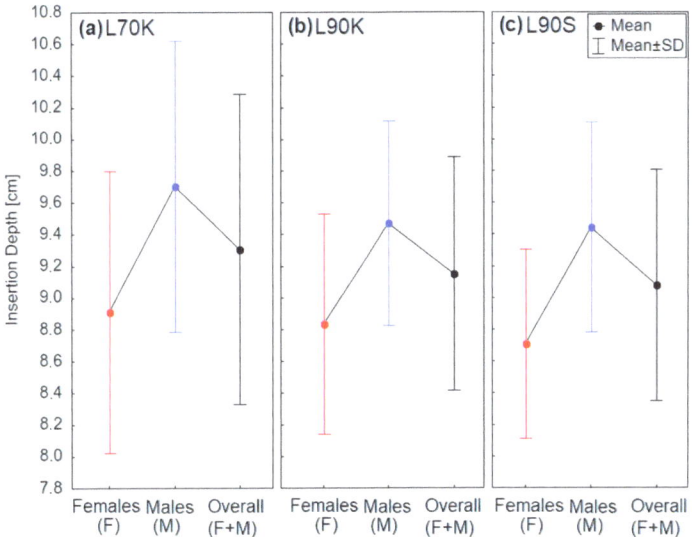

Figure 4. The insertion depth, D_I, of different types of laryngoscopes for females (red), males (blue), and all adults (females plus males, black): (**a**) laryngoscope L70K, (**b**) laryngoscope L90K, and (**c**) laryngoscope L90S.

3.1. Female–Male Differences

The results of the measurements comparing the laryngoscope insertion depths in female and male subjects are provided at the bottom of Table 3. The *t*-test (two-sample test with equal variances) showed that the insertion depth significantly differed between males and females, which was true for all three laryngoscopes used. On average, the insertion depth was 7 mm larger in male than in female subjects (see also Figure 4). The F-test revealed no significant differences in variances of the insertion depth between females and males for any of the laryngoscopes.

3.2. Differences among the Laryngoscopes

Since each subject in Groups 1 and 2 was examined using two different laryngoscopes (L70K and L90S for Group 1; L90K and L90S for Group 2), we could investigate the paired differences in the insertion depth of the laryngoscopes. The results are provided in Table 4. The 70° laryngoscope (L70K) was inserted, on average, about 3 mm deeper into the mouth than the 90° laryngoscope (L90S). The paired *t*-test revealed that this difference fulfilled the significance criterion for females (*p*-value of 0.04), but not for males and the adults (males and females pooled together). Much smaller, insignificant differences of 0.4–0.5 mm were found between the average insertion depths of the two 90° laryngoscopes (L90S and L90K, used for stroboscopy and videokymography, respectively). Hence, in the last column of Table 3, we provide the pooled measurement results for both of the 90° laryngoscopes.

Table 4. Laryngoscope insertion depth: differences among the different laryngoscopes—L70K, L90K, and L90S. Levels of significance were highlighted as *p*-value < 0.05 (*).

Sex	Insertion Depth Differences (cm)			Pair *t*-Test (*p*-Value)			F-Test (*p*-Value)		
	N	L70K–L90S	L90K–L90S	N	L70K vs. L90S	L90K vs. L90S	N	L70K vs. L90S	L90K vs. L90S
Females (F)	20/20	0.28 ± 0.56	0.04 ± 0.38	20/20	0.04 *	0.55	20/20	0.04 *	0.32
Males (M)	20/20	0.25 ± 0.76	0.05 ± 0.38	20/20	0.16	0.72	20/20	0.07	0.39
Adults (F + M)	40/40	0.27 ± 0.67	0.04 ± 0.38	40/40	0.17	0.80	40/40	0.04 *	0.47

The variability of the insertion depth among the subjects was also found to be slightly larger for the 70° than for the 90° laryngoscope (standard deviations of 9 mm versus 6–7 mm, respectively, as shown in Table 3 and by the whiskers in Figure 4). This difference passed the threshold of statistical significance in females and in all adults, as indicated by the *p*-value 0.04 obtained from the F-test (see Table 4).

4. Discussion

The obtained results confirmed our two hypotheses to be true:

1. The laryngoscope insertion depth was larger in male than female patients;
2. The insertion depth was slightly larger for the 70°-view laryngoscope than for the 90°-view laryngoscope.

The specific results and their implications are discussed below.

4.1. Female–Male Differences in Insertion Depth

Our results show that the laryngoscope is inserted deeper in the mouth in males than in females (Table 3). The difference was about 7 mm, and it was found statistically highly significant. This could be related to the significant anatomical differences in the vocal tract length between females and males observed by other authors, with the female vocal tract being shorter [15–20]. It is worth comparing our results specifically to the anatomical measurements of the horizontal length of the vocal tract or of the oral cavity depth reported in the literature. Vorperian [17–19] defined the horizontal length of the vocal tract as the distance from a line tangential to the lips to the posterior pharyngeal wall. Their data reveal these lengths to be 9.26 ± 0.63 cm for females and 9.81 ± 0.96 cm for males. Similar results were found by Goldstein [20], who reported the oral cavity length plus lips to be 9.2 cm for females and 9.7 cm for males. These lengths are only a few millimeters longer than our values for laryngoscope insertion depth provided in Table 3, which is well understandable: when inserted, the tip of the laryngoscope typically does not touch the posterior pharyngeal wall to avoid a gagging reflex. The distance of the scope's tip from the pharyngeal wall may thus account for the differences between our measurements and those of Goldstein [20] and Vorperian et al. [17–19]. The female-to-male differences of 5–6 mm found by Goldstein and Vorperian et al. are close to the 7 mm differences found in our data.

4.2. Insertion Depth Differences among Different Laryngoscopes

Regarding the differences among the laryngoscope types, the results indicate the following:

1. The 70° scope (L70K) was inserted about 3 mm deeper into the mouth, and its insertion depth varied slightly more among the subjects than in the case of the 90° laryngoscope (L90S);
2. The two 90° laryngoscopes (L90S and L90K) could be considered similar in terms of their insertion depth (Table 4).

Although not passing the significance threshold in all cases, the 3 mm larger insertion depth for the 70° laryngoscope type is not surprising given the fact that its construction allows the tip of the laryngoscope to be placed in the oro-pharyngeal cavity slightly lower and closer to the larynx than the 90° laryngoscope [10]. On the other hand, there was a negligible difference of less than 0.5 mm between the two 90° laryngoscopes used here.

Interestingly, the L90K and L90S laryngoscopes were of highly different construction (classical versus chip-on-the-tip design), and they had significantly different positions of the centers of their objective lenses from the tip of the laryngoscope: 6.1 ± 0.1 mm versus 3.0 ± 0.1 mm, respectively (recall Table 2). The more distant position of the lens from the tip was not found to be compensated by deeper insertion of the laryngoscope into the mouth—the 3 mm difference in the lens positions did not appear to have any significant influence on the laryngoscope insertion depth in our study. This suggests that the depth of laryngoscope insertion into the mouth is similar for rigid laryngoscopes of different constructions when they have the same angle of view. Based on these results, we assume the insertion depth to be similar for rigid laryngoscopes of the same type within and among different manufacturers. Verifying this assumption, however, would require a more extensive study with several more laryngoscopes, which exceeded our current possibilities. Nevertheless, considering the ca. ± 7mm variation in the insertion depth found among different subjects, as indicated in Table 3, and only the 0.5 mm difference between the two 90° laryngoscopes, as indicated in Table 4, we could safely assume that the insertion depth differences among different laryngoscopes of the same type are smaller than the depth variation among different subjects.

4.3. Stroboscopy–Videokymography Differences in Insertion Depth

Our study showed negligible differences in the laryngoscope insertion depth between stroboscopy and videokymography (Table 4; p-values above 0.55 for the t-test and above 0.32 for the F-test, columns L90S vs. L90K). We do not find this surprising: the videokymography camera provides a dual image—besides the videokymographic view, there is simultaneously also a full laryngeal view (recall Figure 2b), which is no different from the views provided by the cameras used for laryngeal stroboscopy. This full laryngeal view is used as a basis for adequate laryngoscope insertion. Furthermore, the stroboscopic laryngeal view is identical to the laryngeal view obtained in high-speed laryngeal imaging; the only difference is the number of frames per second (fps) delivered by the video cameras (50–60 fps in stroboscopy versus 2000 fps or more in high-speed imaging). Therefore, there is no principal difference between stroboscopy and the other laryngoscopic methods (videokymography and high-speed videolaryngoscopy) concerning the insertion of the laryngoscope into the mouth. We were able to test the stroboscopy—videokymography differences only with the 90° laryngoscope; nevertheless, we find no logical reasons to assume that the results for the 70° laryngoscope should be different. Hence, we consider the insertion depths measured in stroboscopy to be representative also for videokymography and high-speed videoendoscopy, regardless of the type of rigid laryngoscope used. However, the fact that the stroboscopic device allowed us to use only the camera-integrated 90° laryngoscope and not the 70° laryngoscope is a limitation of this study.

4.4. Rules for Estimating the MTM Distance in Rigid Laryngoscopy

The empirical data on the insertion depth, D_I, can be used to estimate the MTM distance, d, for the laryngoscope-attached microphones. To obtain this distance, it is only necessary to know the horizontal and vertical placement of the microphone with respect to the tip of the laryngoscope (distances a and b, respectively, as indicated in Figures 1 and 3). We measured these distances by using calibrated photographs, but, in principle, they can also be measured directly, using a simple ruler. Once the a and b values are known, the empirical values of D_I listed in Table 3 can be used, and the MTM distance, d, can simply be determined using the Pythagorean theorem, according to the formula

$$d = \sqrt{(a - D_I)^2 + b^2}. \tag{2}$$

Figure 5a,b shows the average MTM distances, d, for the 70° and 90° rigid laryngoscopes in adults (males and females pooled together). These were obtained from Equation (2) for different microphone positions, as defined by the distances a and b from the tip of the laryngoscope. In clinical setups, the values of *a* can be expected to be in the range from ca. 15 cm (in the case when the microphone is attached directly or embedded in the laryngoscope with a short tube) up to ca. 40 cm (in cases of microphones fixed on camera heads attached to long-tubed laryngoscopes). Similarly, the values of *b* can be expected to be in the range from ca. 0.5 cm (in the case when the microphone is attached directly or embedded in the laryngoscope) up to ca. 10 cm (in cases when the microphone is fixed on the top of a bulky camera head). These microphone positions result in the final MTM distances, *d*, between 5 and 33 cm (Figure 5a,b). In 1992, Wendler recommended standardizing the MTM distance during laryngoscopy to 15 cm [9]. Our method allows us to find the specific values of *a* and *b* to obtain the average MTD distance of 15 cm; these values are indicated in Figure 5a,b by dots.

In principle, the distances *a* and *b* could be provided directly by the manufacturer. When not provided (the current state-of-the-art), the distances *a* and *b* can be measured with an uncertainty of 1 mm or smaller by an educated researcher or technician in the clinical institute, using, e.g., a simple ruler.

4.5. Uncertainty of the MTM Distance

Expressing the uncertainties of D_I, *a*, and *b* by the symbols $u(D_I)$, $u(a)$, and $u(b)$, according to International Organization for Standardization [21], we can determine that the overall uncertainty of the MTM distance, *d*, i.e., the possible difference of the true value from the value estimated by the Equation (2), is equal to

$$u(d) = \sqrt{\left(\frac{\partial d}{\partial D_I}\right)^2 u(D_I)^2 + \left(\frac{\partial d}{\partial a}\right)^2 u(a)^2 + \left(\frac{\partial d}{\partial b}\right)^2 u(b)^2}$$
$$= \sqrt{\frac{u(D_I)^2 + u(a)^2 + \left(\frac{b}{a-D_I}\right)^2 u(b)^2}{1 + \left(\frac{b}{a-D_I}\right)^2}}. \quad (3)$$

The scaling factor, $\left(\frac{b}{a-D_I}\right)^2$, in Equation (3) relates the perpendicular and longitudinal distances of the microphone from the mouth. In practice, this ratio is expected to be smaller than 1 in order to keep the vertical angle of the microphone from the mouth less than 45°. This gives less weight to the uncertainty $u(b)$ compared to $u(D_I)$ and $u(a)$ in the numerator of Equation (3). Furthermore, the measurement uncertainties of the microphone position on the endoscope, $u(a)$, the $u(b)$, which are expected to be up to ca. 1 mm, are about 7–9 times smaller than the uncertainty of the insertion depth, $u(D_I)$, resulting from the inter-subject variation (recall the 7–9 mm standard deviations of the insertion depth, Table 3). The overall uncertainty of the MTM distance, $u(d)$, is therefore predominantly determined by the variation in D_I within and among the examined subjects, and the combined uncertainties, $u(a)$ and $u(b)$, contribute to the overall uncertainty by less than ca. 2%. When neglecting the uncertainties $u(a)$ and $u(b)$, Equation (3) can be simplified to the following form:

$$u(d) = \frac{u(D_I)}{\sqrt{1 + \left(\frac{b}{a-D_I}\right)^2}}. \quad (4)$$

Notice that the factor $\left(\frac{b}{a-D_I}\right)^2$ could also be neglected when the vertical position, *b*, of the microphone is much smaller than the horizontal distance of the microphone from the mouth $(a - D_I)$. In that case, the uncertainty of the MTM distance, $u(d)$, becomes approximately equal to the uncertainty of the endoscope insertion depth, $u(D_I)$. This can also be noticed in Figure 5c,d, which depicts the results of Equation (3) graphically. For $b = 0$, the uncertainty, $u(d)$, equals 0.91/0.75 cm in the case of the 70°/90° laryngoscope regardless of the horizontal position of the microphone, *a*. These values are less than 2%

different from the standard deviations of the measured 70°/90° laryngoscope insertion depth, i.e., 0.90/0.74 cm (recall Table 3), as expected.

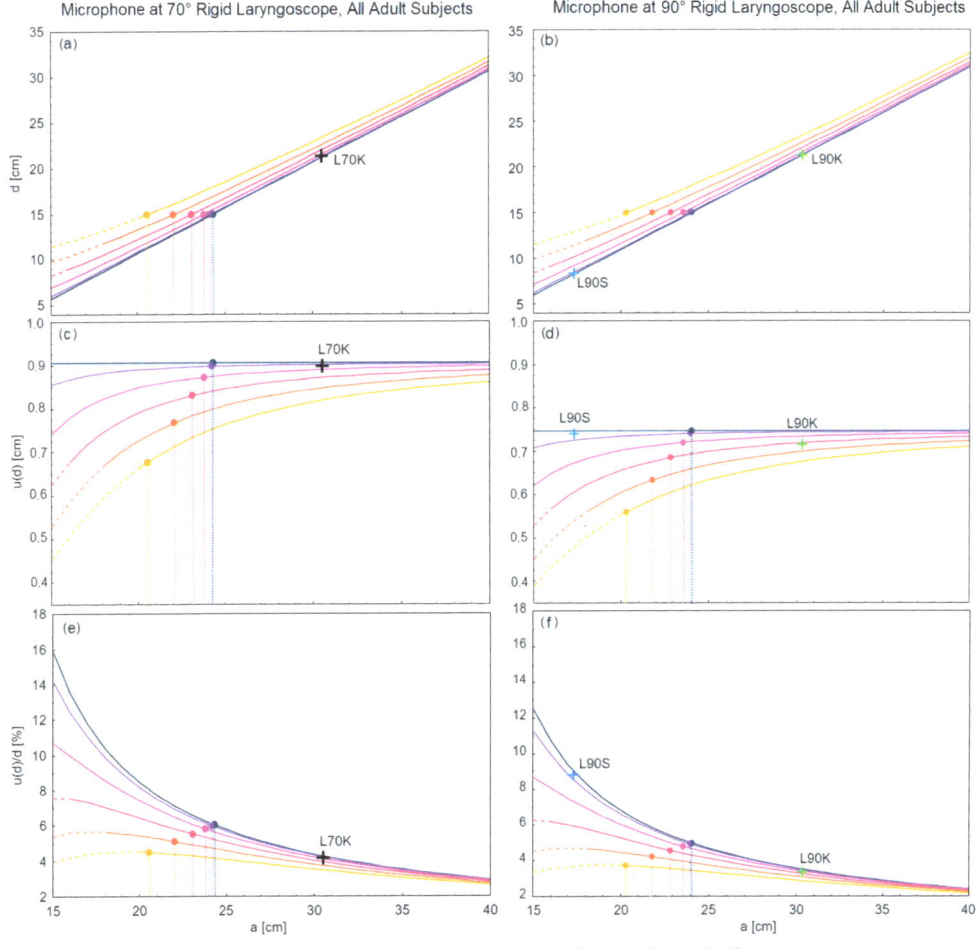

Figure 5. The average MTM distances, d, in adults (males and females pooled together) and their uncertainties $u(d)$ for different microphone positions with respect to the tip of the laryngoscope (distances a and b indicated in Figures 1 and 3). The results for the 70° laryngoscope are on the left (panels **a,c,e**) and for the 90° laryngoscope on the right (panels **b,d,f**). (**a,b**) MTM distance, d; (**c,d**) uncertainty of MTM distance, $u(d)$; and (**e,f**) relative MTM distance uncertainty, $u(d)/d$. Crosses indicate results for the specific locations of the microphones used in this study. Dots indicate the standard MTM distance of 15 cm recommended by Wendler [9] for different values of a and b. For the separate female and male results, see Figures A1 and A2 in the Appendix A.

Figure 5e,f show the relative uncertainty, $\frac{u(d)}{d}$, for the varying positions of the microphone with respect to the tip of the laryngoscope. We see that the relative uncertainty decreases with the increasing distance, a. For a given a, the largest relative uncertainty is found for the microphone vertically placed at the closest proximity to the laryngoscope tube ($b = 0$ cm). In this case, the relative uncertainty of the MTM distance ranges from ca. 16% at $a = 15$ cm down to ca. 2% at $a = 40$ cm.

4.6. MTM Distances for L70K, L90K, and L90S Laryngoscopes

Finally, Table 5 provides information on the resulting MTM distances, *d*, for the three laryngoscope-fixed microphones used in this study. Recall that, in the case of L90S, the microphone was embedded in the laryngoscope (Figure 3c), whereas, in the case of the L70K and L90K laryngoscopes, the microphone position was at the proximal top edge of the camera head (Figure 3a,b). These microphone placement differences cause substantial differences in the MTM distance during laryngoscopy (ca. 21–22 cm for L70K and L90K versus ca. 8–9 cm for L90S, as indicated in Table 5).

Table 5. Mouth-to-microphone distances (*d*) and their uncertainties for the three laryngoscope-fixed microphones utilized in this study. The results were obtained by Formulas (1) and (2), using the microphone position characteristics *a* and *b* listed in Table 2 and the corresponding D_I values listed in Table 3.

Type of Laryngoscope	*d* Adults (cm)	*d* Females (cm)	*d* Males (cm)
L70K	21.38 ± 0.89	21.77 ± 0.86	20.99 ± 0.89
L90K	21.28 ± 0.72	21.59 ± 0.68	20.96 ± 0.63
L90S	8.33 ± 0.74	8.71 ± 0.63	7.95 ± 0.65

4.7. Representativeness of the Sample Size in Relation to the Broader Population and Study Limitations

Our data are based on investigations of adult clients visiting the clinical outpatient center in Prague. Out of these, 119 self-reported to be White and 1 self-reported to be Hispanic. Previous studies found some differences in the volume of the oral and pharyngeal cavities among subjects of different ethnicities and races, but no significant differences were found in the lengths of these cavities [22,23]. Since the length dimensions are most relevant for our study, based on these findings, our results may be assumed representative for adults regardless of ethnicity and race. Nevertheless, more studies are welcome to verify this assumption further, as well as to verify our measurements with more laryngoscopes.

Our results are limited to adult subjects only. The laryngoscope insertion depth is expected to be smaller and age-dependent in children since the volume and length of the oral cavity increases with age during childhood [17–19]. More research is therefore needed to find a universal formula to determine the MTM distance in children. Nevertheless, rigid laryngeal endoscopy is less preferred to be used in children, often being replaced by flexible naso-laryngeal endoscopy [24].

Our study applies to rigid laryngeal endoscopes only; the results cannot simply be transferred to flexible naso-laryngeal endoscopes that are sometimes preferred over the rigid ones for laryngeal examination. In the flexible case, we recommend head-mounted or stand-mounted microphones to be used instead of endoscope-mounted microphones for capturing the sound of voice, so that the microphone position is not dependent on the depth of the insertion of the endoscope into the nasal and vocal tract. Recommendations on the positioning of these microphone types with respect to the mouth were provided in other studies [7,8].

5. Practical Recommendations and Conclusions

The laryngoscope insertion depths determined here allow clinicians to specify the MTM distance in adults, avoiding the need to specifically measure this distance on patients during laryngoscopic examinations. It is applicable for microphones attached either to rigid laryngoscopes or to camera heads mounted on the rigid laryngoscopes.

To specify the MTM distance using our method, one should take the following steps:

1. Measure the position of the microphone with respect to the tip of the rigid endoscope (the distances *a* and *b*; Figures 1 and 3);
2. Use the table value of the laryngoscope insertion depth, D_I (i.e., 9.7/9.4 cm for men, 8.9/8.7 cm for women, or 9.3/9.0 cm for all adults for 70°/90° endoscopes, respectively);

3. Calculate the typical MTM distance for that endoscope by using the Equation (2). These steps were used for specifying the MTM distances of the three microphones reported in Table 5 that can be considered typical case examples.

A single educated person or a technician could accomplish these tasks. It is recommended to mention the MTM distance when reporting the acoustic measurements of voice obtained during laryngoscopy. For instance, when the MTM distance was calculated to be 15 cm, and the SPL was found to be 80 dB(A), one could specify it as SPL@15 cm = 80 dB(A) [8].

One should be aware that the MTM distance obtained via this method is approximate; it will vary slightly among examined subjects. In our results, this is taken into account by specifying the distance uncertainty, calculated by using Equation (3). How much the MTM distance is expected to vary is specified in Figure 5c,d and in Figures A1c,d and A2c,d in the Appendix A. The largest standard uncertainty of the MTM distance determined using our method is 0.91/0.75 cm for 70°/90° endoscopes, respectively (recall Figure 5c,d). This results in the relative uncertainty of ca. 3%/2.5% for microphones placed at the distance a = 40 cm from the tip of the endoscope, and it increases up to ca. 16%/12.5% when the a distance is decreased to 15 cm, for 70°/90° endoscopes, respectively (recall Figure 5e,f). Such uncertainties, especially those for longer a distances, are deemed acceptable. Importantly, the method offers the possibility of determining the MTM distance and its uncertainty already by the manufacturers of laryngoscopes. To achieve the standard laryngoscopic MTM distance of 15 cm recommended by Wendler [9], one should position the microphone at the a and b distances between 25 and 20 cm and between 0 and 10 cm, respectively, from the tip of the rigid laryngoscope (recall Figure 5 for the specific values). Specifying and reporting the MTM distance is relevant for properly interpreting the recorded voice and is helpful for better reproducibility and repeatability of laryngeal exams.

Author Contributions: Conceptualization, J.G.Š.; methodology, D.V. and J.G.Š.; validation, J.G.Š.; formal analysis, D.V. and J.G.Š.; investigation, J.V. and D.V.; resources, J.G.Š. and J.V.; data curation, D.V.; writing—original draft preparation, D.V.; writing—review and editing, J.G.Š., D.V. and J.V.; supervision, J.G.Š.; project administration, J.G.Š. and J.V. All authors have read and agreed to the published version of the manuscript.

Funding: This research was funded by a grant from the Technology Agency of the Czech Republic, TH04010422 "VKG. 3.0" (Vydrová J. and Švec J.G.); a grant from the Palacký University in Olomouc, IGA_PrF_2021_017 (Švec J.G.); and a scholarship from the Palacký University in Olomouc, IGA_PrF_2023_023, IGA_PrF_2022_029, IGA_PrF_2021_017 (Valášková D.).

Institutional Review Board Statement: The study was conducted in accordance with the Declaration of Helsinki and approved by the Ethics Committee of the Voice and Hearing Centre Prague, Medical Healthcom, Ltd. (protocol code 1/2015; date of approval, 8 July 2015).

Informed Consent Statement: Written informed consent was obtained from the patient(s) to publish this paper.

Data Availability Statement: The data presented in this study are available upon request from the corresponding author.

Acknowledgments: We thank R. Domagalská from the Voice and Hearing Centre Prague for her help with organizational issues and to the participants who voluntarily decided to contribute to this research.

Conflicts of Interest: J. Vydrová J. and J. Švec have received a grant from the Technology Agency of the Czech Republic. J. Vydrová is the Head of the Voice and Hearing Centre Prague, Medical Healtcom, Ltd. J. Švec received a grant from the Palacký University in Olomouc, is the Head of the Voice Research Laboratory at Palacký University in Olomouc, serves as an associate research scientist at the Voice and Hearing Centre Prague, Medical Healtcom, Ltd. and is the inventor of the method of videokymography.

Appendix A. MTM Distances for Females and Males

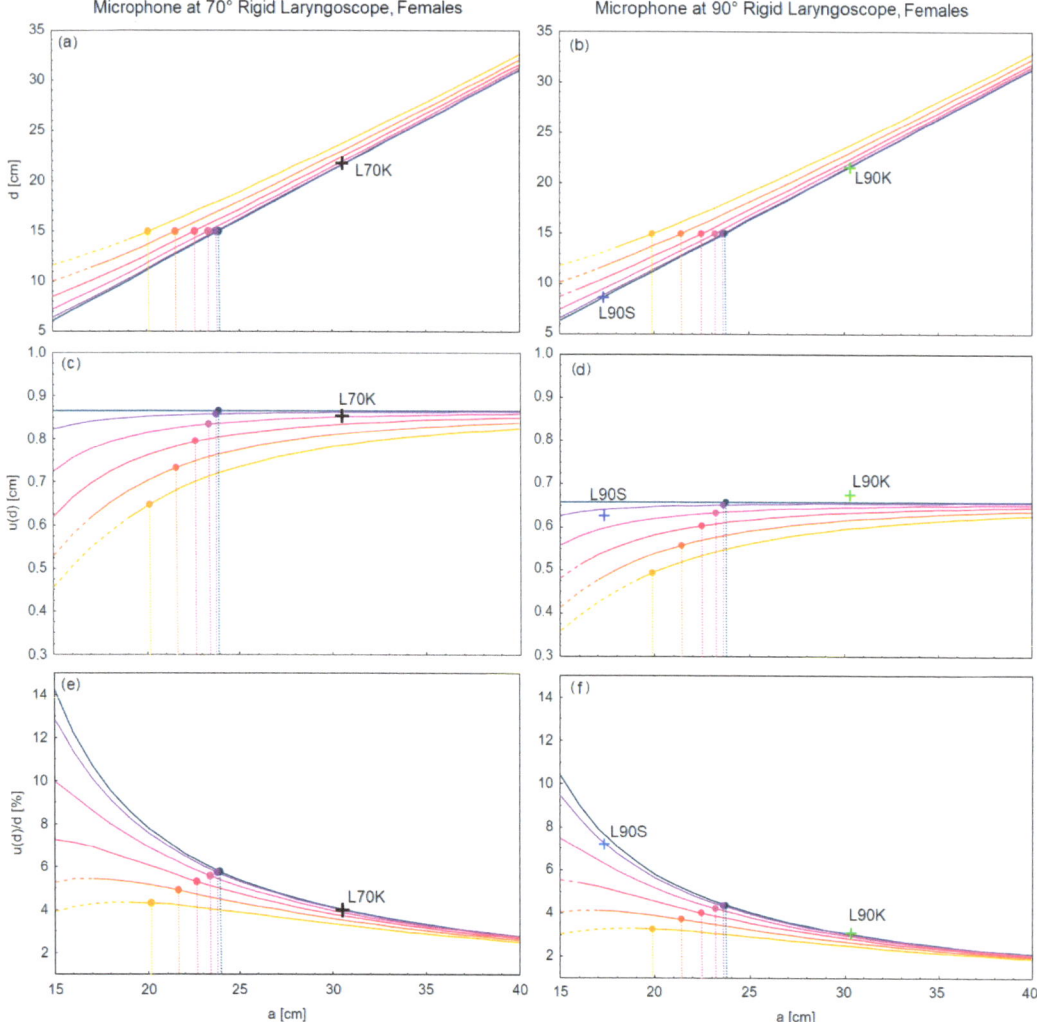

Figure A1. The average MTM distances, d, in females and their uncertainties $u(d)$ for different microphone positions with respect to the tip of the laryngoscope (distances a and b indicated in Figures 1 and 3). The results for the 70° laryngoscope are on the left (panels **a,c,e**) and for the 90° laryngoscope on the right (panels **b,d,f**). For the 90° laryngoscopes (**right** panels), the colored lines correspond to the pooled results from both the laryngoscopes, whereas the crosses indicate the results for the two laryngoscopes (L90K and L90S) separately. (**a,b**) MTM distance, d; (**c,d**) uncertainty of MTM distance, $u(d)$; and (**e,f**) relative MTM distance uncertainty, $u(d)/d$. Crosses indicate results for the specific locations of the microphones used in this study. Dots indicate the standard MTM distance of 15 cm recommended by Wendler [9] for different values of a and b.

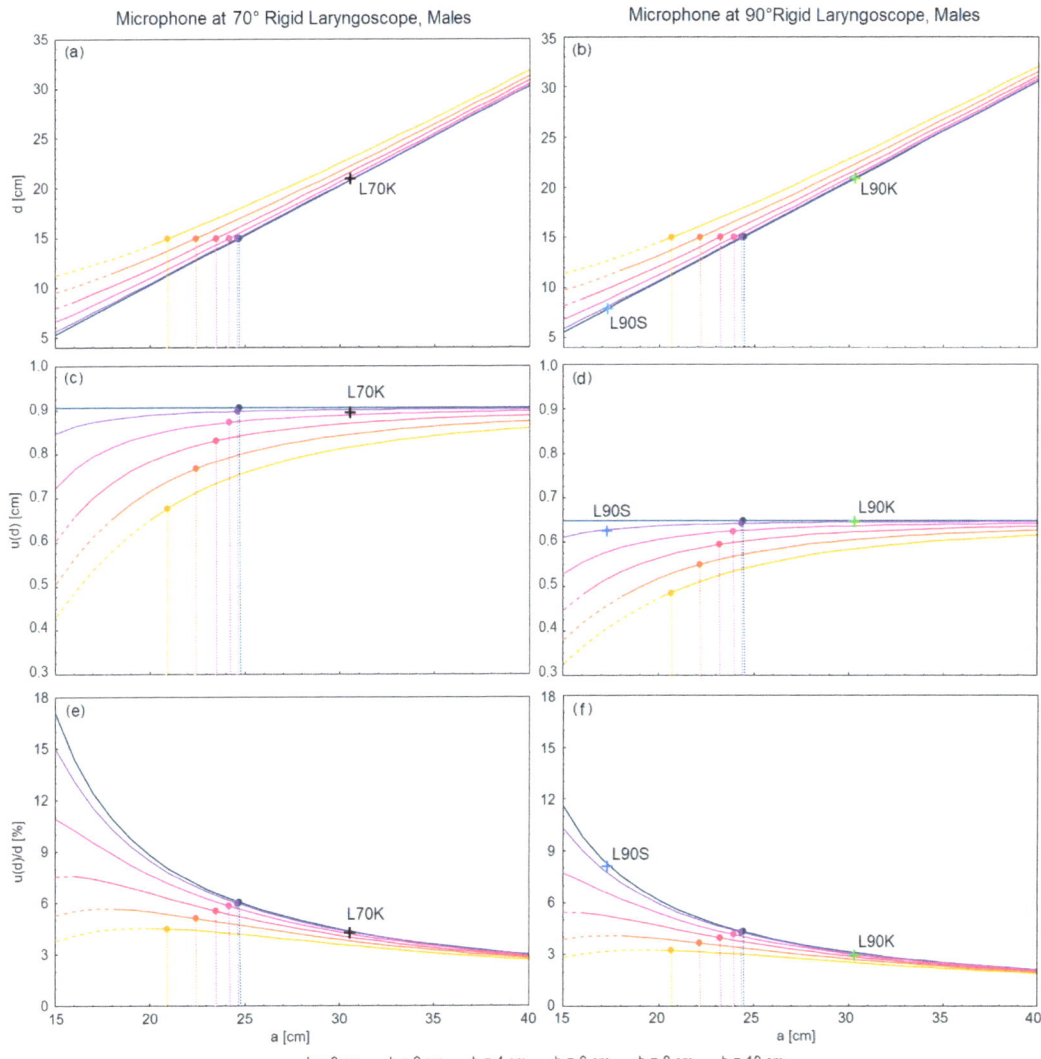

Figure A2. The average MTM distances, d, in males and their uncertainties $u(d)$ for different microphone positions with respect to the tip of the laryngoscope (distances a and b indicated in Figures 1 and 3). The results for the 70° laryngoscope are on the left (panels **a,c,e**) and for the 90° laryngoscope on the right (panels **b,d,f**). For the 90° laryngoscopes (**right** panels), the colored lines correspond to the pooled results from both laryngoscopes, whereas the crosses indicate the results for the two laryngoscopes (L90K and L90S) separately. (**a**,**b**) MTM distance, d; (**c**,**d**) uncertainty of MTM distance, $u(d)$; and (**e**,**f**) relative MTM distance uncertainty, $u(d)/d$. Crosses indicate results for the specific locations of the microphones used in this study. Dots indicate the standard MTM distance of 15 cm recommended by Wendler [9] for different values of a and b.

References

1. Angerstein, W.; Baracca, G.; Dejonckere, P.; Echternach, M.; Eysholdt, U.; Fussi, F.; Geneid, A.; Hacki, T.; Karmelita-Katulska, K.; Haubrich, R.; et al. Diagnosis and Differential Diagnosis of Voice Disorders. In *Phoniatrics I: Fundamentals–Voice Disorders–Disorders of Language and Hearing Development*; Zehnhoff-Dinnesen, A.A., Wiskirska-Woznica, B., Neumann, K., Nawka, T., Eds.; Springer: Berlin/Heidelberg, Germany, 2020; pp. 349–430.
2. Woo, P. Objective Measures of Laryngeal Imaging: What Have We Learned Since Dr. Paul Moore. *J. Voice* **2014**, *28*, 69–81. [CrossRef] [PubMed]
3. Bless, D.M.; Patel, R.R.; Connor, N. Laryngeal Imaging: Stroboscopy, High-Speed Digital Imaging, and Kymography. In *The Larynx*; Fried, M.P., Ferlito, A., Eds.; Plural Publishing: San Diego, CA, USA, 2009; pp. 181–210.
4. Švec, J.G.; Schutte, H.K. Kymographic Imaging of Laryngeal Vibrations. *Curr. Opin. Otolaryngol. Head Neck Surg.* **2012**, *20*, 458–465. [CrossRef] [PubMed]
5. Woo, P. Objective Measures of Stroboscopy and High-Speed Video. *Adv. Oto-Rhino-Laryngol.* **2020**, *85*, 25–44. [CrossRef]
6. Kumar, S.P.; Švec, J.G. A Simple Method to Obtain Basic Acoustic Measures from Video Recordings as Subtitles. *J. Speech Lang. Hear. Res.* **2018**, *61*, 2196–2204. [CrossRef] [PubMed]
7. Patel, R.R.; Awan, S.N.; Barkmeier-Kraemer, J.; Courey, M.; Deliyski, D.; Eadie, T.; Paul, D.; Švec, J.G.; Hillman, R. Recommended Protocols for Instrumental Assessment of Voice: American Speech-Language-Hearing Association Expert Panel to Develop a Protocol for Instrumental Assessment of Vocal Function. *Am. J. Speech Lang. Pathol.* **2018**, *27*, 887–905. [CrossRef] [PubMed]
8. Švec, J.G.; Granqvist, S. Tutorial and Guidelines on Measurement of Sound Pressure Level in Voice and Speech. *J. Speech Lang. Hear. Res.* **2018**, *61*, 441–461. [CrossRef] [PubMed]
9. Wendler, J. Stroboscopy. *J. Voice* **1992**, *6*, 149–154. [CrossRef]
10. Shao, J.; Stern, J.; Wang, Z.-M.; Hanson, D.; Jiang, J. Clinical Evaluation of 70° and 90° Laryngeal Telescopes. *Arch. Otolaryngol. Neck Surg.* **2002**, *128*, 941. [CrossRef] [PubMed]
11. Junaid, M.; Roohullah, M.; Uddin, I.; Hussain, A.; Khan, M.A. Comparative Evaluation of 70° And 90° Rigid Endoscope In Successful Visualization of The Hidden Areas of Larynx. *J. Med. Sci.* **2021**, *29*, 243–246. [CrossRef]
12. Holm, S. A Simple Sequentially Rejective Multiple Test Prodecure. *Scand. J. Stat.* **1979**, *6*, 65–70.
13. Valášková, D. Variability of Distance of a Laryngoscope-Attached Microphone from the Mouth in Laryngoscopic Examinations. Bachelor's Thesis, Palacký University, Olomouc, Czechia, 2018.
14. Valášková, D. Depth of Laryngoscope Insertion in the Mouth during Laryngoscopic Examinations: Implications for Measurements of Sound Pressure Level by a Microphone Attached to the Laryngoscope. Master's Thesis, Palacký University, Olomouc, Czechia, 2020.
15. Fitch, W.T.; Giedd, J. Morphology and Development of the Human Vocal Tract: A Study Using Magnetic Resonance Imaging. *J. Acoust. Soc. Am.* **1999**, *106*, 1511–1522. [CrossRef] [PubMed]
16. Barbier, G.; Boë, L.-J.; Captier, G.; Laboissière, R. Human Vocal Tract Growth: A Longitudinal Study of the Development of Various Anatomical Structures. In Proceedings of the Interspeech 2015-16th Annual Conference of the International Speech Communication Association, Dresden, Germany, 10 September 2015; pp. 364–368.
17. Vorperian, H.K.; Wang, S.; Michael Schimek, E.; Durtschi, R.B.; Kent, R.D.; Gentry, L.R.; Chung, M.K. Developmental Sexual Dimorphism of the Oral and Pharyngeal Portions of the Vocal Tract: An Imaging Study. *J. Speech Lang. Hear. Res.* **2011**, *54*, 995–1010. [CrossRef] [PubMed]
18. Vorperian, H.K.; Wang, S.; Chung, M.K.; Schimek, E.M.; Durtschi, R.B.; Kent, R.D.; Ziegert, A.J.; Gentry, L.R. Anatomic Development of the Oral and Pharyngeal Portions of the Vocal Tract: An Imaging Study. *J. Acoust. Soc. Am.* **2009**, *125*, 1666–1678. [CrossRef] [PubMed]
19. Vorperian, H.K.; Schimek, E.M.; Wang, S.; Chung, M.K.; Kent, R.D.; Ziegert, A.J.; Gentry, L.R. Anatomic Development of the Vocal Tract during the First Two Decades of Life: Evidence on Prepubertal Sexual Dimorphism from MRI and CT Studies. *J. Acoust. Soc. Am.* **2007**, *122*, 3031. [CrossRef]
20. Goldstein, U.G. An Articulatory Model for the Vocal Tracts of Growing Children. Doctoral Dissertation, Massachusetts Institue of Technology, Cambridge, MA, USA, 1980.
21. *ISO/IEC Guide 98:1993*; Guide to the Expression of Uncertainty in Measurement (GUM). International Organization for Standardization: Geneva, Switzerland, 1993.
22. Xue, S.A.; Hao, G.J.P.; Mayo, R. Volumetric Measurements of Vocal Tracts for Male Speakers from Different Races. *Clin. Linguist. Phon.* **2006**, *20*, 691–702. [CrossRef] [PubMed]
23. Xue, S.A.; Hao, J.G. Normative Standards for Vocal Tract Dimensions by Race as Measured by Acoustic Pharyngometry. *J. Voice* **2006**, *20*, 391–400. [CrossRef] [PubMed]
24. Wolf, M.; Primov-Fever, A.; Amir, O.; Jedwab, D. The Feasibility of Rigid Stroboscopy in Children. *Int. J. Pediatr. Otorhinolaryngol.* **2005**, *69*, 1077–1079. [CrossRef] [PubMed]

Disclaimer/Publisher's Note: The statements, opinions and data contained in all publications are solely those of the individual author(s) and contributor(s) and not of MDPI and/or the editor(s). MDPI and/or the editor(s) disclaim responsibility for any injury to people or property resulting from any ideas, methods, instructions or products referred to in the content.

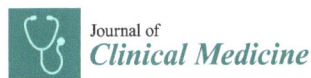

Systematic Review

"Do You Hear What I Hear?" Speech and Voice Alterations in Hearing Loss: A Systematic Review

Arianna Di Stadio [1,*], Jake Sossamon [2,†], Pietro De Luca [3,†], Iole Indovina [4,5], Giovanni Motta [1], Massimo Ralli [6], Michael J. Brenner [7,*], Elliot M. Frohman [8] and Gordon T. Plant [9]

1. Otolaryngology Department, Vanvitelli University, 80138 Naples, Italy; giovannimotta95@yahoo.it
2. Medical University of South Carolina, Charleston, SC 29425, USA; sossamon@musc.edu
3. Department of Otolaryngology, Fatebenefratelli-Isola Hospital, 00186 Rome, Italy; dr.dlp@hotmail.it
4. Department of Systems Medicine, Centre for Space BioMedicine, University of Rome Tor Vergata, 00133 Rome, Italy; i.indovina@hsantalucia.it
5. Laboratory of Neuromotor Physiology, IRCCS Foundation Santa Lucia, 00179 Rome, Italy
6. International Medical University UNICAMILLUS, 00131 Rome, Italy; massimo.ralli@unicamillus.org
7. Department of Otolaryngology—Head and Neck Surgery, University of Michigan Medical School, Ann Arbor, MI 48109, USA
8. Neuroimmunology Laboratory of Professor Lawrence Steinman, Stanford University School of Medicine, Palo Alto, CA 94305, USA; elliotfrohman123@gmail.com
9. Department of Brain Repair and Neurorehabilitation, University College London, London WC1E 6BT, UK; g.plant@ucl.ac.uk
* Correspondence: ariannadistadio@hotmail.com or arianna.distadio@unicampania.it (A.D.S.); mbren@med.umich.edu (M.J.B.)
† These authors contributed equally to this work.

Abstract: Background: Although hearing loss influences voice characteristics, such changes may be under-recognized during clinical consultations. This systematic review examines voice alterations in adults with post-lingual hearing loss, considering diagnostic and rehabilitative implications. **Methods**: A comprehensive search of PubMed, Scopus, and Google Scholar was conducted following PRISMA guidelines, targeting studies reporting quantitative data on vocal parameters in adults with sensorineural hearing loss. Exclusion criteria included pre-lingual hearing loss and non-English studies. Data extraction focused on pitch, loudness, and prosody, with study quality assessed using NIH tools. **Results**: Eleven case–control studies, involving 594 patients with sensorineural hearing loss and 326 control patients, were analyzed. Patients with untreated hearing loss exhibited elevated fundamental frequency, F_0 (males: 158–169 Hz; females: 206–251 Hz) and loudness levels (males: 79–96 dB; females: 89–116 dB) compared to controls (F_0—males: 75–150 Hz; females: 150–300 Hz; loudness—males: 30–70 dB; females: 40–68 dB). Alterations in jitter, shimmer, and maximum phonation time (MPT) contributed to the distinct "hearing loss voice". Cochlear implants (CIs) and hearing aids improved vocal parameters, with CIs reducing F_0 by approximately 12–15 Hz. Continuous hearing aid use normalized pitch and loudness within four months. Prosody alterations, such as monotone speech, were reported in long-term cases. In noisy environments, individuals with hearing loss exhibited exaggerated increases in pitch and loudness, indicative of compensatory mechanisms. **Conclusions**: Post-lingual hearing loss disrupts the central regulation of voice, altering pitch, loudness, and other vocal parameters. Recognizing these changes, particularly in noisy environments, could facilitate the early diagnosis and timely rehabilitation of hearing deficits, potentially mitigating associated risks of cognitive decline.

Keywords: hearing loss; pitch; loudness; cochlear implant; auditory rehabilitation; voice modulation; compensatory mechanisms; age-related hearing loss; presbycusis

1. Introduction

Hearing loss is a pervasive but often underdiagnosed condition with significant consequences. Untreated hearing loss has been strongly associated with cognitive decline, dementia, and social isolation, making early detection and intervention critical. Despite its deleterious effects on quality of life and long-term health, hearing loss frequently remains unrecognized in clinical practice, in part due to the subtlety and variability of its early manifestations [1]. One underexplored avenue for early identification is through the analysis of voice and speech characteristics, which are known to change with hearing loss. These changes often go unnoticed during routine clinical consultations. Many neurological conditions manifest with voice or speech-related symptoms, such as dysarthria and dysphonia, which can complicate diagnosis and interpretation [2–4]. Paying close attention to voice characteristics, particularly in individuals with severe bilateral hearing loss (HL), can provide diagnostic clues about underlying auditory deficits [5]. Both the severity and duration of hearing loss have been shown to influence voice quality [6].

While it is well-recognized that hearing loss can alter voice, the characteristics of these changes in patients with post-lingual, acquired hearing loss remain poorly understood. Existing research highlights the influence of the severity and duration of hearing loss on voice quality, yet a systematic understanding of these relationships has not been established [6]. This gap in knowledge limits the ability of clinicians to leverage vocal changes as diagnostic clues for hearing loss, particularly in patients with severe bilateral hearing loss. Each human has distinct pitch, volume, and timbre that have potential to be altered in hearing loss [7]. The human ear easily detects changes in these parameters when the listener is paying attention to alterations. The pitch is a function of the fundamental frequency (F_0) that is generated by vocal cord (VC) vibrations. Pitch is measured in Hertz (Hz), with high tones corresponding to high-frequency VC vibrations and low tones to low-frequency VC vibrations. Loudness, measured in decibel (dB), is the measure of voice volume and can vary depending on the context of communication and emotional states [8,9]. Timbre, which is shaped by the resonance structures above the larynx, arises from harmonic frequencies (F1 and F2) that are multiples of F_0. Timbre contributes to the voice's tonal quality [8]. Speech prosody refers to the rhythm and intonation patterns of speech; it allows speakers to convey meaning and emotional nuance, helping listeners distinguish between questions, statements, and subtler psychological cues [10].

While clinicians cannot directly perceive a patient's subjective hearing loss, they can readily discern altered vocal characteristics. These signs of hearing loss, easily observable during clinical consultations, create an opportunity for clinicians to identify auditory deficits early. Recognizing and quantifying these changes could not only enhance detection but also facilitate timely rehabilitation, potentially mitigating the associated risks of cognitive decline and social isolation [1]. In this systematic review, we aim to address this gap by identifying changes in pitch and loudness among patients with post-lingual acquired hearing loss. Such insights can advance our understanding of how hearing loss alters vocal characteristics and promote early detection and intervention for hearing loss.

2. Materials and Methods

This study was conducted in accordance with the Preferred Reporting Items for Systematic Reviews and Meta-Analyses (PRISMA) guidelines (Figure 1). Ethical approval from the Institutional Review Board was not required for this systematic review.

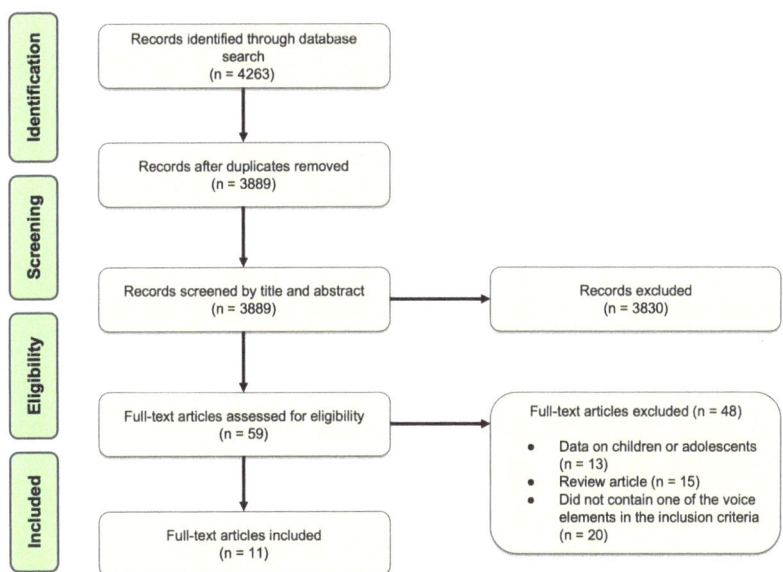

Figure 1. PRISMA Flow chart illustrating the process of our systematic review.

2.1. Search Strategy

Two researchers (JS and PDL), under the supervision of ADS, performed a comprehensive literature search on PubMed, Scopus, and Google Scholar without geographical or time restrictions. The search incorporated a combination of MeSH terms and free-text keywords, such as "Voice and Hearing Loss", "Speech and Hearing Loss", "Speech and Deafness", "Voice and Deafness", "Hearing Loss and Vocal Characteristics", "Communication and Hearing Loss", and "Voice Characteristics and Hearing Loss". Boolean operators (AND, OR) were applied strategically to refine the searches, ensuring sensitivity and specificity.

Abstracts of all extracted articles were independently screened, and duplicate entries were identified and systematically removed using reference management software. Articles were then cross-checked for consistency, and disagreements on the inclusion or exclusion of studies were resolved through structured discussions and iterative consensus meetings involving all three researchers (JS, PDL, and ADS). To ensure methodological transparency and reproducibility, the systematic review adhered strictly to the PRISMA guidelines, with a PRISMA flow diagram developed to track the selection process. Reference lists of included studies were manually reviewed to identify additional relevant articles that may have been overlooked in the database searches.

2.2. Study Selection Criteria

The inclusion and exclusion criteria were pre-specified to ensure a rigorous selection process. Pre-lingual cases were excluded to avoid confounding effects from developmental factors, such as delayed auditory or speech rehabilitation, which can result in persistent voice alterations unrelated to the acquired loss of hearing.

Inclusion Criteria:
- Studies providing quantitative data on at least one of the following parameters: fundamental frequency (F_0)/pitch, loudness, or prosody in patients with sensorineural hearing loss.
- Studies published in peer-reviewed journals.
- Studies involving adult patients with post-lingual sensorineural hearing loss.

- Articles published in English.

Exclusion Criteria:
- Studies involving children or adolescents under 18 years old.
- Studies focusing exclusively on pre-lingual hearing loss.
- Studies lacking data on the specified vocal parameters (F_0/pitch, loudness, or prosody).
- Non-peer-reviewed articles, conference abstracts, or opinion pieces.

2.3. Data Extraction

Data extraction was independently performed by two researchers (ADS and PDL) to ensure accuracy and minimize bias. A structured data extraction form was developed and piloted before use. The following key information was systematically recorded for each study: author name, year of publication, study design, country of origin, sample size, patient demographics, hearing loss characteristics, specific vocal and speech parameters assessed (including pitch, loudness, or prosody), and any additional outcomes related to voice or communication characteristics. To maintain data integrity, all extracted information was cross-verified by the supervising investigator (ADS) in biweekly review sessions. Any discrepancies identified during data extraction were resolved through discussion or, if necessary, consultation with an external expert in systematic reviews.

The extracted data were organized in a detailed spreadsheet for quantitative synthesis and qualitative analysis. This approach facilitated the identification of trends, gaps, and potential sources of bias across the included studies.

2.4. Risk of Bias Assessment

The National Institutes of Health (NIH) quality assessment tools for case–control studies were used to assess the risk of bias, as these checklists are designed for various study designs (National Heart, Lung, and Blood Institute. Study Quality Assessment Tools. (2014). Available at: https://www.nhlbi.nih.gov/health-topics/study-quality-assessment-tools, accessed on 14 November 2024). Studies were categorized as poor, fair, or good based on their quality, with special consideration given to phonological analyses. Incomplete phonological data were considered a source of bias, and studies were rated fair even if they were unbiased and fully described. Two authors (ADS and PDL) independently scored each article, and disagreements were resolved by consensus. The results are summarized in Table 1.

Table 1. Results of the quality assessment performed on the included papers.

References	Design of the Study	Overall Quality Rating Consensus
Higgins [11]	Prospective case–control	Good
Weatherley et al. [12]	Prospective case–control	Fair
Lee [13]	Prospective case–control	Fair
Ubrig et al. [14]	Prospective case–control	Good
Akil et al. [6]	Prospective case–control	Fair
Hengen et al. [15]	Prospective case–control	Good
Zamani et al. [16]	Prospective case–control	Fair
Aria-Vergara et al. [17]	Prospective case–control	Good
Albera et al. [18]	Prospective case–control	Fair
Cardella et al. [19]	Prospective study	Fair
Mora et al. [4]	Prospective case–control	Good

3. Results

A total of 11 articles were included in this study (Figure 1) [5,6,11–19]. The studies included 594 patients with sensorineural hearing loss who were compared with 326 control subjects without hearing loss (Figure 2). Four articles (36.4%) specifically stated that the studies were conducted on individuals with post-lingual auditory deficits. In the remaining cases (63.6%), the patients were adults with sensorineural hearing loss. The cause of sensorineural hearing loss was not defined in any of the studies.

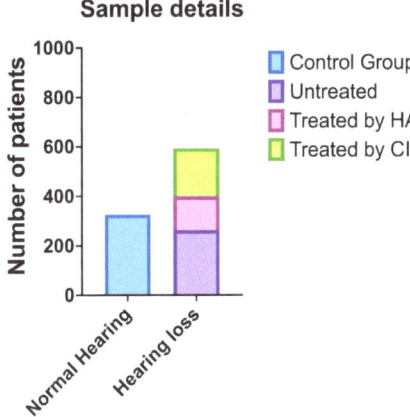

Figure 2. The graph shows the sample distribution between control (normal hearing) and patients with hearing loss. The latter are represented with different colors based on the treatment used/not used (HA = hearing aid; CI = cochlear implant).

All included studies were prospective observational case–control studies. Three were conducted in Italy (27.7%), while the others were conducted in the United States, Australia, Taiwan, Brazil, Iran, Turkey, Sweden, and Germany (Table 2).

In five studies (45.4%), voice characteristics were analyzed only at baseline without the use of hearing aids. Four studies (36.3%) examined the voice at baseline and after cochlear implant rehabilitation, and two studies (18.3%) assessed the voice at baseline and after using hearing aids (Table 2 and Figure 2).

In one article (9%), data on pitch, loudness, and prosody were available. Three papers (27%) reported both pitch and loudness, while the remaining seven articles (64%) provided data only on pitch (Table 2).

We summarized the results of the quality assessment performed on the studies included in this systematic review in Table 2. Five studies (45.5%) received quality rating consensus of good quality, while the remaining six (54.5%) received a rating of fair.

F_0 was consistently increased in the presence of hearing loss; however, the use of hearing aids (cochlear implant or traditional hearing prosthesis) allowed for a reduction in F_0. The voice loudness of people with hearing loss also increased when compared to loudness in individuals with normal hearing (data reported in four studies only). Prosody, reported in only one study, was reduced in patients with hearing loss when compared to individuals with normal hearing.

Table 2. The table shows the articles included in the systematic review and the voice findings that were available to be analyzed.

Author, Year, Country	Study Type	Sample Size	Sample Characteristic (Age and Sex)	Affected	Control *	Treatment (Yes/No, Type of Hearing Treatment)	Voice Characteristic			Method of Voice Analysis
							Pitch/F_0 (Hz)	Loudness (dB)	Prosody (rhythm)	
Higgins, 1994, United States [11]	POCCS	11	4 M, 7 F; mean age 42 yr	11	5	None		Females, 223.8 ± 53.2; Males, 158.5 ± 22.6		APM
Weatherley et al., 1997, Australia [12]	POCCS	40	gender n/a; mean age 74.5 yr	40	21	None	Females /a/ 189.68 Females /i/ 211.72 Females /u/ 205.78 Males /a/ 127.46 Males /i/ 135.25 Males /u/ 135.02	Maximum loudness level 96.44		APM
Lee, 2012, Taiwan [13]	POCCS	23	17 M, 6 F; mean age 66 yr	23	14	None	vF_0% 2.71 ± 2.37	79.0 ± 7.7 SNHL vs. 83.9 ± 7.8 control		APM
Ubrig et al., 2010, Brazil [14]	POCCS	40 postlingual	20 M, 20 F; mean age 44.5 yr	40	12	CI	Male pre-CI, 154.2 ± 54.52; Male post-CI, 148.1 ± 58.18; Female pre-CI, 206.1 ± 43.01; Female post-CI, 199.9 ± 39.26			APM
Akil et al., 2017, Turkey [6]	POCCS	50	24 M, 26 F;	50	20	None	141 ± 24			APM
Hengen et al., 2018, Sweden [15]	POCCS	110 non-HA users + 110 HA users	non-HA users, 70 M, 40 F; mean age 70 yr/HA users, 59 M, 51F; mean age 74 yr	220	70	HA + none	Male non-HA users, 142.1 ± 28.2 Male HA users, 140.6 ± 31.8 Female non-HA users, 193.8 ± 29.1 Female HA users, 188.9 ± 26.5			APM
Zamani et al., 2021, Iran [16]	POCCS	48 post-lingual	17 M, 31 F; mean age 36.5 yr	48	50	CI	1st-on 166.2 ± 26.1 Off 169.2 ± 28.4 2nd on 166.1 ± 27.9			APM

Table 2. *Cont.*

Author, Year, Country	Study Type	Sample Size	Sample Characteristic (Age and Sex)	Affected	Control *	Treatment (Yes/No, Type of Hearing Treatment)	Voice Characteristic			Method of Voice Analysis
Aria-Vergara et al., 2022, Germany [17]	POCCS	74 post-lingual	37 M, 27 F: mean age 66 yr	74	72	CI	134 ± 26	Mean SPL 69 / Mean Std SPL 15	Mean Std Voc (ms) 96 / Mean Std Con (ms) 79	APM
Albera et al., 2022, Italy [18]	POCCS	32, 16 prelingual/16 postlingual	16 M, 16 F; mean age 49.7 yr	32	32	CI	Male, CI off 156.5 ± 40 / Male, CI on 150.8 ± 42 / Female, CI off 251.2 ± 54 / Female, CI on 218.4 ± 52	CI off 82.5 ± 11 dB / CI on 80.9 ± 13 dB		APM
Cardella, 2023, Italy [19]	POCCS	26	18 M, 8 F; mean age 71 yr	26	0	HA	Males before HA 130.1 ± 10.9 / Males after HA 132.8 ± 8.8 / Female before HA 212.4 ± 20.1 / Female after HA 197.1 ± 21.1			APM
Mora et al., 2012 [5]	POCCS	30 with HL; 30 healthy	60 M; 30 HL (35–53) and 30 control (38–51)	30	30	None	Male affected 137 vs. 120 Control			MDVP

POCCS: prospective observational case–control study; CI: cochlear implant; HA: hearing aids; APM: ambulatory phonation monitor; MDVP: Multimensional Voice Program; HZ: hertz; dB: decibel; Std: standard deviation. *: including untreated patients in case of treatment vs. untreated patient studies.

4. Discussion

The results of this systematic review reveal that patients with moderate to severe hearing loss exhibit higher pitch (F_0) and louder volume compared to gender-matched controls. Furthermore, the extent of change correlated with the severity of sensory auditory loss. In addition, other vocal parameters, such as jitter, shimmer, soft phonation index, and maximum phonation time, were also altered in individuals with hearing loss. Together, these findings define a distinct "hearing loss voice". These parameters can be detected during speaking; jitter and shimmer are perceived as roughness, breathiness, or hoarseness in a patient's voice. Soft phonation index and time are also perceived as slight roughness and reduced time of phonation (<10 s).

4.1. Methodological Variations and Its Implications

The studies had heterogeneity in the reporting of hearing impairment, the vocal parameters studied, and the methodologies used to assess them. In 83.3% of the studies (Table 2), researchers employed ambulatory phonation monitors, whereas the remaining researchers used the Multidimensional Voice Program (MDVP) [20]. MDVP is a software tool that analyzes several vocal characteristics beyond F_0, including jitter, shimmer, noise-to-harmonic ratio (NHR), soft phonation index (SPI), degree of voice break (DVB), degree of voicelessness (DUV), and peak amplitude variation (vAm) (Table 3).

Table 3. The definition of the relevant voice characteristics that are analyzed by MDVP.

Jitter	Measures cycle-to-cycle frequency variations, where cycle means opening and closure of vocal folds
Shimmer	Measures amplitude of sound wave variation
Soft phonation index	Measures approximation of vocal folds. High values correlate with incomplete vocal fold adduction
Maximum phonation time	The maximum amount of time a person can sustain phonation of "ah" is timed (typical range of 15 to 25 s in women and 25 to 35 s in men

While MDVP provides a more comprehensive analysis of voice characteristics, allowing researchers to define a clearer "hearing loss voice", its use is limited in clinical settings. Additionally, MDVP assessments are typically performed for a brief period, not capturing the patient's voice in everyday conditions. In contrast, ambulatory phonation monitors [21] are simpler to use. When used as portable devices [22], they have the advantage of being wearable throughout the day, enabling voice analysis in real-life contexts. However, these devices are more limited in the range of vocal characteristics they can assess compared to MDVP (Figure 3).

Mora et al. [5] used MDVP to compare the voices of people with hearing loss to those of healthy individuals. They found that, in addition to a rise in fundamental frequency (137.2 Hz vs. 120.0 Hz), there were significant differences in jitter (1.93% vs. 0.67%), shimmer (6.67% vs. 3.81%), NHR (0.19 vs. 0.10), SPI (12.9 vs. 8.76), DVB (2.12% vs. 0.01%), DUV (9.53% vs. 0.51%), and vAm (23.12% vs. 12.06%). All these parameters tended to worsen as the degree of hearing loss increased.

Akil et al. [6] compared adults with normal auditory thresholds to those with mild-to-moderate bilateral sensorineural hearing loss (average: 25–60 dB) and moderate-to-profound sensorineural hearing loss (average: 60–90 dB). This study analyzed males and females separately and found significant differences in F_0, variable F_0 (vF_0), absolute jitter, shimmer, SPI, and maximum phonation time (MPT) between healthy individuals and those with hearing loss. Men with hearing deficits exhibited the most significant changes in the vocal parameters studied. Individuals with mild-to-moderate hearing loss tended to become higher-pitched (acute F_0) and louder. People with hearing loss exhibit escalated voice volume, with roughness, breathiness, or hoarseness of the voice. They also present a reduced time of phonation that is generally under 10 s that is punctuated by the need to stop and breathe before the resumption of speech.

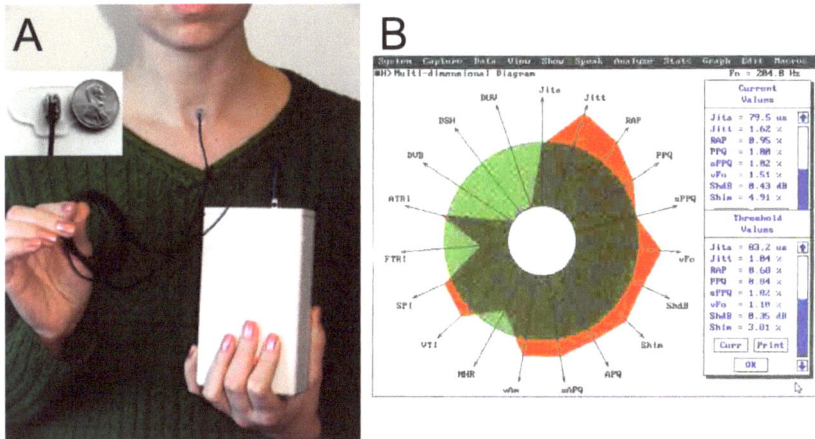

Figure 3. (**A**) The image shows the portable device to analyze the voice characteristics used in some of the studies included in the review. (**B**) The graph shows how the results of MDPV visually appear to the operator during the analysis of voice.

4.2. Association of Interventions with Voice Characteristics

Studies of patients with hearing loss who were treated with cochlear implants (CIs) demonstrated improvements in F_0 (reduced) and loudness (reduced) when the device was activated, compared to when it was switched off [18]. CI have a receiver and an electrode that through electronic stimulation within the cochlea facilitates listening and the accuracy of sound interpretation. The stimulation of the auditory cortex and laryngeal motor cortex [23] allows for effective and accurate sequential timing pattern commands to the larynx and vocal cords. In patients treated by CI, the voice exhibited can be indistinguishable from normal [18].

In patients with age-related moderate-to-severe hearing loss, using hearing aids continuously for at least four months resulted in reductions in both pitch and loudness, indicating that voice parameters can return to normal with proper prosthetic use [19]. The central control of vocal pitch and volume is complex and heavily influenced by auditory function, highlighting the interdependence of sensory input and motor output within and across sensory channels. This process involves interactions between diverse sensory modalities, culminating in sensory–motor integration. Beyond hearing and listening, such integration shapes our overall sensory experience and can give rise to synesthesia through the higher-order merging of information from distinct but interconnected sensory inputs.

4.3. Neurological Mechanisms Underlying Vocal Adjustments

Dichter et al. used high-density cortical recordings from the human brain to investigate the encoding of vocal pitch during natural speech [23]. They found that neural populations in the bilateral dorsal laryngeal motor cortex (dLMC) selectively encoded produced pitch but not non-laryngeal articulatory movements. The dLMC controlled short pitch accents to express prosodic emphasis on words within sentences [23]. Speaking and listening require sensorimotor integration. The impulse to speak is initiated first, followed by listening, with pitch adjustments occurring during conversation. In individuals with hearing impairment, reduced auditory input likely disrupts this balance, contributing to an increase in pitch [24] (Figure 4).

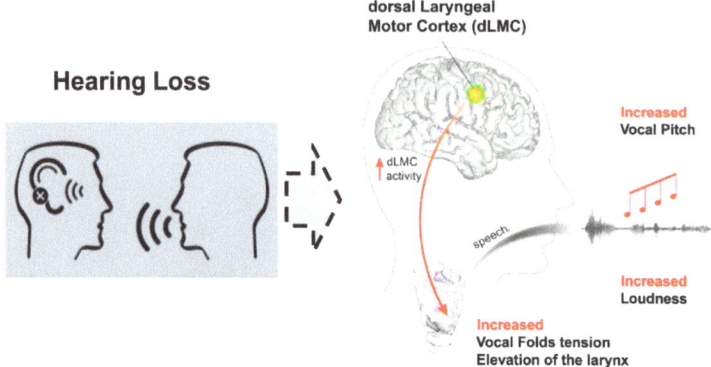

Figure 4. The drawing summarizes the mechanism that causes the increase in loudness and pitch in patients with hearing loss. We use the term "hearing loss voice" to summarize a high-pitch and high-volume voice. The image was modified from the original [23].

4.4. Clinical Relevance and Role for Early Intervention

Patients with hearing loss tend to speak with a louder voice and exhibit escalated high-pitch intonation (high F_0/pitch). In noisy environments, both parameters increase further [13]. These changes can be tested during clinical consultations by introducing noise (such as crumpling paper or tapping a pen on a desk) while asking questions to observe if the patient raises the volume and/or pitch in response. Generally, people without hearing deficits tend to maintain the same volume, whereas people with hearing loss rapidly transition to augmented speech volume and pitch.

In addition, due to the diminished ability of the auditory system to detect sound frequency distributions over time in hearing loss [25], patients with longstanding hearing loss may lose prosody [26] and develop a monotone voice. Therefore, earlier identification and treatment of hearing loss can produce disease modifying effects. While the diminished capacity of the auditory system to detect and effectively parse sound frequencies can result in the loss of prosody (i.e., the melodic aspects of speech) and a monotone voice, auditory rehabilitation could potentially prevent, delay, or even partly reverse these changes.

4.5. Limitations and Future Directions

This review has limitations relating to the limited evidence base and limited standardization of data reporting. All included studies were either case–control or observational studies. Randomized clinical trials evaluating the effect of hearing interventions on voice characteristics in individuals with hearing impairment would clarify causality and potential effects on cognitive performance.

Future research should prioritize longitudinal studies to better understand the progression of vocal changes in hearing loss and the potential for recovery with timely intervention. Innovative tools, such as machine learning algorithms and wearable technologies, could be developed to identify subtle vocal changes as early markers of auditory decline, enabling earlier diagnosis and intervention. These findings underscore the critical need for clinicians, researchers, and policymakers to work together in raising awareness of the vocal signs of hearing loss and integrating routine voice assessments into clinical practice. By doing so, we can ensure that individuals receive interventions sooner, preventing long-term complications and improving overall quality of life.

5. Conclusions

Hearing loss is associated with distinct changes to voice such as increased pitch and loudness, which are often compensatory mechanisms for impaired auditory feedback. These alterations become more pronounced as the severity and duration of hearing loss increase. Despite their diagnostic potential, these vocal changes are under-recognized during clinical consultations. The early identification of the "hearing loss voice" through attentive listening could provide a simple yet effective screening tool for clinicians. Such observations not only facilitate timely diagnosis and rehabilitation but also offer an opportunity to mitigate the broader cognitive and social consequences of untreated hearing loss [27]. Moreover, because untreated hearing loss is associated with neuroinflammation and neurodegeneration, the proactive use of hearing aids might slow or prevent such changes [28].

Author Contributions: Conceptualization, A.D.S.; methodology, A.D.S., P.D.L. and M.J.B.; formal analysis, A.D.S., J.S. and P.D.L.; investigation, J.S. and P.D.L.; resources, A.D.S. and M.J.B.; data curation, A.D.S., M.J.B., I.I., E.M.F. and G.T.P.; writing—original draft preparation, A.D.S., E.M.F., G.T.P. and M.J.B.; writing—review and editing, M.R., G.M. and I.I.; supervision, A.D.S., G.T.P. and E.M.F. All authors have read and agreed to the published version of the manuscript.

Funding: This research received no external funding.

Data Availability Statement: Data are available upon reasonable request to the corresponding authors.

Conflicts of Interest: The authors declare no conflicts of interest.

Abbreviations

The following abbreviations are used in this manuscript:

F_0	Fundamental frequency
PRISMA	Preferred Reporting Items for Systematic Reviews and Meta-Analyses
MDVP	Multidimensional Voice Program
CI	Cochlear implant
NHR	Noise-to-harmonic ratio
SPI	Soft phonation index
DUV	Degree of voicelessness
DVB	Degree of voice break
vAm	Peak amplitude variation
vF_0	Variable F_0
MPT	Maximum phonation time

References

1. Tsai Do, B.S.; Bush, M.L.; Weinreich, H.M.; Schwartz, S.R.; Anne, S.; Adunka, O.F.; Bender, K.; Bold, K.M.; Brenner, M.J.; Hashmi, A.Z.; et al. Clinical Practice Guideline: Age-Related Hearing Loss. *Otolaryngol. Head Neck Surg.* **2024**, *170* (Suppl. S2), S1–S54. [CrossRef] [PubMed]
2. Wijdicks, E.F.M. The neurologic consultation: Pointers and takeaways for intensivists. *Intensive Care Med.* **2020**, *46*, 1267–1270. [CrossRef] [PubMed]
3. Fuller, G. *Neurological Examination Made Easy*, 6th ed.; Elsevier: Amsterdam, The Netherlands, 2020.
4. Abdo, W.F.; van de Warrenburg, B.P.; Burn, D.J.; Quinn, N.P.; Bloem, B.R. The clinical approach to movement disorders. *Nat. Rev. Neurol.* **2010**, *6*, 29–37. [CrossRef] [PubMed]
5. Mora, R.; Crippa, B.; Cervoni, E.; Santomauro, V.; Guastini, L. Acoustic features of voice in patients with severe hearing loss. *J. Otolaryngol. Head Neck Surg.* **2012**, *41*, 8–13. [PubMed]

6. Akil, F.; Yollu, U.; Ozturk, O.; Yener, M. Differences of the Voice Parameters Between the Population of Different Hearing Tresholds: Findings by Using the Multi-Dimensional Voice Program. *Clin. Exp. Otorhinolaryngol.* **2017**, *10*, 278–282. [CrossRef]
7. Lee, Y.; Kreiman, J. Acoustic voice variation in spontaneous speech. *J. Acoust. Soc. Am.* **2022**, *151*, 3462. [CrossRef]
8. Saggio, G.; Costantini, G. Worldwide Healthy Adult Voice Baseline Parameters: A Comprehensive Review. *J. Voice* **2022**, *36*, 637–649. [CrossRef]
9. Scherer, K.R. Voice, Stress, and Emotion. In *Dynamics of Stress*; Appley, M.H., Trumbull, R., Eds.; The Plenum Series on Stress and Coping; Springer: Boston, MA, USA, 1986. [CrossRef]
10. Legris, E.; Henriques, J.; Aussedat, C.; Aoustin, J.M.; Robier, M.; Bakhos, D. Emotional prosody perception in presbycusis patients after auditory rehabilitation. *Eur. Ann. Otorhinolaryngol. Head Neck Dis.* **2021**, *138*, 163–168. [CrossRef] [PubMed]
11. Higgins, M.B.; Carney, A.E.; Schulte, L. Physiological assessment of speech and voice production of adults with hearing loss. *Speech Hear. Res.* **1994**, *37*, 510–521. [CrossRef]
12. Weatherley, C.C.; Worrall, L.E.; Hickson, L.M. The effect of hearing impairment on the vocal characteristics of older people. *Folia Phoniatr. Logop.* **1997**, *49*, 53–62. [CrossRef]
13. Lee, G.S. Variability in voice fundamental frequency of sustained vowels in speakers with sensorineural hearing loss. *J. Voice* **2012**, *26*, 24–29. [CrossRef] [PubMed]
14. Ubrig, M.T.; Goffi-Gomez, M.V.; Weber, R.; Menezes, M.H.; Nemr, N.K.; Tsuji, D.H.; Tsuji, R.K. Voice analysis of postlingually deaf adults pre- and postcochlear implantation. *J. Voice* **2011**, *25*, 692–699. [CrossRef] [PubMed]
15. Hengen, J.; Hammarström, I.L.; Stenfelt, S. Perceived Voice Quality and Voice-Related Problems Among Older Adults with Hearing Impairments. *J. Speech Lang. Hear. Res.* **2018**, *61*, 2168–2178. [CrossRef] [PubMed]
16. Zamani, P.; Bayat, A.; Saki, N.; Ataee, E.; Bagheripour, H. Post-lingual deaf adult cochlear implant users' speech and voice characteristics: Cochlear implant turned-on versus turned-off. *Acta Otolaryngol.* **2021**, *141*, 367–373. [CrossRef]
17. Arias-Vergara, T.; Batliner, A.; Rader, T.; Polterauer, D.; Högerle, C.; Müller, J.; Orozco-Arroyave, J.R.; Nöth, E.; Schuster, M.J. Adult Cochlear Implant Users Versus Typical Hearing Persons: An Automatic Analysis of Acoustic-Prosodic Parameters. *Speech Lang. Hear. Res.* **2022**, *65*, 4623–4636. [CrossRef]
18. Albera, A.; Puglisi, G.E.; Astolfi, A.; Riva, G.; Cassandro, C.; Mozzanica, F. Canale A Ambulatory Phonation Monitoring in Prelingual and Postlingual Deaf Patients after Cochlear Implantation. *Audiol. Neurootol.* **2023**, *28*, 52–62. [CrossRef]
19. Cardella, A.; Ottaviani, F.; Luzi, L.; Albera, A.; Schindler, A.; Mozzanica, F. Daily speaking time and voice intensity before and after hearing aids rehabilitation in adult patients with hearing loss. *Folia Phoniatr. Logop.* **2024**, *76*, 440–448. [CrossRef]
20. Nicastri, M.; Chiarella, G.; Gallo, L.V.; Catalano, M.; Cassandro, E. Multidimensional Voice Program (MDVP) and amplitude variation parameters in euphonic adult subjects. Normative study. *Acta Otorhinolaryngol. Ital.* **2004**, *24*, 337–341.
21. Nacci, A.; Fattori, B.; Mancini, V.; Panicucci, E.; Ursino, F.; Cartaino, F.M.; Berrettini, S. The use and role of the Ambulatory Phonation Monitor (APM) in voice assessment. *Acta Otorhinolaryngol. Ital.* **2013**, *33*, 49–55.
22. Han, Y.; Wang, C.-T.; Li, J.-H.; Lai, Y.-H. Ambulatory Phonation Monitoring Using Wireless Headphones with Deep Learning Technology. *IEEE Syst. J.* **2023**, *17*, 4752–4762. [CrossRef]
23. Dichter, B.K.; Breshears, J.D.; Leonard, M.K.; Chang, E.F. The Control of Vocal Pitch in Human Laryngeal Motor Cortex. *Cell* **2018**, *174*, 21–31.e9. [CrossRef] [PubMed]
24. Liu, P.; Chen, Z.; Jones, J.A.; Huang, D.; Liu, H. Auditory feedback control of vocal pitch during sustained vocalization: A cross-sectional study of adult aging. *PLoS ONE* **2011**, *6*, e22791. [CrossRef] [PubMed]
25. Brownell, W.E. How the ear works—Nature's solutions for listening. *Volta. Rev.* **1997**, *99*, 9–28. [PubMed]
26. Karimi-Boroujeni, M.; Dajani, H.R.; Giguère, C. Perception of Prosody in Hearing-Impaired Individuals and Users of Hearing Assistive Devices: An Overview of Recent Advances. *J. Speech Lang. Hear. Res.* **2023**, *66*, 775–789. [CrossRef] [PubMed]
27. Bisogno, A.; Scarpa, A.; Di Girolamo, S.; De Luca, P.; Cassandro, C.; Viola, P.; Ricciardiello, F.; Greco, A.; Vincentiis, M.; Ralli, M.; et al. Hearing Loss and Cognitive Impairment: Epidemiology, Common Pathophysiological Findings, and Treatment Considerations. *Life* **2021**, *11*, 1102. [CrossRef]
28. Di Stadio, A.; Ralli, M.; Roccamatisi, D.; Scarpa, A.; Della Volpe, A.; Cassandro, C.; Ricci, G.; Greco, A.; Bernitsas, E. Hearing loss and dementia: Radiologic and biomolecular basis of their shared characteristics. A systematic review. *Neurol. Sci.* **2021**, *42*, 579–588. [CrossRef]

Disclaimer/Publisher's Note: The statements, opinions and data contained in all publications are solely those of the individual author(s) and contributor(s) and not of MDPI and/or the editor(s). MDPI and/or the editor(s) disclaim responsibility for any injury to people or property resulting from any ideas, methods, instructions or products referred to in the content.

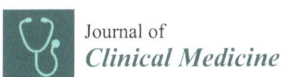

Article

The Impact of Protective Face Coverings on Acoustic Markers in Voice: A Systematic Review and Meta-Analysis

Ben Barsties v. Latoszek [1,*], Viktoria Jansen [1], Christopher R. Watts [2] and Svetlana Hetjens [3]

1. Speech-Language Pathology, SRH University of Applied Health Sciences, 40210 Düsseldorf, Germany
2. Harris College of Nursing & Health Sciences, Texas Christian University, Fort Worth, TX 76109, USA
3. Department for Medical Statistics and Biomathematics, Medical Faculty Mannheim, University of Heidelberg, 68165 Mannheim, Germany
* Correspondence: benjamin.barstiesvonlatoszek@srh.de

Abstract: Background: Wearing respiratory protective masks (RPMs) has become common worldwide, especially in healthcare settings, since the onset of the COVID-19 pandemic. Hypotheses have suggested that sound transmission could be limited by RPMs, which possibly affects the characteristics of acoustic energy and speech intelligibility. The objective of this study was to investigate the effect of RPMs on acoustic measurements through a systematic review with meta-analysis. Methods: Five database searches were conducted, ranging from their inception to August 2023, as well as a manual search. Cross-sectional studies were included that provided data on widely used gender-independent clinical acoustic voice quality measures (jitter, shimmer, HNR, CPPS, and AVQI) and habitual sound pressure level (SPL). Results: We found nine eligible research studies with a total of 422 participants who were compared both without masks and with different types of masks. All included studies focused on individuals with vocally healthy voices, while two of the studies also included those with voice disorders. The results from the meta-analysis were related to medical/surgical and FFP2/(K)N95 masks. None of the acoustic measurements showed significant differences between the absence and presence of masks ($p > 0.05$). When indirectly comparing both mask types, statistical significance was identified for parameters of jitter, HNR, CPPS and SPL ($p < 0.001$). Conclusions: The present meta-analysis indicates that certain types of RPMs have no significant influence on common voice quality parameters and SPL compared to recordings without masks. Nevertheless, it is plausible that significant differences in acoustic parameters might exist between different mask types. Consequently, it is advisable for the clinical practice to always use the same mask type when using RPMs to ensure high comparability and accuracy of measurement results.

Keywords: respiratory protection masks; acoustics; corona pandemic; COVID-19; voice quality; dysphonia

1. Introduction

Multidimensional voice evaluation (e.g., visual analysis, auditory-perceptual judgment, aerodynamic analysis, acoustic analysis, and self-assessment [1]) is essential to determine the degree and type of dysphonia with individual voice complaints in patients with voice disorders. However, in order to provide a high measurement of accuracy to the individual measurement procedures on the one hand, but also to protect the investigator staff and the patients on the other hand, it is necessary to take the appropriate safety precautions. For example, during the coronavirus pandemic from 11 March 2020 to 5 May 2023, without a global emergency [2], the aim was to control and prevent all coronavirus-related diseases and mortality, particularly through hand hygiene, social distancing and nose-and-mouth-covering respiratory protective masks (RPMs). To avoid potential infection through respiratory droplets or airborne transmission, various RPMs such as medical/surgical or FFP2/(K)N95 masks were widely used in everyday life and clinical settings and are still in use today. Research conducted over the past three years has suggested the hypothesis that sound transmission is limited when passing through RPMs, which act as a low-pass filter, attenuating sound in the mid- and high-frequency ranges with consequences on perceptual speech intelligibility and acoustic properties of the voice [3–5]. Face masks might alter people's perception of sound by reducing the perceived loudness and selectively removing certain sound components, particularly the high-frequency elements that are critical for a clear understanding of spoken language. This could be even more evident when a phone is used with a face mask, as the filtering of these important high frequencies is even more impaired, especially in special groups, such as individuals wearing cochlear implants or hearing aids or individuals with communication issues such as dysphonia and aphasia. Thus, the wearers of masks would speak louder, which, therefore, would lead to more effort and the development of vocal fatigue and a potential increase in vocal discomfort. Several systematic reviews or others without meta-analyses have attempted to summarize and examine acoustics, the effects on aerodynamic characteristics, self-reported characteristics of vocal effort and fatigue, vocal tract discomfort, and voice handicap index [6–9]. Overall, the results of these literature reviews did not unanimously show that the results of acoustic markers such as habitual intensity [6,8], formant frequencies of F2 and F3 [6], harmonics-to-noise-ratio [6,8] and mean spectral values in high-frequency levels (1000–8000 Hz) [6–8] may be influenced by wearing face masks; however, there is a lack of a clear statement of the expected distribution when an overall significant effect was statistically demonstrated across the single studies.

Acoustic measurements for voice quality and vocal function analyses have a main part in the clinical examination routine of laryngology, evaluating the degree and type of dysphonia. If this RPM effect significantly impacts acoustic voice analysis assessing voice quality parameters and vocal function parameters such as loudness/intensity, these effects must be taken into account in the recording procedure and analysis since they would influence measurement accuracy (e.g., threshold values). Therefore, the present study is, to our knowledge, the first study that investigated the effect of RPMs on the outcome of gender-independent acoustic parameters of voice quality and vocal function in a meta-analysis.

2. Materials and Methods

2.1. Data Sources and Searches

We utilized the reporting guideline provided by the Preferred Reporting Items for Systematic Reviews and Meta-Analyses (PRISMA) to systematically search five databases (MEDLINE, CENTRAL, LIVIVO, Speechbite, and Google Scholar) from their inception until 2 August 2023. A combination of different keywords such as "face mask", "acoustic", and "voice quality" was used, and a comprehensive list of these keywords can be found in Table S1 of the Supplementary Materials.

Potential articles were initially identified based on their titles and abstracts. Furthermore, a manual search of the grey literature sources was conducted. This involved examining the bibliographies of the included studies to identify additional relevant articles. The process of hand searching was carried out for scientific reports published in both German and English languages, and those included in the databases were considered for the meta-analysis.

2.2. Study Selection

The present study included cross-sectional studies that investigated the effect on acoustic parameters with and without RPMs (i.e., medical/surgical masks and FFP2/(K)N95). To minimize variation in specifications and reliability caused by the use of different acoustic software packages, we considered only studies that performed acoustic measurements with Praat (developed by Paul Boersma and David Weenink at the Institute of Phonetic Sciences, University of Amsterdam, The Netherlands: http://www.praat.org/ accessed on 13 August 2023). This meta-analysis included widely used quantitative acoustic measures from an internationally recognized set of gender-independent voice quality measurements encompassing key clinical parameters such as jitter (Jit%) [1], shimmer (Shim%) [1], harmonics-to-noise ratio (HNR) [10], smoothed cepstral peak prominence (CPPS) [10], and Acoustic Voice Quality Index (AVQI) [11]. Furthermore, habitual sound intensity level or sound pressure level (SPL) as a vocal function parameter and relevant for a voice diagnostic battery was also considered [1].

To be included in this meta-analysis, studies had to include at least one of these acoustic measures assessing habitual voice production of sustained vowel /a:/ (jitter, shimmer, HNR, CPPS, and sound intensity level) or the standardized concatenation of continuous speech and sustained vowel /a:/ for AVQI in voice evaluation.

2.3. Risk of Bias Assessment

The risk of bias assessment of the included studies was determined using the checklist for cross-sectional studies of 11 items from the Agency for Healthcare Research and Quality (AHRQ) [12]. For a better interpretation, a high quality with a low risk of bias was assessed when $\geq 75\%$ were answered with "yes". A moderate risk of bias was present when 50% to 75% of items received a confirmation, and a high risk of bias was provided below 50% replies with "yes" for all items. Items marked with "unclear" reduces the total number of 11 items for the individual study.

2.4. Data Extraction

Two reviewers (B.B.v.L. and V.J.) extracted the data. Any discrepancies were resolved through discussion. Information collected from the selected studies included details such as article attributes (authors, publication year, journal, article title), study characteristics (research design, sample size, participants with voice disorders compared with vocally healthy individuals, acoustic data processing methodology, results with and without face masks), patient demographics (age and gender), and outcomes (jitter, shimmer, HNR, CPPS, AVQI, and SPL).

2.5. Statistics

The statistical analyses were conducted using MedCalc software (version 19.6) and SAS software (version 9.4).

First, the differences between the mean values of study parameters $\bar{x}_{without\ mask} - \bar{x}_{mask}$ and standard errors (SE) were calculated SE $= \frac{(S_1+S_2)/2}{\sqrt{n}}$.

Second, meta-analyses were performed using MedCalc software version 19.6 for the six parameters: Jit%, Shim%, CPPS, HNR, AVQI and SPL. For each parameter, the mean difference (MD) was calculated along with a 95% confidence interval (CI) for each individual study. To present the results of the meta-analyses visually, a forest plot was used. An I^2 index was used to assess heterogeneity between studies included in the analysis. According to Higgins definition [13], $I^2 = 0\%$: there is no observed heterogeneity; $I^2 > 0\%$ and $\leq 25\%$: there is insignificant heterogeneity; $I^2 > 25\%$ and $\leq 50\%$: there is low heterogeneity; $I^2 > 50\%$ and $\leq 75\%$: There is moderate heterogeneity; and $I^2 > 75\%$: there is high heterogeneity. Since in the meta-analysis there are differences in the characteristics of the population or in other factors, leading to heterogeneity or dissimilarity in the results, the random effect model was used so that heterogeneity between studies was accounted for. The weighting, according to DerSimonian and Laird [14], was used.

Third, an indirect comparison between medical/surgical masks and (K)N95/FFP2 was calculated. For this purpose, the two confidence intervals were compared using Welch's *t*-test. A confidence interval is the estimate of the basic population and contains more information than a direct comparison. A *p*-value of <0.05 was considered statistically significant.

3. Results
3.1. Study Characteristics

During our searches, we encountered 64 unique papers (see Figure 1). Of these, nine studies met the criteria for inclusion in the current review. The study details of these selected papers can be obtained in Table 1 [15–23]. In total, 422 volunteers were investigated without and with different types of masks, ranging from seven to one hundred and fifty-nine participants in the studies. All studies included vocally healthy individuals, and two studies also included different types of voice disorders and severity degrees of dysphonia. The risk of bias assessment is shown in Table S2 of the Supplementary Materials, in which most cases have a moderate risk of bias, and in two cases [17,21], a low risk of bias was assessed.

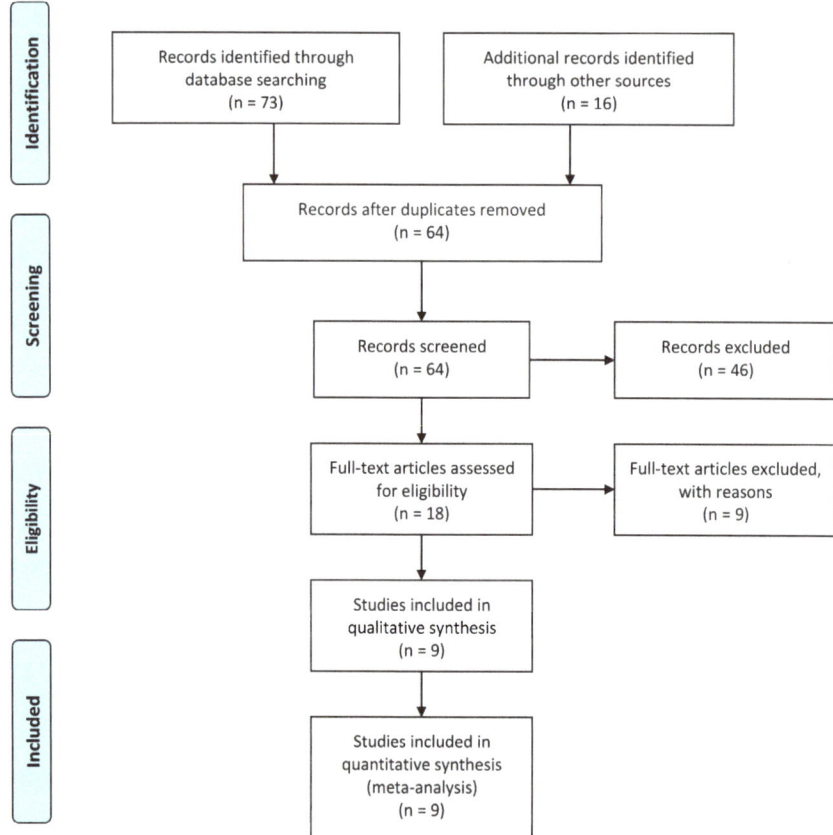

Figure 1. Prisma flow diagram.

Table 1. Characteristics of cross-sectional trials in the meta-analysis.

Study	Sample Size	Voice Status	Age (Mean/Range in Years)/Gender	Types of Masks	Acoustic Parameters
Maggee et al. (2020) [15]	Total: $n = 7$	Vocally-healthy	28.1 (21–39) F/M = 3/4	No mask; surgical/medical mask; N95; Cloth mask	Jit%; Shim%; HNR; CPPS; SPL
Cavallaro et al. (2021) [16]	Total: $n = 50$	Vocally-healthy	47.0 (26–69) F/M = 30/20	No mask; surgical/medical mask	Jit%; Shim%; HNR
Nguyen et al. (2021) [17]	Total: $n = 16$	Vocally-healthy	43.0 (24–61) F/M = 12/4	No mask; surgical/medical mask; KN95;	HNR; CPPS; SPL
Lin et al. (2022) [18]	Total: $n = 159$	Vocally healthy ($n = 53$); VFBL ($n = 59$); IGC ($n = 27$); ESGC ($n = 20$)	Vocally healthy 42.62 (20–85) F/M = 28/25 Voice-disordered 47.7 (24–70) F/M = 49/57	No mask; surgical/medical mask	CPPS; SPL
Lehnert et al. (2022) [19]	Total: $n = 31$	Vocally healthy	Age unknown F/M = 18/13	No mask; surgical/medical mask; FFP2	AVQI
Fiorella et al. (2023) [20]	Total: $n = 60$	Vocally healthy	47.0 (26–69) F/M = 36/24	No mask; surgical/medical mask	Jit%; Shim%; HNR; SPL
Maryn et al. (2023) [21]	Total: $n = 50$	Vocally healthy ($n = 12$); VVD ($n = 38$)	44.9 (10–77) F/M = 29/21	No mask; surgical/medical mask; FFP2; transparent mask	Jit%; Shim%; HNR; CPPS; AVQI; SPL
Joshi et al. (In Press) [22]	Total: $n = 19$	Vocally-healthy	35.0 (18–67) F/M = 10/9	No mask; surgical/medical mask; KN95; Cloth mask; Face shield	CPPS; SPL
Gao et al. (In Press) [23]	Total: $n = 30$	Vocally-healthy	23.26 (20–40) F/M = 15/15	No mask; surgical/medical mask; N95	Jit%; Shim%; HNR; SPL

F: Female; M: Male; VFBL: vocal fold benign lesions; IGC: insufficient glottal closure; ESGC: early stage glottic carcinoma; VVD: various voice disorders; Jit%: jitter; Shim%: shimmer; HNR: harmonics-to-noise ratio; CPPS: cepstral peak prominence smooth; AVQI: Acoustic Voice Quality Index; SPL: sound pressure level, habitual sound intensity level.

3.2. Meta-Analysis

Figures 2–4 and Table 2 show the results for the six parameters: Jit%, Shim%, CPPS, HNR, AVQI, and SPL. The mean difference between without mask and medical/surgical mask was negative for parameters Jit%, Shim%, HNR and SPL and positive for CPPS and AVQI. The findings from the meta-analysis, along with heterogeneity statistics and assessments of publication bias, revealed no publication bias in all parameters and no heterogeneity in Jit% and HNR, low heterogeneity in Shim% and SPL, and moderate heterogeneity in CPPS and AVQI.

In the analysis between without mask and FFP2/(K)N95, the mean difference was negative for the parameters Shim% and HNR and positive for Jit%, CPPS, AVQI, and SPL. No publication bias was present in all parameters. Furthermore, no heterogeneity was revealed in Jit%, Shim%, and SPI, low heterogeneity in CPPS, moderate heterogeneity in HNR, and high heterogeneity in AVQI was found.

None of the parameters were significant when comparing acoustic measurements with and without masks ($p > 0.05$; see Table 2).

Table 2. Meta-analysis by Treatment and by Voice Measures (Random Effects Model).

Comparison between Masks and Without	Parameter	n	Mean Difference (95% CI)	p-Value	I²	p-Value from Begg's Test
Medical/Surgical masks vs. without	Jit%	197	−0.02% (−0.04% to 0.003%)	0.086	6.17%	0.573
	Shim%	197	−0.06% (−0.20% to 0.08%)	0.414	35.48%	0.851
	HNR	213	−0.17 dB (−0.69 dB to 0.35 dB)	0.522	0.22%	0.293
	CPPS	251	0.28 dB (−0.36 dB to 0.91 dB)	0.396	64.79%	0.174
	AVQI	81	0.06 dB (−0.47 dB to 0.60 dB)	0.824	71.58%	0.317
	SPL	341	−0.35 dB (−1.04 dB to 0.34 dB)	0.316	41.71%	0.152
FFP2/(K)N95 masks vs. without	Jit%	87	0.01% (−0.02% to 0.03%)	0.716	0.00%	0.602
	Shim%	87	−0.07% (−0.18% to 0.05%)	0.240	0.00%	0.602
	HNR	103	−1.37 dB (−2.79 dB to 0.05 dB)	0.059	59.48%	0.497
	CPPS	92	0.003 dB (−0.69 dB to 0.69 dB)	0.994	38.96%	0.050
	AVQI	81	0.05 (−0.70 to 0.79)	0.905	85.30%	0.317
	SPL	122	0.36 dB (−0.59 dB to 1.31 dB)	0.460	13.18%	0.348

Jit%: jitter; Shim%: shimmer; HNR: harmonics-to-noise ratio; CPPS: cepstral peak prominence smooth; AVQI: Acoustic Voice Quality Index; SPL: sound pressure level, habitual sound intensity level.

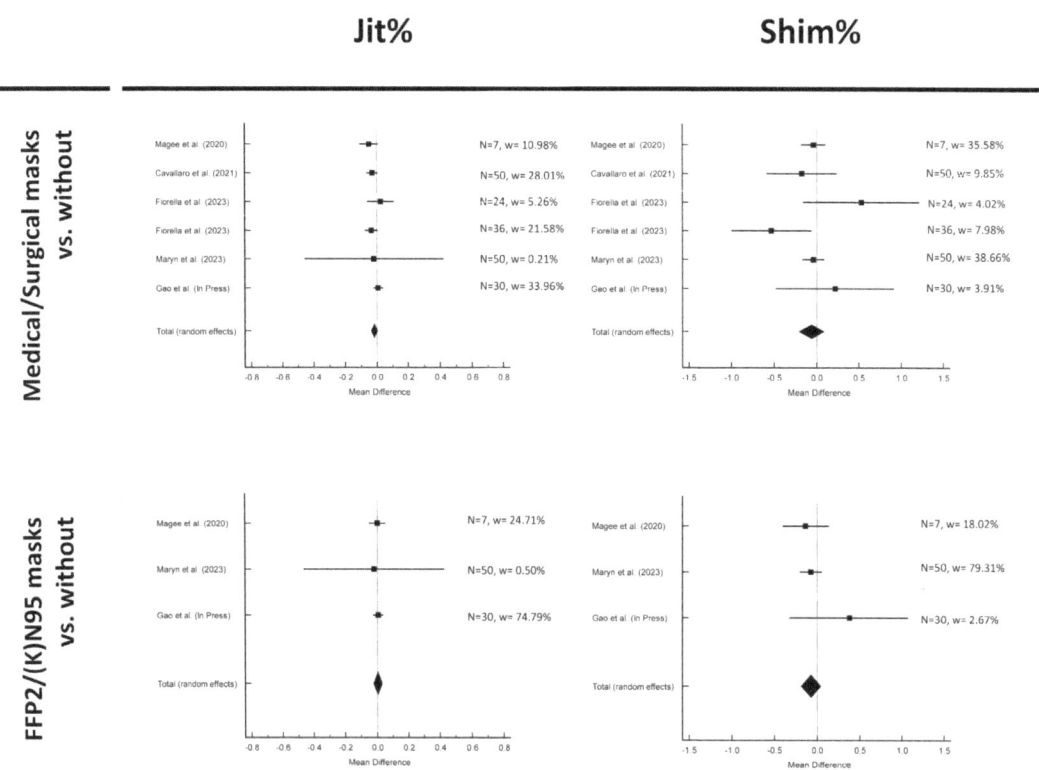

Figure 2. Forest plots of measurements Jit% and Shim% [15,16,20,21,23].

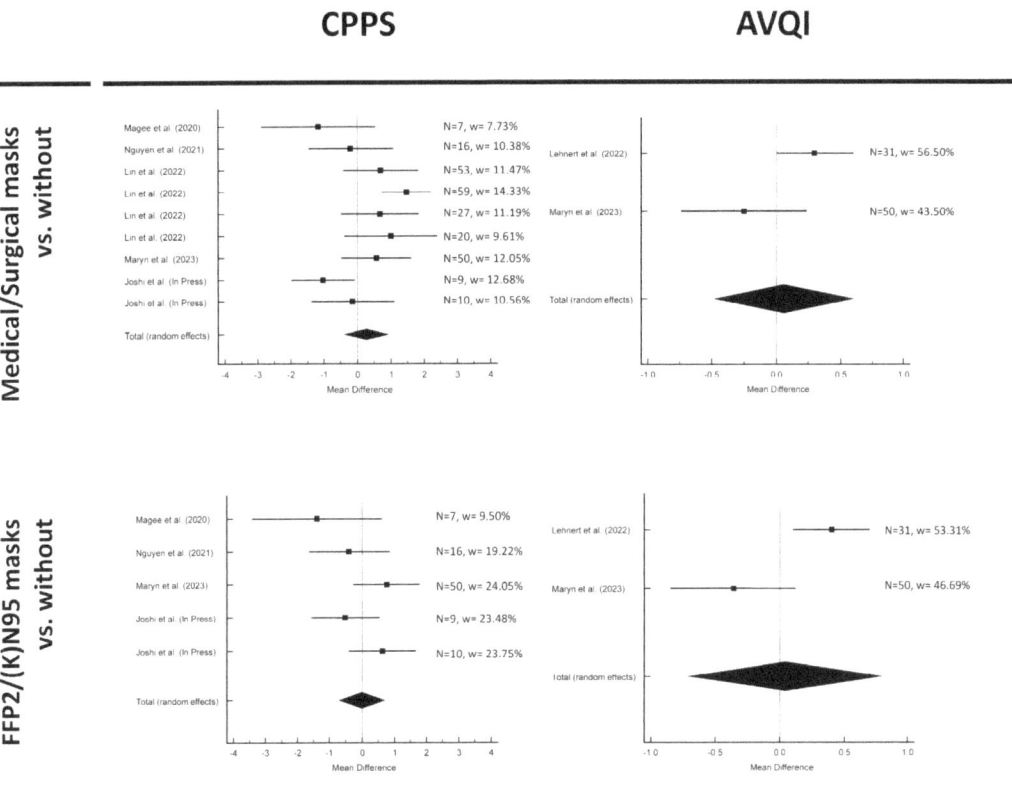

Figure 3. Forest plots of measurements CPPS and AVQI [15,17–19,21,22].

3.3. Indirect Comparison between the Two Mask Types

The comparison between FFP2/(K)N95 and medical/surgical masks showed significance for the parameters Jit%, HNR, CPPS, and SPL ($p < 0.001$). The pooled difference of the Jit% parameter for medical/surgical mask was larger than FFP2/(K)N95 (MD (without mask–medical/surgical mask): −0.02 and MD (without mask–FFP2/(K)N95 mask): 0.01). For the parameter HNR, the pooled difference for FFP2/(K)N95 was larger than for medical/surgical mask (MD (without mask–medical/surgical mask): −0.17 and MD (without mask–FFP2/(K)N95): −1.37). For the parameter CPPS, the pooled difference for medical/surgical mask was larger than for FFP2/(K)N95 (MD (without mask–medical/surgical mask): 0.28 and MD (without mask–FFP2/(K)N95): 0.003). For the parameter SPL, the two signs were contradictory (MD (without mask–medical/surgical mask): −0.35 and MD (without mask–FFP2/(K)N95 mask): 0.36).

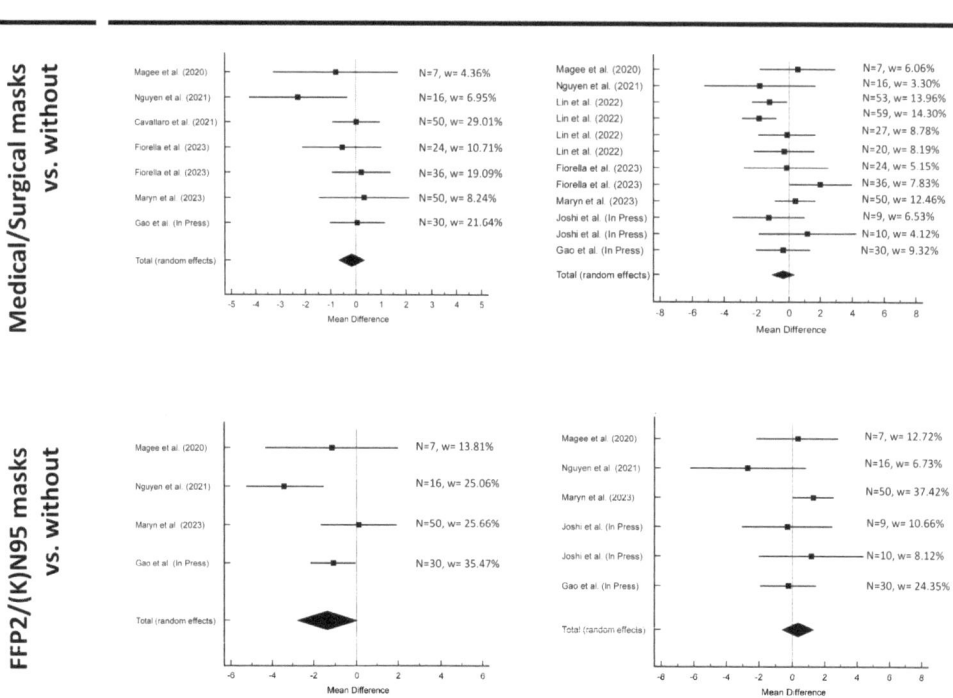

Figure 4. Forest plots of measurements HNR and SPL [15–18,20–23].

4. Discussion

The aim of this study was to examine how RPMs impact six gender-independent acoustic parameters connected to voice quality and vocal function among vocally healthy and voice-disordered individuals. For six acoustic parameters, there was no significant effect detected when comparing measurements with or without a RPM. However, there were differences between mask types, which led to recommendations of caution in the clinical routine when masks have to be used. The included publications had mostly a moderate risk of bias, while two of the nine studies revealed a low risk of bias. The heterogeneity ranged from no to high, but eight out of twelve analyses yielded no or low heterogeneity. Just one outcome presented a high heterogeneity for AVQI, which was twice investigated. There was no evidence of imprecision, publication bias, or indirectness.

The present meta-analysis was useful to assess an overall picture of the possible impact on the outcome of acoustic measurements based on RPMs. Although some systematic reviews and further single studies noted for HNR [6,8,17,23–25], Jitter [26], Shimmer [24,26], CPPS [18,21], SPL [6,8,18,26], and AVQI [21] significantly effects by RPMs, the present evaluation of this meta-analysis did not support these findings using the software Praat for the signal processing of the included acoustic measures. Further studies that were not included in the present meta-analysis (based on different signal processing methods of the acoustic parameters or other mask types) also concluded that for the same acoustic measures for vocally healthy and voice-disordered individuals, no significant differences between wearing a RPM or not [27–29]. Moreover, it must be taken into account that voice physiology and voice characteristics may differ between different speakers and between single or multiple voice recordings for consistency of sound measurements [30,31]. Although studies asked speakers to produce the same utterances while wearing a mask and while not wearing or changing masks, a fluctuation of voice is presented, at least to a small extent and should be controlled by the investigator groups. Due to minimal changes in the outcomes of the acoustic parameters between the recordings, a clinical significance could not be clearly observed. Although wearing masks for a prolonged period of time may cause observable self-perceived changes (e.g., breathing difficulties, increased effort of speaking, greater perception of symptoms of vocal fatigue and discomfort and changes in speaking behavior) in wearers [32–35], this influence remains unexplained in the present study, notwithstanding the fluctuations in multiple recordings of the voice analyses. To verify mask effects after prolonged wearing, it should be further investigated in future studies. Moreover, the possibility of individuals adjusting their speaking behavior when wearing masks is, in this context, also valuable to investigate and assess the potential impact of the validity of the acoustic measurements. Another confounding factor with a significant impact on the present results could be the recording hardware from the different studies. There are standards defined for instrumental assessments of voice recordings for vocal function to minimize bias and increase the comparability of studies [36]. A quick check revealed that some included studies could have deviations with regard to these recording standards [15,17,18,22].

The only significant effect demonstrated by the current meta-analysis was a measurable, significant difference in most of the included parameters based on mask type. Thus, it is recommended, for a clinical routine in laryngological practice, to always use the same mask type and not change. This will allow for comparability in the results between mask-wearing and without, and no systematic error in intra- or inter-individual comparison of patients' recordings and their analyses is present. In real-world clinical practice, facilities utilize the same face mask vendors, so this recommendation is likely to be followed without problem.

The limitations of this meta-analysis not only relate to the applicability of its results but also offer insights for future studies. First, only two types of masks were evaluated. These two types were the most often compared in the literature, which facilitated the ability to apply meta-analysis to the data. Further mask types, such as cloth masks or face shields, are missing in the present meta-analysis. Furthermore, one study also investigated the combination of wearing several types of masks at the same time (e.g., N95 plus face shield) [22], which is also commonly used in medical practice [37–39]. Second, the majority of the nine included studies were found to be at moderate risk of bias (only two were at low risk of bias). Third, the signal processing is limited to the software Praat. Studies that used other software, such as the Multi Dimensional Voice Program or Analysis of Dysphonia in Speech and Voice from Pentax Medical or Dr. Speech, were excluded based on specification and reliability differences due to the application of different acoustic software packages. Fourth, the most evaluated voices were vocally healthy. A minority of voice-disordered voice samples were also included, but these types of voices reveal a high fluctuation and abnormality in the outcomes of the voice measures, which can have an influence on the variability of the measures for the present study. Fifth, the search strategy for relevant papers in this study was conducted in two languages, excluding other languages such as Asian languages, Spanish, or French that might have contained relevant publications. Sixth, the present meta-analysis evaluated mainly acoustic markers which are dedicated to voice quality. Other acoustic aspects for speech intelligibility, such as formant frequencies and spectral analysis, were not part of the present meta-analysis and have to be analyzed in the future as well. Seventh, the long-term effects of wearing masks will need to be studied in the future. There is some indication that the voice may change in acoustic voice quality markers after prolonged wearing of a mask evaluated in a longitudinal investigation over two years [40].

5. Conclusions

The present meta-analysis mainly included vocally healthy individuals without sufficient data from the clinical population because only two out of nine included studies considered participants with dysphonia. However, this study demonstrated no impact of RPMs on five acoustic voice quality parameters and SPL. However, mask type effects on acoustic parameters did differ significantly. In the current study, this was confirmed for Jit%, HNR, CPPS, and SPL. Thus, for clinical laryngology practice, it is recommended that if RPMs are used, then the same mask type should always be applied and not changed to keep the comparability and accuracy of the measurement results high.

Supplementary Materials: The following supporting information can be downloaded at https://www.mdpi.com/article/10.3390/jcm12185922/s1, Table S1: Search strategies for systematic review; Table S2: Risk of Bias analyzed with AHRQ Methodology Checklist for cross-sectional studies. References [15–23] are cited in the Supplementary Materials.

Author Contributions: Conceptualization, B.B.v.L., V.J. and C.R.W.; methodology, B.B.v.L., C.R.W., V.J. and S.H.; software, S.H.; formal analysis, B.B.v.L., V.J. and S.H.; writing—original draft preparation, B.B.v.L., V.J. and S.H.; writing—review and editing, C.R.W. All authors have read and agreed to the published version of the manuscript.

Funding: This research received no external funding.

Institutional Review Board Statement: Not applicable.

Informed Consent Statement: Not applicable.

Data Availability Statement: The original contributions presented in the study are included in the article; further inquiries can be directed to the corresponding author.

Conflicts of Interest: The authors declare no conflict of interest.

References

1. Dejonckere, P.H.; Bradley, P.; Clemente, P.; Cornut, G.; Crevier-Buchman, L.; Friedrich, G.; Van De Heyning, P.; Remacle, M.; Woisard, V.; Committee on Phoniatrics of the European Laryngological Society (ELS). A basic protocol for functional assessment of voice pathology, especially for investigating the efficacy of (phonosurgical) treatments and evaluating new assessment techniques. Guideline elaborated by the Committee on Phoniatrics of the European Laryngological Society (ELS). *Eur. Arch. Otorhinolaryngol.* **2001**, *258*, 77–82. [CrossRef] [PubMed]
2. Coronavirus Disease (COVID-19) Pandemic. Available online: https://www.who.int/europe/emergencies/situations/covid-19 (accessed on 5 August 2023).
3. Corey, R.M.; Jones, U.; Singer, A.C. Comparison of the acoustic effects of face masks on speech. *Hear. J.* **2021**, *74*, 36–39. [CrossRef]
4. Sönnichsen, R.; Llorach Tó, G.; Hochmuth, S.; Hohmann, V.; Radeloff, A. How face masks interfere with speech understanding of normal-hearing individuals: Vision makes the difference. *Otol. Neurotol.* **2022**, *43*, 282–288. [CrossRef]
5. Oren, L.; Rollins, M.; Gutmark, E.; Howell, R. How face masks affect acoustic and auditory perceptual characteristics of the singing voice. *J. Voice* **2023**, *37*, 515–521. [CrossRef] [PubMed]
6. Gama, R.; Castro, M.E.; van Lith-Bijl, J.T.; Desuter, G. Does the wearing of masks change voice and speech parameters? *Eur. Arch. Otorhinolaryngol.* **2022**, *279*, 1701–1708. [CrossRef] [PubMed]
7. Badh, G.; Knowles, T. Acoustic and perceptual impact of face masks on speech: A scoping review. *PLoS ONE* **2023**, *18*, e0285009. [CrossRef]
8. Shekaraiah, S.; Suresh, K. Effect of face mask on voice production during COVID-19 pandemic: A systematic review. *J. Voice* **2021**, in press. [CrossRef]
9. Francis, R.; Leavitt, M.; McLelland, C.; Hamilton, D.F. The influence of facemasks on communication in healthcare settings: A systematic review. *Disabil. Rehabil.* **2023**, in press. [CrossRef]
10. Barsties V. Latoszek, B.; Mayer, J.; Watts, C.R.; Lehnert, B. Advances in Clinical Voice Quality Analysis with VOXplot. *J. Clin. Med.* **2023**, *12*, 4644. [CrossRef]
11. Barsties V. Latoszek, B.; Mathmann, P.; Neumann, K. The cepstral spectral index of dysphonia, the acoustic voice quality index and the acoustic breathiness index as novel multiparametric indices for acoustic assessment of voice quality. *Curr. Opin. Otolaryngol. Head Neck Surg.* **2021**, *29*, 451–457. [CrossRef]
12. Quality Assessment Forms. Available online: https://www.ncbi.nlm.nih.gov/books/NBK35156/ (accessed on 5 August 2023).
13. Higgins, J.P.; Thompson, S.G.; Deeks, J.J. Altman DG. Measuring inconsistency in meta-analyses. *BMJ* **2003**, *327*, 557–560. [CrossRef] [PubMed]
14. DerSimonian, R.; Laird, N. Meta-analysis in clinical trials. *Control Clin. Trials.* **1986**, *7*, 177–188. [CrossRef] [PubMed]

15. Magee, M.; Lewis, C.; Noffs, G.; Reece, H.; Chan, J.C.S.; Zaga, C.J.; Paynter, C.; Birchall, O.; Rojas Azocar, S.; Ediriweera, A.; et al. Effects of face masks on acoustic analysis and speech perception: Implications for peri-pandemic protocols. *J. Acoust. Soc. Am.* **2020**, *148*, 3562. [CrossRef] [PubMed]
16. Cavallaro, G.; Di Nicola, V.; Quaranta, N.; Fiorella, M.L. Acoustic voice analysis in the COVID-19 era. *Acta Otorhinolaryngol. Ital.* **2021**, *41*, 1. [CrossRef] [PubMed]
17. Nguyen, D.D.; McCabe, P.; Thomas, D.; Purcell, A.; Doble, M.; Novakovic, D.; Chacon, A.; Madill, C. Acoustic voice characteristics with and without wearing a facemask. *Sci. Rep.* **2021**, *11*, 5651. [CrossRef]
18. Lin, Y.; Cheng, L.; Wang, Q.; Xu, W. Effects of medical masks on voice quality in patients with voice disorders. *J. Speech Lang. Hear. Res.* **2022**, *65*, 1742–1750. [CrossRef] [PubMed]
19. Lehnert, B.; Herold, J.; Blaurock, M.; Busch, C.J. Reliability of the Acoustic Voice Quality Index AVQI and the Acoustic Breathiness Index (ABI) when wearing COVID-19 protective masks. *Eur. Arch. Otorhinolaryngol.* **2022**, *279*, 4617–4621. [CrossRef]
20. Fiorella, M.L.; Cavallaro, G.; Di Nicola, V.; Quaranta, N. Voice differences when wearing and not wearing a surgical mask. *J. Voice* **2023**, *37*, 467.e1–467.e7. [CrossRef]
21. Maryn, Y.; Wuyts, F.L.; Zarowski, A. Are acoustic markers of voice and speech signals affected by nose-and-mouth-covering respiratory protective masks? *J. Voice* **2023**, *37*, 468.e1–468.e12. [CrossRef]
22. Joshi, A.; Procter, T.; Kulesz, P.A. COVID-19: Acoustic measures of voice in individuals wearing different facemasks. *J. Voice* **2021**, *in press*. [CrossRef]
23. Gao, Y.; Feng, Y.; Wu, D.; Lu, F.; He, H.; Tian, C. Effect of wearing different masks on acoustic, aerodynamic, and formant parameters. *J. Voice* **2023**, *in press*. [CrossRef] [PubMed]
24. Gojayev, E.K.; Büyükatalay, Z.Ç.; Akyüz, T.; Rehan, M.; Dursun, G. The effect of masks and respirators on acoustic voice analysis during the COVID-19 pandemic. *J. Voice* **2021**, *in press*. [CrossRef] [PubMed]
25. McKenna, V.S.; Kendall, C.L.; Patel, T.H.; Howell, R.J.; Gustin, R.L. Impact of face masks on speech acoustics and vocal effort in healthcare professionals. *Laryngoscope* **2022**, *132*, 391–397. [CrossRef] [PubMed]
26. Lin, Y.; Cheng, L.; Wang, Q.; Xu, W. Effects of medical masks on voice assessment during the COVID-19 pandemic. *J. Voice* **2021**, *in press*. [CrossRef] [PubMed]
27. Lee, S.J.; Kang, M.S.; Park, Y.M.; Lim, J.Y. Reliability of acoustic measures in dysphonic patients with glottic insufficiency and healthy population: A COVID-19 perspective. *J. Voice in press.* **2022**. [CrossRef] [PubMed]
28. Ho, G.Y.; Kansy, I.K.; Klavacs, K.A.; Leonhard, M.; Schneider-Stickler, B. Effect of FFP2/3 Masks on voice range profile measurement and voice acoustics in routine voice diagnostics. *Folia Phoniatr. Logop.* **2022**, *74*, 335–344. [CrossRef] [PubMed]
29. Yu, M.; Jin, Q.; Zhang, W.; Sun, X.; Sun, Y.; Xie, Q. Effects of different medical masks on acoustic and aerodynamic voice assessment during the COVID-19 pandemic. *Medicine* **2023**, *102*, e34470. [CrossRef] [PubMed]
30. Leong, K.; Hawkshaw, M.J.; Dentchev, D.; Gupta, R.; Lurie, D.; Sataloff, R.T. Reliability of objective voice measures of normal speaking voices. *J. Voice* **2013**, *27*, 170–176. [CrossRef]
31. Pierce, J.L.; Tanner, K.; Merrill, R.M.; Shnowske, L.; Roy, N. A field-based approach to establish normative acoustic data for healthy female voices. *J. Speech Lang. Hear. Res.* **2021**, *64*, 691–706. [CrossRef]
32. Priya, K.; Vaishali, P.N.A.; Rajasekaran, S.; Balaji, D.; Navin, R.B.N. Assessment of effects on prolonged usage of face mask by ENT professionals during COVID-19 pandemic. *Indian. J. Otolaryngol. Head Neck Surg.* **2022**, *74*, 3173–3177. [CrossRef]
33. Ribeiro, V.V.; Dassie-Leite, A.P.; Pereira, E.C.; Santos, A.D.N.; Martins, P.; Irineu, R.A. Effect of wearing a face mask on vocal self-perception during a pandemic. *J. Voice* **2022**, *36*, 878.e1–878.e7. [CrossRef] [PubMed]
34. Karagkouni, O. The effects of the use of protective face mask on the voice and its relation to self-perceived voice changes. *J. Voice* **2022**, *in press*. [CrossRef] [PubMed]
35. Hamdan, A.L.; Jabbour, C.; Ghanem, A.; Ghanem, P. The impact of masking habits on voice in a sub-population of healthcare workers. *J. Voice* **2022**, *in press*. [CrossRef]
36. Patel, R.R.; Awan, S.N.; Barkmeier-Kraemer, J.; Courey, M.; Deliyski, D.; Eadie, T.; Paul, D.; Švec, J.G.; Hillman, R. Recommended protocols for instrumental assessment of voice: American Speech-Language-Hearing Association expert panel to develop a protocol for instrumental assessment of vocal function. *Am. J. Speech Lang. Pathol.* **2018**, *27*, 887–905. [CrossRef] [PubMed]
37. Tabah, A.; Ramanan, M.; Laupland, K.B.; Buetti, N.; Cortegiani, A.; Mellinghoff, J.; Conway Morris, A.; Camporota, L.; Zappella, N.; Elhadi, M.; et al. Personal protective equipment and intensive care unit healthcare worker safety in the COVID-19 era (PPE-SAFE): An international survey. *J. Crit. Care* **2020**, *59*, 70–75. [CrossRef] [PubMed]
38. Becker, K.; Gurzawska-Comis, K.; Brunello, G.; Klinge, B. Summary of European guidelines on infection control and prevention during COVID-19 pandemic. *Clin. Oral Implant. Res.* **2021**, *32*, 353–381. [CrossRef] [PubMed]
39. Lammers, M.J.W.; Lea, J.; Westerberg, B.D. Guidance for otolaryngology health care workers performing aerosol generating medical procedures during the COVID-19 pandemic. *J. Otolaryngol. Head Neck Surg.* **2020**, *49*, 36. [CrossRef] [PubMed]
40. Tunç-Songur, E.; Gölaç, H.; Önen, Ç.; Duyar, T.R.; Yılmaz, M.; Kemaloğlu, Y.K. How does long term use of surgical face mask affect the voice in normophonic Subjects? *J. Voice* **2023**, *in press*. [CrossRef]

Disclaimer/Publisher's Note: The statements, opinions and data contained in all publications are solely those of the individual author(s) and contributor(s) and not of MDPI and/or the editor(s). MDPI and/or the editor(s) disclaim responsibility for any injury to people or property resulting from any ideas, methods, instructions or products referred to in the content.

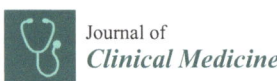
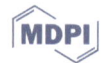

Article

A Pilot Study of the Effect of a Non-Contact Boxing Exercise Intervention on Respiratory Pressure and Phonation Aerodynamics in People with Parkinson's Disease

Christopher R. Watts [1,*], Zoë Thijs [2], Adam King [3], Joshua C. Carr [3] and Ryan Porter [3]

1. Davies School of Communication Sciences & Disorders, Texas Christian University, Fort Worth, TX 76109, USA
2. Department of Communication Sciences & Disorders, Molloy University, Rockville Centre, New York, NY 11570, USA; zthijs@molloy.edu
3. Department of Kinesiology, Texas Christian University, Fort Worth, TX 76109, USA; a.king@tcu.edu (A.K.); joshua.carr@tcu.edu (J.C.C.); r.porter@tcu.edu (R.P.)
* Correspondence: c.watts@tcu.edu

Abstract: This study investigated the effects of a non-contact boxing exercise program on maximum expiratory pressure and aerodynamic voice measurements. Methods: Eight adult males diagnosed with Parkinson's disease participated in the study. Individuals participated in twice-weekly exercise classes lasting one hour across 12-months. Dependent variables were measured on three baseline days and then at six additional time points. A pressure meter acquired maximum expiratory pressure, and a pneumotachograph system acquired transglottal airflow and subglottal air pressure. Results: Measures of average maximum expiratory pressure significantly increased after 9- and 12- months of exercise when compared to baseline. There was an increasing trend for these measures in all participants, with a corresponding large effect size. Measures of transglottal airflow and subglottal pressure did not change over the course of 9- or 12-months, although their stability may indicate that the exercise program influenced maintenance of respiratory-phonatory coordination during voicing. Conclusions: A non-contact boxing exercise program had a significant effect on maximum expiratory pressure in people with Parkinson's disease. The aerobic nature of the program and challenges to the respiratory muscles potentially explain the "ingredient" causing this effect. The small sample size of this pilot study necessitates future research incorporating larger and more diverse participants.

Keywords: dysphonia; Parkinson's disease; respiration

1. Introduction

Over 90% of all people with Parkinson's Disease (PWPD) are affected by impairments in their vocal function (i.e., dysphonia). PD dysphonia results in changes to vocal intensity, voice quality, and communication intelligibility that negatively impact activities of daily living and quality of life. The primary intervention for PD dysphonia is intensive exercise-based voice therapy, centered on increasing vocal intensity and delivered on a short-term (e.g., four weeks) high frequency (e.g., four times per week) schedule. Impairment of respiratory physiology is also a ubiquitous finding in PWPD and can contribute to the morbidity risk associated with aspiration pneumonia in later stages of the disease [1,2]. Even in the early stages, respiratory function can show impairment when measured in the context of maximum performance tasks such as expiratory and inspiratory pressure [3,4]. Decreases in maximum inspiratory pressure (MIP) and maximum expiratory pressure (MEP) in PD are thought to be associated with underlying respiratory muscle weakness and changes to central nervous system regulation of respiratory physiology. The generation of expiratory pressures is critical in airway safety associated with deglutition (e.g., for cough reflex subsequent to laryngeal penetration with or without aspiration) and also in voice production.

Voiced sounds are created through the conversion of respiratory and aerodynamic forces into sound energy. During vocal communication, activation of the respiratory muscles represents the initiation of a coordinated process of respiratory-laryngeal-vocal tract activity leading to the generation of subglottal pressure, transglottal airflow, and phonation to produce voiced acoustic energy [5]. Subglottal pressure and transglottal airflow are negatively impacted by PD and contribute to the characteristic hypophonia exemplified by low volume and breathy voice quality [6,7]. This dysphonia can be present in mild form at disease onset, but typically transitions to greater levels of severity as the disease progresses over time and will eventually impact over 70% of all people with PD (PWPD) [8,9].

Rehabilitative interventions can be effective for treating the diminished respiratory function and dysphonia of PWPD. Strong evidence has been associated with exercise-based interventions such as LSVT LOUD and a related approach, SPEAK OUT!, both of which require multiple sets and repetitions of different voice exercises over a prescribed high-intensity schedule lasting multiple weeks [10–12]. Another intervention utilizing the SpeechVive prosthetic device includes a form of daily exercise consisting of oral reading for 30 consecutive minutes while the device emits noise [13]. Research has found that all three of these interventions can elicit improvement of hypophonia in PD, and both LSVT LOUD and the SpeechVive device are associated with treatment-related changes in respiratory patterns and/or the aerodynamic forces underlying phonation [13–15].

Despite the neurodegenerative nature of the disease, people with PD retain the ability to positively adapt to the imposed demands of exercise. Consequently, exercise may promote neuroplasticity allowing the recovery or improvement in certain motor functions [16]. Exercise-based interventions hold the potential for meaningful disease modification of PD beyond impacts on voice and speech. In animal models, acute exercise resulted in neurogenesis, increased dopamine synthesis and release, and increased dopamine in the striatum [17]. Increased corticomotor excitability, elevated levels of brain-derived neurotrophic factors, and improved striatal dopamine receptor binding potential have been reported for individuals with PD who engage in long-term exercise interventions [18]. Sustained exercise over time also appears to facilitate changes in synaptic plasticity, preservation of dopaminergic cell bodies and terminals, while also bolstering levodopa efficacy [19,20]. Collectively, the functional improvements associated with exercise suggest the presence of neuroplasticity in motor-related circuitry and the ability of the brain to learn new behaviors through modification of existing neural networks. The sum of the cellular and molecular adaptations in PWPD is ultimately expressed through adaptations in the volitional neural drive during motor activity [21]. This may explain why exercise-based voice interventions modify neuromotor control of the respiratory and laryngeal subsystems underlying sound production, and why those modifications demonstrate long-term sustainability even when the formal exercise-based intervention period ends [10].

Exercise-based voice interventions are characterized by training specificity (voice-based exercises to improve voice production) which target respiratory, phonatory, and articulatory physiology [10,22,23]. Many other exercise-based interventions for PWPD, which are not specific to voice production or respiratory support for voice, have been developed for motor rehabilitation including cycling, dance, interval training, and, recently, non-contact boxing programs [23–26]. Non-contact boxing exercise programs may be ideally suited for PWPD because they incorporate multidimensional motor challenges that target the impairments of PD, including respiratory function (i.e., sustained aerobic activity requiring exertion of the respiratory muscles), speed of movement (i.e., speed bag punching drills), balance (i.e., footwork drills), strength (i.e., resistant training incorporated into the program), executive functions (i.e., sensory awareness of body positions), and they can be adapted to the physical abilities of the individual.

Evidence has shown that voice-based exercise interventions for PWPD can have carry-over or "spread" effects on swallowing function, even when swallowing is not specifically targeted [27]. However, we have limited knowledge as to whether other exercise intervention programs for PWPD, which are not specific to voice production, also demonstrate similar carryover effects on respiratory support and phonation physiology. To address this problem, the purpose of this pilot study was to investigate the effects of a non-contact boxing exercise program, called "Punching Out Parkinson's" (PoP), on measures of maximum expiratory pressure, subglottal air pressure, and transglottal airflow in PWPD. A longitudinal case series design was employed to follow participants who were new to participating in the exercise program across nine consecutive months and then again at twelve months. Our hypotheses were that the specificity of the non-contact boxing exercise program would show direct effects on maximum respiratory pressure and also show carryover effects on measures of subglottal air pressure and transglottal airflow during voice production.

2. Materials and Methods

Participants: Eight men with idiopathic Parkinson's disease (PD) served as participants for this study. All participants were diagnosed by a neurologist and were currently receiving dopamine-replacement therapy. At study onset, no participant had a neurological diagnosis other than PD, and none had participated in a non-contact boxing exercise program during the past six months. No participants were receiving speech-language therapy, all were ambulatory, and all were living at home in their communities. For inclusion, clearance by a physician to perform physical exercise was required in addition to screening with the Mini-Mental State examination (MMSE). Each participant also had to verify that they were able to attend two exercise classes per week in Fort Worth, TX. Participants were asked to schedule lab visits for assessment and measurement during times when their medication was effective (e.g., not close to the next dosage cycle).

Intervention: Participants engaged in a non-contact boxing exercise program ("Punching Out Parkinson's"—https://punchingoutparkinsons.org/) (accessed on 15 April 2022) developed by a former world champion professional boxer and adapted to meet the needs and abilities of people with PD at different levels of physiological impairment. The methodology of this program was the same as that reported by Salvatore et al., with each exercise session organized into seven stations across 60 min, with the duration of each station approximately the same [28]. The station components included warm up and cool down, resistance training, and aerobic exercise. The specific stations were warm up including stretching, footwork, heavy bag, hand mitts (manipulated by trainer), speed bag, resistance training, and a cool-down period. Participants engaged in each session as a group, and, other than warm-up and cool-down, the order of stations was rotated between participants. Each participant completed two exercise sessions every week across 12 consecutive months for a total of 120 exercise minutes per week, 480 min per month, and 5750 min total. The aerobic exercise component of each session has been estimated by Salvatore et al. at approximately 30 min per session, or one-half of the total exercise minutes [28].

Measurement Schedule: The study methodology was organized into four different stages (Figure 1): baseline (pre-intervention), an intervention onset period (months 1–2), an intervention maintenance period (months 3–9), and a follow-up period (month 12). All dependent variables were measured on three different baseline days prior to the start of intervention. Once the intervention was initiated, each participant was measured during the intervention onset stage at the end of months 1 and 2. During the intervention maintenance stage, participants were measured at the end of months 3, 6, and 9, and then again at month 12 for the follow-up period. This resulted in a total of 9 unique measurement periods (3 at baseline, 2 at intervention onset, 3 at intervention maintenance, and 1 at follow-up).

Data Acquisition: Measurement sessions for data acquisition were completed in a research laboratory on a university campus on non-exercise days. An assessment battery was employed to acquire data across multiple domains. These included:

- Respiratory pressure: Respiratory support for voice production was assessed via measures of maximum expiratory pressure (MEP), in cmH$_2$O, using the MicroRPM Pressure Meter (Micro Direct, Lewiston, ME). Participants were asked to maximally inhale to total lung capacity and then exhale hard and fast into the mouthpiece of the device while wearing a nose clip. Five consecutive trials were attempted. As this was a maximum performance task, the single maximum pressure from the five trials was recorded.

- Phonation (voicing) aerodynamics: Phonation aerodynamics were assessed via measures of transglottal airflow and subglottal pressure during speech tasks, using the Phonatory Aerodynamic System (PAS, Pentax Medical, Montvale, NJ, USA). For measures of transglottal airflow (in mL/s), voice waveforms were recorded while participants produced connected speech (the all-voiced sentence "We were away a year ago") at a self-reported comfortable pitch and loudness. For measures of subglottal pressure (in cmH_2O), participants repeated the syllable "pa" at a rate of approximately 1.5 syllables per second, at a self-reported comfortable pitch and loudness. Five trials of each transglottal airflow and subglottal pressure stimulus were recorded. The mean measurement for the five trials of each stimulus was calculated.

Analyses: Graphical visual inspection and effect size estimates were applied to the data sets of the three dependent variables separately (MEP, subglottal pressure, and transglottal airflow). For effect size, means and standard deviations of the 15 trials across the three baseline conditions were compared to the same measures of the trials across the intervention maintenance period (months 3, 6, and 9). For graphical analysis, each participant was treated as a single subject and their performance across the longitudinal study was graphed as a trend line representing that participant's unique data set. Non-parametric Wilcoxon signed-rank tests were applied to the data sets, with an alpha level of 0.05 for statistical significance. For each dependent variable, an ad-hoc effect size analysis comparing mean baseline measurements to those at the follow-up period (month 12) was also conducted to determine continuous maintenance or improvement of any potential gains.

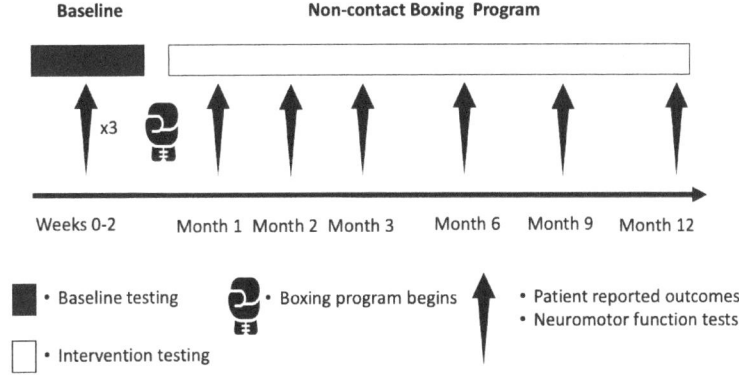

Figure 1. Visual form of study methodology and stages.

3. Results

Demographic information at study baseline associated with the eight male participants is reported in Table 1. Time since diagnosis ranged between 1 to 15 years with disease severity based on Hoehn and Yahr staging, ranging from stage 1 to stage 3. All participants were currently medicated with dopamine replacement, and none were currently enrolled in voice therapy nor had received voice therapy in the recent past. All participants were naive to the boxing exercise intervention program.

Table 1. Participant characteristics at study baseline (pre-intervention).

Participant	Current Age	Age at Diagnosis	MMSE Score	HY Stage	Dopamine Replacement	Current Speech Tx
1	66	66	25	2	Yes	No
2	64	59	30	1	Yes	No
3	82	81	28	3	Yes	No
4	74	62	27	3	Yes	No
5	64	58	28	1	Yes	No
6	63	62	30	3	Yes	No
7	66	51	30	3	Yes	No
8	62	57	25	1	Yes	No

Figures 2–4 illustrate individual participant data graphed together across all measurement intervals for measures of MEP, transglottal airflow, and subglottal pressure, respectively. At the end of 9 months of regular non-contact boxing exercise, all participants demonstrated an increase in MEP and maintained those gains above baseline at follow-up (Figure 2). While baseline performance was highly variable, Figure 2 shows a clear pattern of steady increase across exercise months for most participants. Similar baseline variability was present in transglottal airflow (Figure 3) and subglottal pressure (Figure 4), without any substantial increase or decrease for individual participants. For these two variables, the graphic data suggested that baseline performance was maintained at 9 months and also at the follow-up 12-month period.

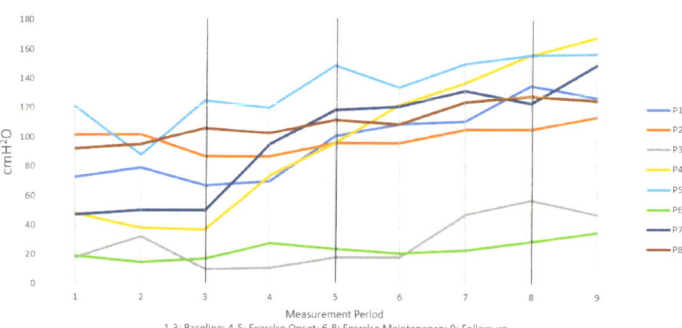

Figure 2. Longitudinal trends in measures of maximum expiratory pressure (MEP).

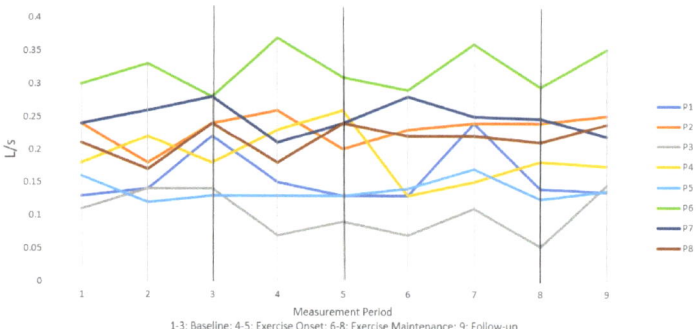

Figure 3. Longitudinal trends in measures of transglottal airflow.

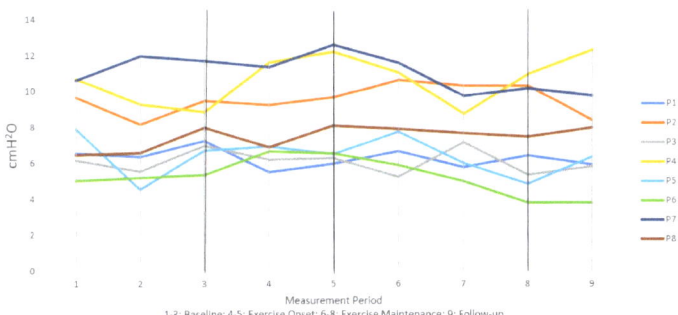

Figure 4. Longitudinal trends in measures of subglottal pressure.

Table 2 shows effect size measurements and significance of Wilcoxon signed-rank tests. At the 9-month period there was a significant effect of exercise on MEP with a large effect size. This increase over baseline was maintained with statistical significance at the 12-month follow-up period, again with a large effect size. Effect sizes for phonation physiology measures of transglottal airflow and subglottal pressure were small and not statistically significant at either the 9-month or 12-month period. This supported the notion that phonation physiology did not change, but performance was maintained, across 12 months of exercise.

Table 2. Means and standard deviations (in parentheses) for dependent variables at baseline, maintenance, and follow-up periods. Effect size data (d) are related to comparisons of baseline (mean of three baseline measurement days) to maintenance periods (mean of measurements at months 3, 6, and 9).

Dependent Variable	Baseline Days 1–3	Maintenance Months 3, 6, 9	Effect Size (d)	Significance	Follow-Up Month 12	Effect Size (d)
Respiratory Pressure (cmH_2O)	63.25 (36.7)	101.99 (45.12)	0.94	$p = 0.01$	115.25 (49.27)	1.19
Transglottal Airflow (L/s)	0.20 (0.05)	0.19 (0.07)	0.16	$p = 0.91$	0.20 (0.07)	0.01
Subglottal Pressure (cmH_2O)	8.03 (2.86)	7.76 (2.29)	0.10	$p = 0.99$	7.54 (2.65)	0.17

4. Discussion

The purpose of this pilot study was to investigate the effects of a non-contact boxing exercise program, called "Punching Out Parkinson's" (PoP), on measures of maximum expiratory pressure and phonation physiology measures of subglottal air pressure and transglottal airflow in PWPD. At 9-months of continuous exercise at a dose of 120 min per week, we found that all participants demonstrated increases in the ability to generate MEP, and those increases were maintained at 12-months while continuing the exercise program. While there were no changes in the aerodynamics of phonation, the stability of these measures at 9-month and 12-month periods in relation to baseline abilities may be a positive finding, as phonation physiology is known to change as PD progresses over time.

The positive impact of a non-contact boxing exercise program on respiratory function may have practical significance as a non-pharmacological intervention for PD. Respiratory dysfunction in the form of inhalation and exhalation muscle weakness is a common manifestation of the disease and is strongly associated with mortality in people with PD via a connection with pneumonia [29,30]. A recent metanalysis comparing 253 PWPD to 181 controls across seven studies found significantly and substantially lower MEP in those with PD. The same metanalysis reported significantly lower measures of peak cough flow, which is associated with the ability to clear foreign material from the lower respiratory tract, in PWPD compared to controls [31]. Expected normal values of MEP in adult males is at or above 80 cmH$_2$O [31,32]. Across the eight participants in the present study, average MEP at baseline was at 63 cmH$_2$O and increased to over 100 cmH$_2$O after 9 months of exercise, which was maintained at the 12-month period. This finding suggests that the non-contact boxing exercise program may directly address the underlying respiratory muscle weakness that is a substantial health risk factor in people with PD.

The "ingredients" of the specific exercise program studied in this investigation provides a potential explanation for the reported positive effect on respiratory function. Non-contact boxing presents an aerobic challenge to the cardiovascular system [28]. This challenge requires engagement of respiratory muscles to alter breathing cycles via faster and deeper breaths. The resistance training element specific to the PoP exercise program may have also facilitated adaptation in the respiratory muscles through increased activation of inspiratory and expiratory muscles during pushing/pulling movements. The frequency (two times per week), intensity (1-h sessions), and duration (9 months) of the PoP program was enough to elicit large increases in MEP through specific targeting of the muscles responsible for baseline respiratory weakness.

This study did not find changes to measures of phonation physiology. Both transglottal airflow and subglottal pressure varied little among the participants across the 12-month study period. While this suggests that the non-contact boxing exercise program did not have any carryover effects on voice production, it should also be noted that the PoP program was not specific to vocal function. That is, voicing and voice exercises were not a component of the exercise program, which may explain the lack of significant effect. On the other hand, it is important to note that neither measure deteriorated from baseline in any substantial way for any participant. While further research is needed to investigate this supposition, the physical challenges of the PoP exercise program may have supported maintenance of respiratory-phonatory coordination as measured with transglottal airflow and subglottal pressure. In this way, non-contact boxing may have been disease modifying for MEP (increasing motor ability) and phonation physiology (maintaining motor ability).

There are a number of limitations to this study which necessitate guarded generalizations. While the experimental design demonstrated significant increases in respiratory power associated with the exercise intervention, we did not control for other physical activities outside of the exercise program that could have also impacted respiratory function. Because exercise has been shown to consistently impact motor abilities in PWPD, activities outside of the intervention should be controlled for or considered in future studies. Each individual was also measured using the same procedures on nine different occasions, which could have facilitated learning effects and the subsequent data set. While no individuals were receiving voice therapy, we also did not control for the amount of talking/voicing that each participant engaged in during activities of daily living, and it is possible that non-voice and non-exercise activities could have influenced study results. The sample size of eight participants was very small and, although we realized strong statistical power, the sample may not be representative of the larger population of PWPD. We also only studied male participants, and whether females with PD respond in the same way to non-contact boxing exercise will need further study. In addition, we did not control for medication timing during exercise. While laboratory measurements were obtained at self-reported times of medication effectiveness, we do not know if medication timing influenced exercise activity (e.g., exertion levels) during individual sessions, and if that potential effect may have influenced results.

5. Conclusions

This study found that a non-contact boxing exercise program, PoP, had a significant effect on MEP in eight males with PD. While there was no effect on measures of phonation physiology, there were also no declines in those measures across the 9-month and 12-month time periods. After 9-months of exercise, the average MEP elevated from below normal thresholds to above normal thresholds, with an increasing trend of MEP was found for all eight participants. The positive results of this pilot study may inform future research seeking to investigate the effects of physical exercise on motor and non-motor abilities of people with PD.

Author Contributions: Conceptualization, C.R.W., Z.T., A.K., J.C.C. and R.P.; supervision, C.R.W.; methodology, C.R.W., Z.T., A.K., J.C.C. and R.P.; Project administration, C.R.W. and Z.T.; Data curation, C.R.W. and Z.T.; formal analysis, C.R.W. and Z.T.; writing—original draft preparation, C.R.W. and Z.T.; writing—review and editing, A.K., J.C.C. and R.P. All authors have read and agreed to the published version of the manuscript.

Funding: This research received no external funding.

Institutional Review Board Statement: The study was conducted in accordance with the Declaration of Helsinki and approved by the Institutional Review Board (or Ethics Committee) of Texas Christian University (protocol code TCU IRB# 2021-108; approved 11 February 2021).

Informed Consent Statement: Informed consent was obtained from all subjects involved in the study.

Data Availability Statement: The original contributions presented in the study are included in the article; further inquiries can be directed to the corresponding author.

Acknowledgments: The authors would like to acknowledge the following research assistants who assisted in data collection for this study: Caleb Voskuil, Malia Shipsey, Emily Watts, and Kuanting Chen.

Conflicts of Interest: The authors declare no conflict of interest.

References

1. Guilherme, E.M.; Moreira, R.D.F.C.; de Oliveira, A.; Ferro, A.M.; Di Lorenzo, V.A.P.; Gianlorenço, A.C.L. Respiratory Disorders in Parkinson's Disease. *J. Park. Dis.* **2021**, *11*, 993–1010. [CrossRef]
2. Akbar, U.; Dham, B.; He, Y.; Hack, N.; Wu, S.; Troche, M.; Tighe, P.; Nelson, E.; Friedman, J.H.; Okun, M.S. Incidence and mortality trends of aspiration pneumonia in Parkinson's disease in the United States, 1979–2010. *Park. Relat. Disord.* **2015**, *21*, 1082–1086. [CrossRef] [PubMed]
3. Zhang, W.; Zhang, L.; Zhou, N.; Huang, E.; Li, Q.; Wang, T.; Ma, C.; Li, B.; Li, C.; Du, Y.; et al. Dysregulation of Respiratory Center Drive (P0.1) and Muscle Strength in Patients with Early Stage Idiopathic Parkinson's Disease. *Front. Neurol.* **2019**, *10*, 724. [CrossRef] [PubMed]
4. Baille, G.; Perez, T.; Devos, D.; Deken, V.; Defebvre, L.; Moreau, C. Early occurrence of inspiratory muscle weakness in Parkinson's disease. *PLoS ONE* **2018**, *13*, e0190400. [CrossRef] [PubMed]
5. Watts, C.R.; Awan, S.N. *Laryngeal Function and Voice Disorders: Basic Science to Clinical Practice*; Thieme Medical Publishers: New York, NY, USA, 2019.
6. Matheron, D.; Stathopoulos, E.T.; Huber, J.E.; Sussman, J.E. Laryngeal Aerodynamics in Healthy Older Adults and Adults with Parkinson's Disease. *J. Speech Lang. Hear. Res.* **2017**, *60*, 507–524. [CrossRef]
7. Burk, B.R.; Watts, C.R. The Effect of Parkinson Disease Tremor Phenotype on Cepstral Peak Prominence and Transglottal Airflow in Vowels and Speech. *J. Voice* **2018**, *33*, 580.e11–580.e19. [CrossRef]
8. Watts, C.R.; Zhang, Y. Progression of Self-Perceived Speech and Swallowing Impairment in Early Stage Parkinson's Disease: Longitudinal Analysis of the Unified Parkinson's Disease Rating Scale. *J. Speech Lang. Hear. Res.* **2022**, *65*, 146–158. [CrossRef]
9. Hartelius, L.; Svensson, P. Speech and swallowing symptoms associated with Parkinson's disease and multiple sclerosis: A survey. *Folia Phoniatr. Logop.* **1994**, *46*, 9–17. [CrossRef]
10. Ramig, L.; Halpern, A.; Ma, C.J.S.; Fox, C.; Freeman, K. Speech treatment in Parkinson's disease: Randomized controlled trial (RCT). *Mov. Disord.* **2018**, *33*, 1777–1791. [CrossRef]
11. Behrman, A.; Cody, J.; Elandary, S.; Flom, P.; Chitnis, S. The Effect of SPEAK OUT! and The LOUD Crowd on Dysarthria Due to Parkinson's Disease. *Am. J. Speech-Lang. Pathol.* **2020**, *29*, 1448–1465. [CrossRef]
12. Watts, C.R. A Retrospective Study of Long-Term Treatment Outcomes for Reduced Vocal Intensity in Hypokinetic Dysarthria. *BMC Ear Nose Throat Disord.* **2016**, *16*, 2. [CrossRef]
13. Richardson, K.; Huber, J.E.; Kiefer, B.; Kane, C.; Snyder, S. Respiratory Responses to Two Voice Interventions for Parkinson's Disease. *J. Speech Lang. Hear. Res.* **2022**, *65*, 3730–3748. [CrossRef] [PubMed]
14. Stathopoulos, E.T.; Huber, J.E.; Richardson, K.; Kamphaus, J.; DeCicco, D.; Darling, M.; Fulcher, K.; Sussman, J.E. Increased vocal intensity due to the Lombard effect in speakers with Parkinson's disease: Simultaneous laryngeal and respiratory strategies. *J. Commun. Disord.* **2013**, *48*, 1–17. [CrossRef] [PubMed]
15. Ramig, L.O.; Dromey, C. Aerodynamic mechanisms underlying treatment-related changes in vocal intensity in patients with Parkinson disease. *J. Speech Lang. Hear. Res.* **1996**, *39*, 798–807. [CrossRef]

16. Johansson, H.; Hagströmer, M.; Grooten, W.J.A.; Franzén, E. Exercise-Induced Neuroplasticity in Parkinson's Disease: A Metasynthesis of the Literature. *Neural Plast.* **2020**, *2020*, 8961493. [CrossRef]
17. Meeusen, R.; De Meirleir, K. Exercise and brain neurotransmission. *Sports Med.* **1995**, *20*, 160–188. [CrossRef] [PubMed]
18. Mak, M.; Wong-Yu, I.S.; Shen, X.; Chung, C.L.-H. Long-term effects of exercise and physical therapy in people with Parkinson disease. *Nat. Rev. Neurol.* **2017**, *13*, 689–703. [CrossRef]
19. Tillerson, J.; Caudle, W.; Reverón, M.; Miller, G. Exercise induces behavioral recovery and attenuates neurochemical deficits in rodent models of Parkinson's disease. *Neuroscience* **2003**, *119*, 899–911. [CrossRef]
20. Muhlack, S.; Welnic, J.; Woitalla, D.; Müller, T. Exercise improves efficacy of levodopa in patients with Parkinson's disease. *Mov. Disord.* **2007**, *22*, 427–430. [CrossRef]
21. Helgerud, J.; Thomsen, S.N.; Hoff, J.; Strandbråten, A.; Leivseth, G.; Unhjem, R.J.; Wang, E. Maximal strength training in patients with Parkinson's disease: Impact on efferent neural drive, force generating capacity, and functional performance. *J. Appl. Physiol.* **2020**, *129*, 683–690. [CrossRef] [PubMed]
22. Tamplin, J.; Morris, M.E.; Marigliani, C.; Baker, F.A.; Noffs, G.; Vogel, A.P. ParkinSong: Outcomes of a 12-Month Controlled Trial of Therapeutic Singing Groups in Parkinson's Disease. *J. Park. Dis.* **2020**, *10*, 1217–1230. [CrossRef] [PubMed]
23. Stegemöller, E.L.; Radig, H.; Hibbing, P.; Wingate, J.; Sapienza, C. Effects of singing on voice, respiratory control and quality of life in persons with Parkinson's disease. *Disabil. Rehabil.* **2016**, *39*, 594–600. [CrossRef] [PubMed]
24. Domingos, J.; Radder, D.; Riggare, S.; Godinho, C.; Dean, J.; Graziano, M.; de Vries, N.M.; Ferreira, J.; Bloem, B.R. Implementation of a Community-Based Exercise Program for Parkinson Patients: Using Boxing as an Example. *J. Park. Dis.* **2019**, *9*, 615–623. [CrossRef]
25. Combs, S.A.; Diehl, M.D.; Chrzastowski, C.; Didrick, N.; McCoin, B.; Mox, N.; Staples, W.H.; Wayman, J. Community-based group exercise for persons with Parkinson disease: A randomized controlled trial. *Neurorehabilitation* **2013**, *32*, 117–124. [CrossRef]
26. Combs, S.A.; Diehl, M.D.; Staples, W.H.; Conn, L.; Davis, K.; Lewis, N.; Schaneman, K. Boxing training for patients with Parkinson disease: A Case Series. *Phys. Ther.* **2011**, *91*, 132–142. [CrossRef] [PubMed]
27. Miles, A.; Jardine, M.; Johnston, F.; de Lisle, M.; Friary, P.; Allen, J. Effect of Lee Silverman Voice Treatment (LSVT LOUD®) on swallowing and cough in Parkinson's disease: A pilot study. *J. Neurol. Sci.* **2017**, *383*, 180–187. [CrossRef]
28. Salvatore, M.F.; Soto, I.; Kasanga, E.A.; James, R.; Shifflet, M.K.; Doshier, K.; Little, J.T.; John, J.; Alphonso, H.M.; Cunningham, J.T.; et al. Establishing Equivalent Aerobic Exercise Parameters Between Early-Stage Parkinson's Disease and Pink1 Knockout Rats. *J. Park. Dis.* **2022**, *12*, 1897–1915. [CrossRef]
29. Bugalho, P.; Ladeira, F.; Barbosa, R.; Marto, J.P.; Borbinha, C.; Salavisa, M.; da Conceição, L.; Saraiva, M.; Fernandes, M.; Meira, B. Motor and non-motor function predictors of mortality in Parkinson's disease. *J. Neural Transm.* **2019**, *126*, 1409–1415. [CrossRef]
30. Fernandez, H.H.; Lapane, K.L. Predictors of mortality among nursing home residents with a diagnosis of Parkinson's disease. *Med. Sci. Monit.* **2002**, *8*, CR241–CR246.
31. McMahon, L.; Blake, C.; Lennon, O. A systematic review and meta-analysis of respiratory dysfunction in Parkinson's disease. *Eur. J. Neurol.* **2023**, *30*, 1481–1504. [CrossRef]
32. Black, L.F.; Hyatt, R.E. Maximal respiratory pressures: Normal values and relationship to age and sex. *Am. Rev. Respir. Dis.* **1969**, *99*, 696–702. [CrossRef] [PubMed]

Disclaimer/Publisher's Note: The statements, opinions and data contained in all publications are solely those of the individual author(s) and contributor(s) and not of MDPI and/or the editor(s). MDPI and/or the editor(s) disclaim responsibility for any injury to people or property resulting from any ideas, methods, instructions or products referred to in the content.

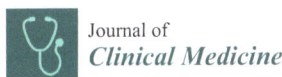

Article

The Efficacy of Different Voice Treatments for Vocal Fold Polyps: A Systematic Review and Meta-Analysis

Ben Barsties v. Latoszek [1,*], Christopher R. Watts [2], Svetlana Hetjens [3,†] and Katrin Neumann [4,†]

1. Speech-Language Pathology, SRH University of Applied Health Sciences, 40210 Düsseldorf, Germany
2. Harris College of Nursing & Health Sciences, Texas Christian University, Fort Worth, TX 76109, USA
3. Department for Medical Statistics and Biomathematics, Medical Faculty Mannheim, University of Heidelberg, 68165 Mannheim, Germany
4. Department of Phoniatrics and Pediatric Audiology, University Hospital Münster, University of Münster, 48149 Münster, Germany; katrin.neumann@uni-muenster.de
* Correspondence: benjamin.barstiesvonlatoszek@srh.de
† These authors contributed equally to this work.

Abstract: Background: Vocal fold polyps (VFP) are a common cause of voice disorders and laryngeal discomfort. They are usually treated by behavioral voice therapy (VT) or phonosurgery, or a combination (CT) of both. However, the superiority of either of these treatments has not been clearly established. Methods: Three databases were searched from inception to October 2022 and a manual search was performed. All clinical trials of VFP treatment were included that reported at least auditory–perceptual judgment, aerodynamics, acoustics, and the patient-perceived handicap. Results: We identified 31 eligible studies (VT: n = 47–194; phonosurgery: n = 404–1039; CT: n = 237–350). All treatment approaches were highly effective, with large effect sizes ($d > 0.8$) and significant improvements in almost all voice parameters (p-values < 0.05). Phonosurgery reduced roughness and NHR, and the emotional and functional subscales of the VHI-30 were the most compared to behavioral voice therapy and combined treatment (p-values < 0.001). Combined treatment improved hoarseness, jitter, shimmer, MPT, and the physical subscale of the VHI-30 more than phonosurgery and behavioral voice therapy (p-values < 0.001). Conclusions: All three treatment approaches were effective in eliminating vocal fold polyps or their negative sequelae, with phonosurgery and combined treatment providing the greatest improvement. These results may inform future treatment decisions for patients with vocal fold polyps.

Keywords: vocal fold polyp; voice treatment; voice therapy; surgery; auditory–perceptual judgment; jitter; shimmer; maximum phonation time; voice handicap index

1. Introduction

Vocal fold polyps (VFP) are functional voice disorders associated with benign tissue changes to the vocal folds. They are commonly unilateral. Their shape can be classified as sessile or peduncular; their morphological characteristics can be classified as gelatinous or translucent, fibrous or organized, and angiomatous or hemorrhagic [1]. Their size can vary from small to medium to large ($<1/4$ of the vocal fold length, $1/4$–$1/3$, $>1/3$) [2]. In some regions, VFP is among the five most common laryngeal diseases, with prevalence figures of 0.4–9% [3–5]. VFP are caused primarily by a coincidence of non-physiologic voice use, i.e., "phonotrauma" (inflammatory response of the vocal fold mucosa to biomechanical stress and deformations during high-effort vibration) often associated with yelling or awkward singing, and other etiological factors such as upper respiratory tract infections, allergies, gastroesophageal reflux, and smoking [1,6]. Patients with VFP can experience significant impairment in phonation and communication, with negative social implications. Usually, voice complaints due to VFP involve dysphonia, increased vocal effort, and decreased vocal stamina. Dysphonia associated with VFP results from complex changes in the vibrational patterns of the vocal folds through alterations in their layered structure and stiffness of tissue. VFP require multidimensional voice assessments (vocal fold imaging, auditory–perceptual judgment, acoustic and aerodynamic measurements, and patients' self-evaluation) [7]. Their results may be influenced by the size, form, mass, and base length of the polyp and the resulting changing area and shape of the glottal gap during phonation [8]. In the treatment of VFPs, phonosurgery is often the first choice [9,10], but behavioral voice therapy (VT) is also recommended as an effective treatment modality, either as a stand-alone treatment or combined with phonosurgery [11]. The efficacy of VT can be explained, in part, by a causal role of hypertension of the laryngeal musculature and, in particular, supraglottic structures in the development of the polyps. Although clinical guidelines recommend treating VFP conservatively first and resecting them secondarily only if results are unsatisfactory, the efficacy of phonosurgery as a primary treatment option for VFP has been confirmed by observational studies [12]. The recurrence rate of VFP after surgery has been reported as low (11%) and not influenced by gender but by age (younger adults have a significantly higher relapse rate than middle-aged or older adults) [13]. The choice of treatment option for VFP is important because either the risks and costs of surgery can be avoided if VT is the treatment of first choice or phonosurgery can lead to the faster recovery of vocal function. Therefore, the aim of this meta-analysis was to compare the efficacy of phonosurgery, VT, and a combination of both (CT) in the treatment of VFP based on multidimensional voice assessments pre- and post-treatment.

2. Materials and Methods

2.1. Data Sources and Searches

We followed the Preferred Reporting Items for Systematic Reviews and Meta-Analyses (PRISMA) guidelines [14] and systematically searched four databases (MEDLINE, CENTRAL, CINAHL, and KoreaScience) from inception to 26 October 2022 (Table S1, Supplementary Materials). Potentially eligible publications, including those published in different languages from the above databases, were identified by title and abstract. In addition, a manual search of congress proceedings, grey literature, and bibliographies was performed.

2.2. Study Selection

All available intervention trials with a pre-post design for VFP using phonosurgery alone, VT alone, or a combination with initial phonosurgery followed by VT were included in the search. According to a preliminary search, the combination of initial VT followed by phonosurgery (investigated minimally in multiple case studies) was low (n = 1); thus, we excluded it from our meta-analysis. The clinical parameters of this meta-analysis included the most commonly used quantitative measures of an internationally agreed battery of voice examinations [7]: auditory–perceptual voice assessment (hoarseness, breathiness, roughness) by at least one examiner using a Likert scale ranging from 0 (no impairment) to 3 (maximum impairment), acoustic (jitter, shimmer, noise-to-harmonics ratio NHR) and aerodynamic (maximum phonation time, MPT) measures, and a standardized questionnaire for the self-assessment of voice handicap. To avoid specification and reliability differences due to the application of different acoustic software packages, only studies that performed acoustic measurements with the Multi-Dimensional Voice Program (Kay Elemetrics Corporation, Lincoln Park, NJ, USA) were included. To make self-assessments of vocal handicap comparable, we included only studies that assessed it with the most widely used international standardized questionnaire, the 30-item Voice Handicap Index (VHI—30) [15], which outputs three subscales with statements on physical (P), functional (F), and emotional (E) domains and a total score (T). Studies eligible for the meta-analysis had to involve at least one of the aforementioned measures.

2.3. Risk of Bias Assessments

The risk of bias assessment of the included studies was determined using the RoB 2 tool [16] for randomized studies (overall risk ranging from low to some concerns to high) and ROBINS-I tool [17] for non-randomized studies (overall risk ranging from low to moderate to serious to critical to no information).

2.4. Statistics

Statistical analyses were completed using MedCalc software (version 19.6) and SAS software, release 9.4 (Cary, NC, USA). At first, the difference between the mean values $\bar{x}_{post} - \bar{x}_{pre}$ and standard error (SE) was calculated as $SE = \frac{(S_1+S_2)/2}{\sqrt{n}}$. Thereafter, the meta-analysis with weighting based on the random effects model was performed using MedCalc software (version 19.6) by treatment and dysphonia measures. The mean pre-post treatment differences of voice measures with a 95% confidence interval (95% CI) per study and pooled analyses are shown in forest plots. The heterogeneity of studies was calculated using the I^2 index (0–25% insignificant, >25–50% low, >50–75% moderate, >75% high heterogeneity) [18]. The random effects model was used to analyze the pooled data, accounting for heterogeneity between studies. Studies were weighted according to DerSimonian and Laird [19]. Potential publication bias was analyzed using Egger's test [20].

To potentially reduce heterogeneity in treatment outcomes and refine them, four subgroup analyses were performed for phonosurgery and CT (fewer studies were available for VT). Subgroup 1 was formed according to the time interval between pre- and postoperative measurements for polyp resection, divided into three follow-up periods: ≤1 month; 1–2 months; ≥3 months. Subgroup 2 was established by the type of three phonosurgical techniques used: cold knife; laser; a combination of cold knife and laser. Subgroup 3 was based on one of two types of surgical techniques combined with VT: cold knife; laser. Subgroup 4 was defined according to one of two durations of VT after phonosurgery: 1–2 weeks; >3 weeks.

A network meta-analysis between treatment approaches was then conducted using SAS software. This involved comparing the pooled mean pre-to-post-treatment differences among the three interventions, along with their confidence intervals, using the Satterthwaite *t*-test. In case of a significant result, the ranking of treatment was based on the highest mean pre- to post-treatment difference in results. Cohen's *d* was calculated as the effect size of treatment approaches and voice measures, whereby convention 0.2–0.5 is considered a small effect, 0.5–0.7 is considered a medium effect, and >0.8 is considered a large effect [21].

3. Results

We identified 234 non-duplicates from our searches (Figure 1). Of these, 31 studies were eligible for inclusion in this review (Table 1) [22–52]. The results of the risk of bias analysis are shown in Table S2, Supplementary Materials. For the randomized trials, the risk of bias was low for one study [42] and some concerns existed for two studies [35,39]. For the observational studies, the overall risk of bias was low for one study [40], moderate for nine studies [28,29,33,37,41,43,50–52], and serious for eighteen studies [22–28,30–32,34,36,44–49]. The results of the meta-analysis with heterogeneity statistics and publication bias analyses are shown in Table S3, Supplementary Materials.

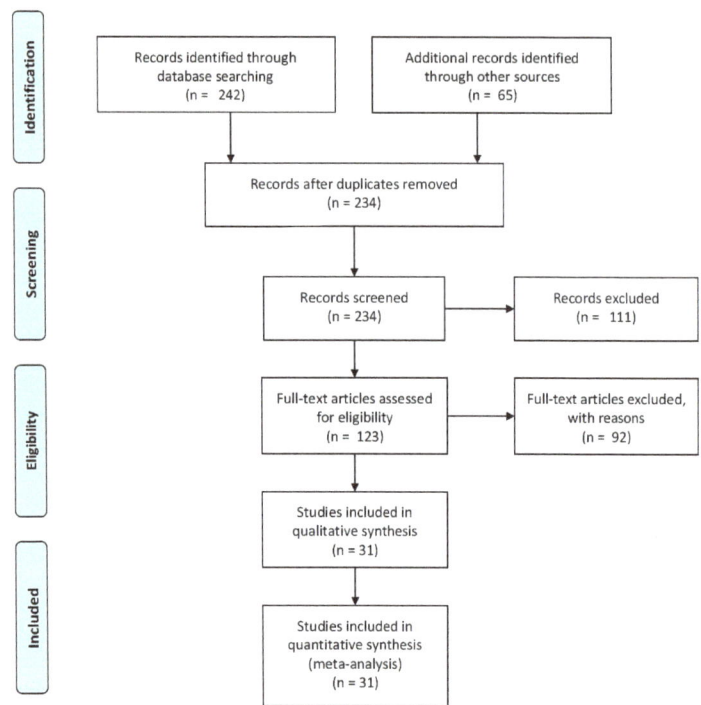

Figure 1. PRISMA flow diagram.

Table 1. Characteristics of clinical trials in the meta-analysis.

Study	Type and Features of VFP	N	Intervention Groups	Interventions with Durations Between Pre- and Post-Treatment	Duration of Voice Therapy in Weeks	Outcome Measures
Kim et al. (1999) [22]	All types and features of VFP	58	Phonosurgery	Treatment method: cold knife Duration: 2 months	n.a.	Jitter Shimmer NHR MPT
Kim & Auo (2008) [23]	All types and features of VFP	62	Phonosurgery	Treatment method: 585 nm pulsed dye laser (office-based) Duration: 2 months	n.a.	Jitter Shimmer NHR G, R, B
Kluch & Olszewski (2008) [24]	All types and features of VFP	16	Combination of phonosurgery and voice therapy	Treatment method: cold knife or CO_2 laser using microlaryngoscopy under general anesthesia, and breathing and voice exercises Duration: > 1 month	4 weeks	G, R, B
Kim et al. (2008) [25]	Unilateral; all sizes and features of VFP	8	Phonosurgery	Treatment method: cold knife Duration: 2–3 months	n.a.	VHI-T
Kluch & Olszewski (2009) [26]	All types and features of VFP	25	Combination of phonosurgery and voice therapy	Treatment method: cold knife or CO_2 laser using microlaryngoscopy under general anesthesia, and breathing and voice exercises Duration: >1 month	4 weeks	G, R, B

Table 1. Cont.

Study	Type and Features of VFP	N	Intervention Groups	Interventions with Durations Between Pre- and Post-Treatment	Duration of Voice Therapy in Weeks	Outcome Measures
Kim et al. (2009) [27]	Small VFP	33	Voice therapy	Treatment method: Vocal hygiene and Seong-Tae Kim's multiple voice therapy technique Duration: >1 month	4 to 16 weeks	Jitter Shimmer NHR MPT
Choi et al. (2011) [28]	All types and features of VFP	128	Phonosurgery	Treatment method: cold knife Duration: >1 month	n.a.	Jitter Shimmer NHR MPT
Petrovic-Lazic et al. (2011) [29]	All types and features of VFP	46	Phonosurgery	Treatment method: cold knife Duration: 3 weeks	n.a.	Jitter Shimmer NHR
Ju et al. (2013) [30]	All types and features of VFP	118	(a) Phonosurgery (n = 63) (b) Combination of phonosurgery and voice therapy (n = 55)	(a) Treatment method: cold knife (a) Duration: 2 months (b) Treatment method: cold knife, vocal hygiene, and resonant voice (b) Duration: 2 months	(a) n.a. (b) 1 week	Jitter Shimmer NHR MPT VHI-T, VHI-P, VHI-F, VHI-E G, R, B
Schindler et al. (2013) [31]	All types and features of gelatinous VFP	20	Voice therapy	Treatment method: vocal hygiene, abdominal breathing, resonant voice, yawn sigh approach, and manual therapy Duration: 1–2 months	1 to 2 months	Jitter Shimmer NHR MPT VHI-T, VHI-P, VHI-F, VHI-E G, R, B
Choe et al. (2013) [32]	Unilateral; no giant VFP but other types and features	41	Combination of phonosurgery and voice therapy (two groups)	Treatment method: CO_2 laser using microlaryngoscopy under general anesthesia or cold knife, vocal hygiene, and resonant voice Duration: 7 weeks	4 weeks	Jitter Shimmer NHR MPT VHI-T, VHI-P, VHI-F, VHI-E
Wang et al. (2013) [33]	Unilateral; hemorrhagic small to medium vocal polyps	36	Phonosurgery (two groups)	Treatment method: KTP laser (office-based) or KTP plus cold knife using microlaryngoscopy under general anesthesia Duration: 6 weeks	n.a.	Jitter Shimmer NHR MPT
Karasu et al. (2014) [34]	All types and features of VFP	51	Phonosurgery (two groups)	Treatment method: diode laser using microlaryngoscopy under general anesthesia or cold knife Duration: 2 months	n.a.	Jitter Shimmer NHR VHI-T, VHI-P, VHI-F, VHI-E
Lin et al. (2014) [35]	Unilateral; all sizes and features of VFP	60	(a) Phonosurgery (n = 30) (b) Combination of phonosurgery and voice therapy (n = 30)	(a) Treatment method: CO_2 laser using microlaryngoscopy under general anesthesia (a) Duration: 5–12 weeks (b) Treatment method: CO_2 laser using microlaryngoscopy under general anesthesia, vocal hygiene, relaxation training, breathing training, yawn sigh approach, chewing approach, and tone sandhi pronunciation (b) Duration: 5–12 weeks	(a) n.a. (b) 4 weeks	Jitter Shimmer NHR MPT VHI-T G, R, B

Table 1. Cont.

Study	Type and Features of VFP	N	Intervention Groups	Interventions with Durations Between Pre- and Post-Treatment	Duration of Voice Therapy in Weeks	Outcome Measures
Wang et al. (2015) [36]	Small to medium sizes and all features of VFP	34	Phonosurgery (two groups)	Treatment method: KTP2 laser (office-based) or cold knife Duration: 6 weeks	n.a.	Jitter Shimmer NHR MPT
Mizuta et al. (2015) [37]	All types and features of VFP	54	Phonosurgery (two groups)	Treatment method: angiolytic laser (office-based) or cold knife Duration: 6 weeks	n.a.	Jitter Shimmer MPT
Petrovic-Lazic et al. (2015) [38]	Medium sizes and all features of VFP	41	Combination of phonosurgery and voice therapy	Treatment method: cold knife and voice therapy Duration: 6 weeks	4 weeks	Jitter Shimmer NHR G, R, B
Zhang et al. (2015) [39]	Bilateral; all sizes and features of VFP	60	Phonosurgery (two groups)	Treatment method: CO_2 laser using microlaryngoscopy under general anesthesia or cold knife Duration: 3 months	n.a.	Jitter Shimmer NHR MPT VHI-T G, R, B
Lee et al. (2016) [40]	Unilateral; all sizes and diffuse or pedunculated growths of VFP	23	Phonosurgery	Treatment method: cold knife Duration: 2 months	n.a.	Jitter Shimmer NHR MPT VHI-T
Zhuge et al. (2016) [41]	Small fusiform translucent bulge unilateral or bilateral VFP located at the junction of 1/3 of the front and the middle of the vocal fold	66	Voice therapy	Treatment method: relaxation training, breathing exercises, vocal function exercises, resonant voice, and vocal hygiene Duration: 3 months	12 weeks	MPT VHI-T, VHI-P, VHI-F, VHI-E
Barillari et al. (2017) [42]	Unilateral; all sizes and features of the VFP at the free edge of the vocal fold	140	(a) Voice therapy (n = 70) (b) Combination of phonosurgery and voice therapy (n = 70)	(a) Treatment method: voice therapy expulsion (a) Duration: 3 months (b) Treatment method: CO_2 laser using microlaryngoscopy under general anesthesia, vocal hygiene, relaxation training, vocal function exercises, and breath support (b) Duration: 6 weeks	(a) 12 weeks (b) 4 weeks	VHI-T G
You et al. (2017) [43]	VFP that were smooth and had translucent pedunculated neoplasm or fusiform translucent smooth neoplasm with a wider base by the free edge of the vocal folds	96	(a) Phonosurgery (n = 41) (b) Combination of phonosurgery and voice therapy (n = 55)	(a) Treatment method: cold knife (a) Duration: 4 months (b) Treatment method: cold knife, vocal hygiene, relaxation training, vocal function exercises, breathing exercises, and resonant voice (b) Duration: 4 months	(a) n.a. (b) 12 weeks	MPT VHI-T, VHI-P, VHI-F, VHI-E
Lin et al. (2018) [44]	All types and features of VFP	90	Phonosurgery (two groups)	Treatment method: KTP laser (office-based) or cold knife Duration: 1–2 months	n.a.	Jitter Shimmer NHR MPT

Table 1. Cont.

Study	Type and Features of VFP	N	Intervention Groups	Interventions with Durations Between Pre- and Post-Treatment	Duration of Voice Therapy in Weeks	Outcome Measures
Sahin et al. (2018) [45]	All types and features of VFP	165	(a) Phonsurgery (n = 138) (b) Voice therapy (n = 27)	(a) Treatment method: cold knife (a) Duration: > 3 months (b) Treatment method: vocal hygiene, relaxation training, vocal function exercises, breathing and posture exercises, and resonant voice (b) Duration: 4 months	(a) n.a. (b) 16 weeks	Jitter Shimmer NHR G, R, B
Oh et al. (2018) [46]	Unilateral; all sizes and features of VFP	130	(a) Phonsurgery (n= 44) (b) Combination of phonosurgery and voice therapy (two groups; n = 86)	(a) Treatment method: cold knife (a) Duration: 1 month (b) Treatment method: cold knife and vocal hygiene or cold knife and relaxation training, vocal function exercises, breathing exercises, resonant voice, and manual therapy (b) Duration: 4 months	(a) n.a. (b) 1–4 weeks	Jitter Shimmer NHR MPT VHI-T, VHI-P, VHI-F, VHI-E G, R, B,
Wang et al. (2019) [47]	Small fusiform translucent bulge VFP's located at the junction of 1/3 of the front and the middle of the vocal fold	69	(a) Phonsurgery (n = 31) (b) Voice therapy (n = 38)	(a) Treatment method: cold knife (a) Duration: 4 months (b) Treatment method: vocal hygiene, relaxation training, breathing and posture training, and vocal acoustic training (b) Duration: 4 months	(a) n.a. (b) 12 weeks	MPT VHI-T, VHI-P, VHI-F, VHI-E
Prasad et al. (2020) [48]	All types and features of VFP	40	Phonosurgery	Treatment method: cold knife Duration: 3 months	n.a.	MPT
Kim et al. (2020) [49]	Unilateral; all sizes and features of VFP	20	Phonosurgery	Treatment method: cold knife Duration: 1 month	n.a.	Jitter Shimmer NHR
Ma et al. (2021) [50]	All types and features of VFP	25	Phonosurgery	Treatment method: KTP laser (office-based) Duration: 3–14 months	n.a.	Jitter Shimmer MPT VHI-T, VHI-P, VHI-F, VHI-E
Lee et al. (In Press) [51]	All types and features of VFP	72	Phonosurgery	Treatment method: cold knife Duration: 10–14 days	n.a.	VHI-T, VHI-P, VHI-F, VHI-E
Kang et al. (In Press) [52]	Unilateral; all sizes and features of VFP	77	Phonosurgery	Treatment method: cold knife Duration: 6 weeks	n.a.	Jitter Shimmer NHR MPT VHI-T, VHI-P, VHI-F, VHI-E G, R, B

VFP: Vocal fold polyp; G: grade/hoarseness; R: roughness; B: breathiness; NHR: noise-to-harmonics ratio; MPT: maximum phonation time; VHI: the 30-item Voice Handicap Index (VHI—30) which outputs three subscales with statements on physical (P), functional (F), and emotional (E) domains and a total score (T).

3.1. Auditory–Perceptual Judgment

This meta-analysis used the G (grade [of dysphonia]), R (roughness), and B (breathiness) parameters of the international GRBAS scale [7]. Its forest plots are shown in Figure 2, The pooled pre- to post-treatment gains of G were −1.256 (95% CI: −1.569−−0.944;

$p < 0.001$) for phonosurgery, -1.223 (95% CI: -2.293–-0.152; $p = 0.025$) for VT, and -1.504 (95% CI: -1.972–-1.037; $p < 0.001$) for CT, indicating that all interventions reduced hoarseness. All Cohen's d values were above 0.8 (Table S4, Supplementary Materials).

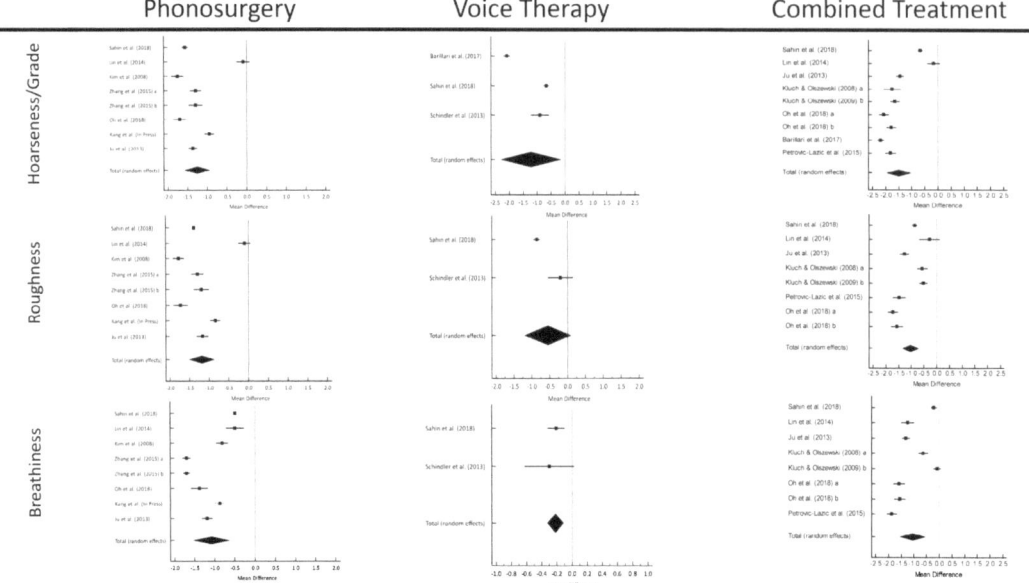

Figure 2. Forest plots of perceived voice quality levels [23,24,26,30,31,35,38,39,42,45,46,52].

There was no significant publication bias for these analyses ($p > 0.05$). Heterogeneity was high (>75%) and persisted in the subgroup analyses (follow-up period and type of phonosurgery) (Table S6, Supplementary Materials). The longer the duration of the follow-up period after phonosurgery, the lower the heterogeneity, but it remained >75%. The mean G reduced the most with CT after 1–2 weeks of follow-up, at -1.638 (95% CI: -1.810–-1.466; $p < 0.001$), and even at a moderate heterogeneity of 64.96%. In the network meta-analysis, G improved more for CT than for phonosurgery alone ($p < 0.001$) or VT ($p < 0.001$), with no significant differences across studies ($p = 0.518$; Table S5, Supplementary Materials). The pooled roughness was -1.189 (95% CI: -1.505–-0.944; $p < 0.001$) for phonosurgery, -0.552 (95% CI: -1.198–-0.093; $p = 0.093$) for VT, and -1.041 (95% CI: -1.361–-0.722; $p < 0.001$) for CT. All Cohen's d values were above 0.8 (Table S4, Supplementary Materials). A significant publication bias was evident for VT ($p < 0.001$). Heterogeneity was high (>75%) but steadily decreased with increasing duration of follow-up, reaching a moderate value of 54.11% $\geq$ 3 months after surgery (Table S6, Supplementary Materials). A network meta-analysis for all treatment modalities showed a significant reduction in roughness, with phonosurgery being the most effective ($p < 0.001$) (Table S5, Supplementary Materials). The pooled breathiness value was -1.080 (95% CI: -1.529–-0.630; $p < 0.001$) for phonosurgery, -0.220 (95% CI: -0.327–-0.113; $p < 0.001$) for VT, and -1.055 (95% CI: -1.557–-0.553; $p < 0.001$) for CT. All Cohen's d values were above 0.8 (Table S4, Supplementary Materials). A significant publication bias was evident for VT ($p < 0.001$) and CT ($p = 0.018$). Heterogeneity was 0% for VT but was high (>75%) for phonosurgery and CT and remained high in subgroup analyses (follow-up period and type of phonosurgery; Table S6, Supplementary Materials).

The network meta-analysis showed significant outcome differences between phonosurgery and VT ($p < 0.001$) and VT and CT ($p < 0.001$) but not between phonosurgery and CT ($p = 0.198$), both of which were most effective (Table S5, Supplementary Materials).

3.2. Acoustics

Forest plots for this meta-analysis are depicted in Figure 3. The pooled pre- to post-treatment jitter differences were −1.266% (95% CI: −1.663−−0.869%; $p < 0.001$) for phonosurgery, −0.494% (95% CI: −0.932−−0.057%; $p < 0.001$) for VT, and −1.457% (95% CI: −1.615−−1.299%; $p < 0.001$) for CT. The pooled pre–post shimmer differences were −2.300% (95% CI: −3.061−−1.539%; $p < 0.001$) for phonosurgery, −1.487% (95% CI: −3.065–0.092%; $p < 0.001$) for VT, and −3.181% (95% CI: −3.950−−2.413%; $p < 0.001$) for CT. The pooled pre-post NRH differences were −0.087 dB (95% CI: −0.113−−0.061 dB; $p < 0.001$) for phonosurgery, −0.068 dB (95% CI: −0.118−−0.017 dB; $p < 0.001$) for VT, and −0.077 dB (95% CI: −0.096−−0.059 dB; $p < 0.001$) for CT. All Cohen's d values were above 0.8 (Table S4, Supplementary Materials).

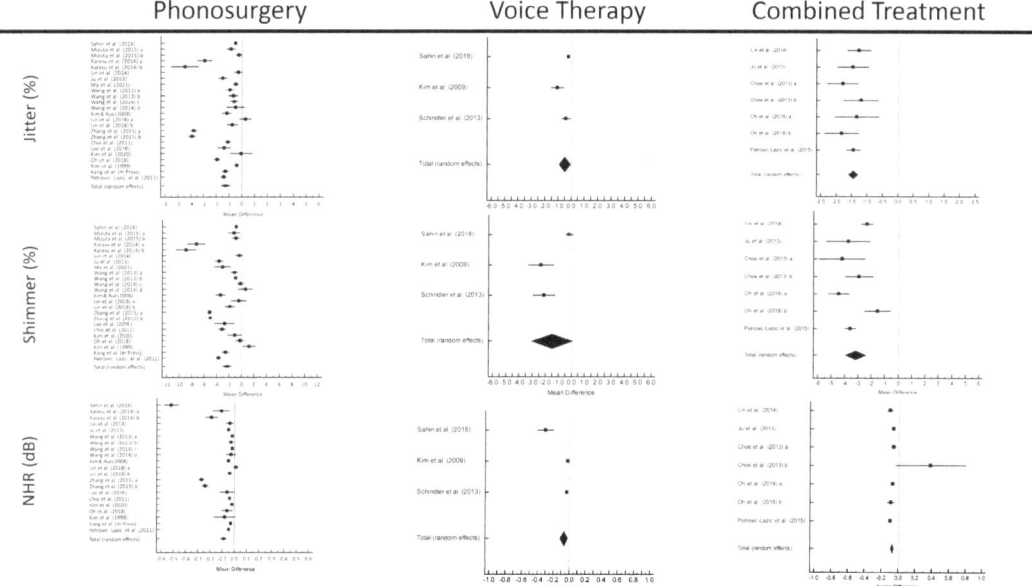

Figure 3. Forests plot of acoustic measures [22,23,27–40,44–46,49,50,52].

For shimmer in the VT analysis and jitter in the phonosurgery analysis, there were significant publication biases ($p = 0.026$ and $p = 0.045$, respectively). Heterogeneity was high for phonosurgery and VT but low for CT (Table S3, Supplementary Materials), with comparable results in the subgroup analyses (Table S7, Supplementary Materials). For jitter, the heterogeneity for CT even reached 0%. For all three parameters, the mean gain after phonosurgery gains was greatest for a follow-up period of ≥3 months: jitter: −2.166% (95% CI: −3.925−−0.408%; $p = 0.016$), NRH: −0.339 dB (95% CI: −0.452−−0.225 dB; $p < 0.001$), shimmer: −2.646% (95% CI: −5.039−−0.252%; $p = 0.030$).

In the network meta-analysis, the pooled pre–post improvements of all three acoustic parameters were significant for all treatment modalities, with jitter and shimmer showing the strongest improvements with CT and NHR showed the strongest improvements with phonosurgery (all $p < 0.001$; Table S5, Supplementary Materials).

3.3. Maximum Phonation Time

The pooled pre- to post-treatment MPT elongations were 3.265 s (95% CI: 2.203–4.328 s; $p < 0.001$) for phonosurgery, 2.561 s (95% CI: 1.355–3.766 s; $p < 0.001$) for VT, and 4.065 s

(95% CI: 2.045–6.084 s; $p < 0.001$) for CT (forest plots in Figure 4). All Cohen's d values were above 0.8 (Table S4, Supplementary Materials).

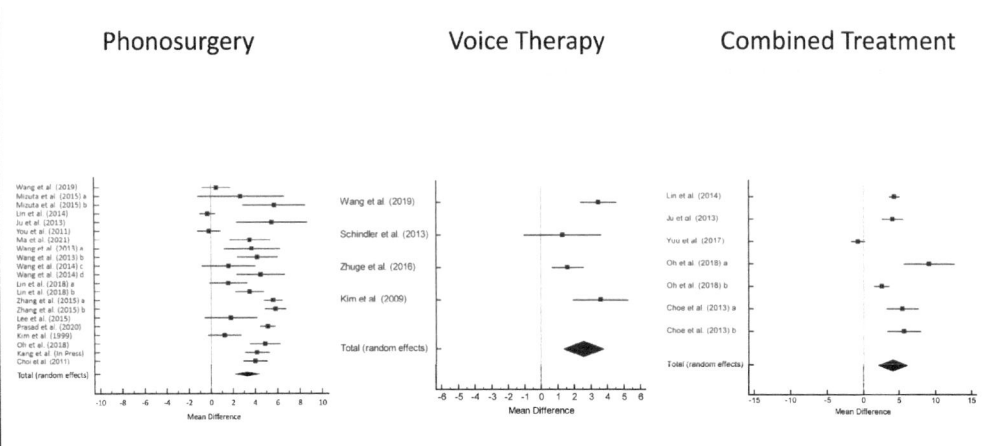

Figure 4. Forest plots of maximum phonation time [22,27,28,30–33,35–37,39–41,43,44,46–48,50,52].

There was no significant publication bias ($p > 0.05$). Heterogeneity was lowest for VT with $I^2 = 65.80\%$. In the subgroup analyses (Table S8, Supplementary Materials), the mean pre–post gain was highest for CT if administered for longer than 3 weeks (4.521 s; 95% CI: 1.436–7.606 s; $p = 0.004$), but heterogeneity was high (95.55%). High pooled MPT gains of 4.468 s (95% CI: 3.632–5.303 s; $p < 0.001$) with insignificant heterogeneity of 7.26% was achieved for CT with phonosurgical laser technology.

In the network meta-analysis, pooled pre–post MPT prolongation was significant for all treatment modalities and highest for CT ($p < 0.001$; Table S5, Supplementary Materials).

3.4. Voice Handicap Index—30

Forest plots are shown in Figure 5. The pooled pre–post improvements of the E (emotional) subscale values were −7.072 (95% CI: −10.786−−3.357; $p < 0.001$) for phonosurgery, −3.093 (95% CI: −4.440−−1.747; $p < 0.001$) for VT, and −6.242 (95% CI: −11.913−−0.571; $p = 0.031$) for CT. The pooled pre–post gains of the F (functional) subscale values were −7.437 (95% CI: −11.389−−3.485; $p < 0.001$) for phonosurgery, −2.731 (95% CI: −4.162−−1.300; $p < 0.001$) for VT, and −5.239 (95% CI: −7.124−−3.354; $p < 0.001$) for CT. The pooled pre-to-post treatment P (physical) subscale enhancements were −10.463 (95% CI: −15.829−−5.096; $p < 0.001$) for phonosurgery, −5.022 (95% CI: −6.569−−3.476; $p < 0.001$) for VT, and −12.200 (95% CI: −16.668−−7.731; $p < 0.001$) for CT. The pooled pre–post T (total) score gains were −22.753 (95% CI: −29.266−−16.240; $p < 0.001$) for phonosurgery, −18.886 (95% CI: −42.996−−5.224; $p = 0.125$) for VT, and −22.896 (95% CI: −33.529−−12.264; $p < 0.001$) for CT. All Cohen's d values were above 0.8 (Table S4, Supplementary Materials).

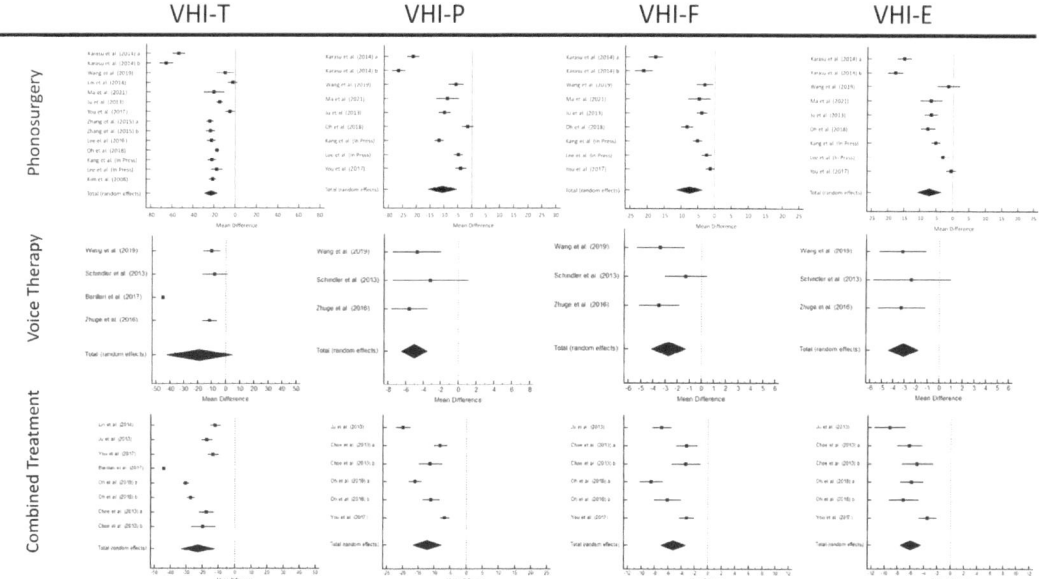

Figure 5. Forest plots of Voice Handicap Index parameters [25,30–32,34,35,39–43,46,47,50–52].

Significant publication biases were evident for the E subscale for CT ($p < 0.001$), P subscale for VT ($p = 0.027$), and T score for VT ($p = 0.017$) and CT ($p < 0.001$). The E, F, and P subscales scores showed low to moderate heterogeneity for VT (0—48.9%). High T score heterogeneity was present for all treatment modalities, with predominantly high heterogeneity in all subgroup analyses of the VHI parameters for CT and phonosurgery (Table S9, Supplementary Materials). For all four parameters, the mean pre- to post-phonosurgery gains were greatest with a follow-up of 1–2 months: E subscale: -11.106 (95% CI: -17.278—-4.935; $p < 0.001$), F subscale: -11.875 (95% CI: -19.680—-4.070; $p = 0.003$), P subscale: -17.370 (95% CI: -24.860—-9.879; $p < 0.001$), T score: -35.674 (95% CI: -52.365—-18.982; $p < 0.001$). Comparing phonosurgery with CT, the network meta-analysis showed significant improvements ($p < 0.001$, Table S5, Supplementary Materials) for all four VHI parameters, except for the T scores ($p = 0.674$).

4. Discussion

This meta-analysis showed that phonosurgery, VT, and a sequential combination of both resulted in significant voice improvements in the treatment of vocal fold polyps, with either phonosurgery alone or phonosurgery followed by VT being the most effective treatment options, with not much difference. Subgroup analyses did not significantly reduce heterogeneity.

To optimize treatment pathways, it would be desirable to include morphologic features of VFP in treatment decisions. We therefore performed an extra subgroup analysis with regard to the morphological characteristics of polyps using the twelve studies available for this purpose. The results are sobering and suggest that further research is needed on this clinical issue. There were six studies that differentiated somewhat in morphologic characteristics but with no common intersection on these characteristics, let alone even two studies per treatment format. These six studies describe the following criteria: bilateral polyps only; unilateral, but no giant polyps; all features and sizes, but polyps must be positioned at the free edge; all types and features of gelatinous polyps; variable sizes; and additional different features in two studies. Six studies further defined the size of the polyp; these studies considered only small to medium-sized polyps. Three studies analyzed voice therapy and phonosurgery and one study analyzed their combination. Thus, no comparative analysis could be performed across all three treatment modalities. By testing VT and phonosurgery in the small to medium polyp sizes, another problem occurred: these six studies did not analyze all 11 of our chosen measures. The only intersection between all studies was maximum phonation time. However, as shown in Table S10, Supplementary Materials, MPT improved on average by the same amount with both methods, namely, by 2.90 s each, with comparable SD. Thus, although the sample was large, with n = 100 patients for each of the two groups examined, there was no clinical difference between phonosurgery and VT in MPT.

Included publications revealed some serious concerns about the risk of bias for many (20 out of 31) studies and high heterogeneity, including in the subgroups. There was imprecision only in the VT group for all voice parameters and publication bias in some cases, but no indirectness.

Our meta-analysis evaluated only the combination of phonosurgery followed by VT, as our search found only one study [45] reporting initial VT followed by phonosurgery if VT did not result in sufficient voice improvement. Nonetheless, the latter treatment modality is recommended in current clinical guidelines for hoarseness [12]. According to our results, VT alone may also be an effective treatment option for VFP, but showed less improvement in voice measures than the other methods. Therefore, the efficiency of initial VT may also be questioned. Moreover, the efficiency of initial or sole VT has been less well studied than that of the other treatment modalities, and the meta-analysis could only rely on a smaller number of participants and less variability in VT. Additionally, it is still unclear which voice exercises in VFP particularly facilitate behavioral changes in voice use or improved voice function. Two recent network meta-analyses identified four VT programs as effective: stretch-and-flow phonation, resonant voice, vocal function exercises, and an eclectic VT program [53,54]. Strong, direct VT concepts for VFP might include VT expulsion [42], Seong-Tae Kim's multiple VT technique [27], vocal function exercises [41–43,45,46], and resonant voice [30–32,41,43,45,46]. Furthermore, polyp characteristics such as small size influence the success of VT and should be considered [2,55]. Further research is needed to clarify the effectiveness of the named VT methods, depending on VFP characteristics. Moreover, vocal hygiene, including environment change (e.g., humidifier in dry air, mask in dusty air, amplification in a noisy environment), behavior change (e.g., avoiding lifting/pushing heavy things, loud coughing, throat clearing, excessive alcohol and caffeine consumption, smoking, late meals, fatty and spicy foods), and vocal habits change (e.g., avoiding shouting, speaking with anger, loud whispering), is imperative after VFP phonosurgery [26,30–32,35,41–43,45–47].

In clinical practice, polyp-like masses of the vocal folds are occasionally not given names when diagnosed by stroboscopy or laryngoscopy because of uncertainty about their histologic nature or dignity (e.g., thin-walled cyst, atypical laryngeal carcinoma); these patients are then referred to a laryngeal surgeon with diagnoses such as "unclear lesion of the vocal fold." In these cases, phonosurgical ablation is the method of choice. Thus, in the cases of VT alone, our meta-analysis carries some uncertainty as to whether polyps were really involved. However, that this possibility may have had only a small impact is shown by the large effect of VT.

Most studies included in our meta-analysis used the VHI-30 as a self-assessment measure, and only seven studies applied the VHI-10, which is also often utilized in routine clinical practice [56]. Of these, five studies were already included in this meta-analysis based on other measures of acoustics, auditory–perceptual judgment, or aerodynamics. For inclusion in a meta-analysis, the VHI-10 would have had to be used in more than one study for all three treatment modalities, a constellation that was not found in our search. Nevertheless, it is useful to consider a VHI that is standardized in terms of its item numbers in clinical and research evaluations of voice treatments, and we encourage readers to invest more in standardized multidimensional voice assessments to achieve better comparability of treatment outcomes.

According to our meta-analysis, phonosurgery is the first option to be considered in VFP treatment, but conservative voice rehabilitation plays a crucial role too. Its duration and type vary widely and post-surgery VT longer than 3 weeks seems to be more effective than shorter VT (see Tables S6—S9, Supplementary Materials). After phonosurgery, patients are usually prescribed vocal rest. However, standards on its reasonable duration and the type of vocal utterances that can be allowed during this period are lacking [57–59]. For optimal vocal outcome, postoperative VT that includes vocal hygiene and a few weeks of VT with vocal function exercises, resonant voice, or other exercise programs described above seems reasonable. A hierarchy of effective voice exercises, starting with a soft voice with little impact on the vocal folds and progressing to a loud voice for robust daily voice use, should be compiled and researched.

5. Conclusions

In our meta-analysis, phonosurgery alone and phonosurgery followed by voice therapy are effective in treating dysphonia due to vocal fold polyps. Both phonosurgery alone and phonosurgery with subsequent voice therapy can result in specific voice-related outcomes; thus, the type of therapy can be chosen according to the results of the assessment parameters after phonosurgery. In particular, additional voice therapy should be considered if a hoarse or unstable voice is still present after phonosurgery. If there is uncertainty in the clinical diagnosis about the possible dignity of the polyp mass, phonosurgery should be performed.

Further research on vocal hygiene and rehabilitation strategies after phonosurgery and on treatment effects according to the size and other morphological characteristics of vocal fold polyps is recommended.

In addition, further studies and meta-analyses are needed to account for polyp size, form, mass, length, and impact on glottic configuration in determining whether phonosurgery, voice therapy, or a combination treatment is most helpful.

Supplementary Materials: The following supporting information can be downloaded at https://www.mdpi.com/article/10.3390/jcm12103451/s1, Table S1: Systematic search strategies; Table S2: Risk of bias analysis of RCT and observational studies; Table S3: Meta-analyses by treatment and by voice measures (random effects model), with heterogeneity index I^2 and Egger's publication bias test; Table S4: Meta-analysis for Cohen's *d* (random effects model); Table S5: Network meta-analysis; Table S6: Subgroup meta-analysis for perceived voice quality level; Table S7: Subgroup meta-analysis for acoustics; Table S8: Subgroup meta-analysis for MPT; Table S9: Subgroup meta-analysis for VHI-30; Table S10: Influence of morphological polyp characteristics on the MPT outcome of both phonosurgery and VT.

Author Contributions: Conceptualization, B.B.v.L., C.R.W. and K.N.; methodology, B.B.v.L., C.R.W., K.N. and S.H.; software, S.H.; formal analysis, B.B.v.L. and S.H.; writing—original draft preparation, B.B.v.L. and S.H.; writing—review and editing, K.N. and C.R.W. All authors have read and agreed to the published version of the manuscript.

Funding: This research received no external funding.

Institutional Review Board Statement: Not applicable.

Informed Consent Statement: Not applicable.

Data Availability Statement: The original contributions presented in the study are included in the article; further inquiries can be directed to the corresponding author.

Conflicts of Interest: The authors declare no conflict of interest.

References

1. Vasconcelos, D.; Gomes, A.O.C.; Araújo, C.M.T. Vocal fold polyps: Literature review. *Int. Arch. Otorhinolaryngol.* **2019**, *23*, 116–124. [CrossRef] [PubMed]
2. Cho, K.J.; Nam, I.C.; Hwang, Y.S.; Shim, M.R.; Park, J.O.; Cho, J.H.; Joo, Y.H.; Kim, M.S.; Sun, D.I. Analysis of factors influencing voice quality and therapeutic approaches in vocal polyp patients. *Eur. Arch. Otorhinolaryngol.* **2011**, *268*, 1321–1327. [CrossRef] [PubMed]
3. Hah, J.H.; Sim, S.; An, S.Y.; Sung, M.W.; Choi, H.G. Evaluation of the prevalence of and factors associated with laryngeal diseases among the general population. *Laryngoscope* **2015**, *125*, 2536–2542. [CrossRef] [PubMed]
4. Van Houtte, E.; Van Lierde, K.; D'Haeseleer, E.; Claeys, S. The prevalence of laryngeal pathology in a treatment-seeking population with dysphonia. *Laryngoscope* **2010**, *120*, 306–312. [CrossRef] [PubMed]
5. Martins, R.H.; do Amaral, H.A.; Tavares, E.L.; Martins, M.G.; Gonçalves, T.M.; Dias, N.H. Voice disorders: Etiology and diagnosis. *J. Voice* **2016**, *30*, 761.e1–761.e9. [CrossRef]
6. Martins, R.H.; Defaveri, J.; Domingues, M.A.; de Albuquerque e Silva, R. Vocal polyps: Clinical, morphological, and immunohistochemical aspects. *J. Voice* **2011**, *25*, 98–106. [CrossRef]
7. Dejonckere, P.H.; Bradley, P.; Clemente, P.; Cornut, G.; Crevier-Buchman, L.; Friedrich, G.; Van De Heyning, P.; Remacle, M.; Woisard, V.; Committee on Phoniatrics of the European Laryngological Society (ELS). A basic protocol for functional assessment of voice pathology, especially for investigating the efficacy of (phonosurgical) treatments and evaluating new assessment techniques. Guideline elaborated by the Committee on Phoniatrics of the European Laryngological Society (ELS). *Eur. Arch. Otorhinolaryngol.* **2001**, *258*, 77–82. [CrossRef]
8. Öcal, B.; Tatar, E.Ç.; Toptaş, G.; Barmak, E.; Saylam, G.; Korkmaz, M.H. Evaluation of voice quality in patients with vocal fold polyps: The size of a polyp matters or does it? *J. Voice* **2020**, *34*, 294–299. [CrossRef]
9. Sulica, L.; Behrman, A. Management of benign vocal fold lesions: A survey of current opinion and practice. *Ann. Otol. Rhinol. Laryngol.* **2003**, *112*, 827–833. [CrossRef]
10. Cohen, S.M.; Pitman, M.J.; Noordzij, J.P.; Courey, M. Management of dysphonic patients by otolaryngologists. *Otolaryngol. Head. Neck Surg.* **2012**, *147*, 289–294. [CrossRef]
11. Cohen, S.M.; Garrett, C.G. Utility of voice therapy in the management of vocal fold polyps and cysts. *Otolaryngol. Head. Neck Surg.* **2007**, *136*, 742–746. [CrossRef] [PubMed]
12. Stachler, R.J.; Francis, D.O.; Schwartz, S.R.; Damask, C.C.; Digoy, G.P.; Krouse, H.J.; McCoy, S.J.; Ouellette, D.R.; Patel, R.R.; Reavis, C.C.W.; et al. Clinical practice guideline: Hoarseness (dysphonia) (update). *Otolaryngol. Head. Neck Surg.* **2018**, *158*, S1–S42. [CrossRef] [PubMed]
13. Lee, M.; Sulica, L. Recurrence of benign phonotraumatic vocal fold lesions after microlaryngoscopy. *Laryngoscope* **2020**, *130*, 1989–1995. [CrossRef] [PubMed]
14. Liberati, A.; Altman, D.G.; Tetzlaff, J.; Mulrow, C.; Gøtzsche, P.C.; Ioannidis, J.P.; Clarke, M.; Devereaux, P.J.; Kleijnen, J.; Moher, D. The PRISMA statement for reporting systematic reviews and meta-analyses of studies that evaluate health care interventions: Explanation and elaboration. *Ann. Intern. Med.* **2009**, *151*, W65–W94. [CrossRef] [PubMed]
15. Herbst, C.T.; Oh, J.; Vydrová, J.; Švec, J.G. DigitalVHI—A freeware open-source software application to capture the Voice Handicap Index and other questionnaire data in various languages. *Logoped Phoniatr. Vocol* **2015**, *40*, 72–76. [CrossRef] [PubMed]
16. Sterne, J.A.C.; Savović, J.; Page, M.J.; Elbers, R.G.; Blencowe, N.S.; Boutron, I.; Cates, C.J.; Cheng, H.Y.; Corbett, M.S.; Eldridge, S.M.; et al. RoB 2: A revised tool for assessing risk of bias in randomised trials. *BMJ* **2019**, *366*, l4898. [CrossRef]
17. Sterne, J.A.; Hernán, M.A.; Reeves, B.C.; Savović, J.; Berkman, N.D.; Viswanathan, M.; Henry, D.; Altman, D.G.; Ansari, M.T.; Boutron, I.; et al. ROBINS-I: A tool for assessing risk of bias in non-randomised studies of interventions. *BMJ* **2016**, *355*, i4919. [CrossRef] [PubMed]
18. Higgins, J.P.; Thompson, S.G.; Deeks, J.J.; Altman, D.G. Measuring inconsistency in meta-analyses. *BMJ* **2003**, *327*, 557–560. [CrossRef]
19. DerSimonian, R.; Laird, N. Meta-analysis in clinical trials. *Control. Clin. Trials* **1986**, *7*, 177–188. [CrossRef]
20. Egger, M.; Davey Smith, G.; Schneider, M.; Minder, C. Bias in meta-analysis detected by a simple, graphical test. *BMJ* **1997**, *315*, 629–634. [CrossRef]
21. Cohen, J. *Statistical Power Analysis for the Behavioral Sciences*; Lawrence Erlbaum Associates: Hillsdale, MI, USA, 1988.
22. Kim, Y.M.; Cho, J.I.; Kim, C.H.; Kim, Y.J.; Ha, H.R. Vocal dynamic studies before and after laryngeal microsurgery. *Korean J. Otolaryngol.* **1999**, *42*, 1174–1178. (In Korean)
23. Kim, H.T.; Auo, H.J. Office-based 585 nm pulsed dye laser treatment for vocal polyps. *Acta Otolaryngol.* **2008**, *128*, 1043–1047. [CrossRef] [PubMed]
24. Kluch, W.; Olszewski, J. Videolaryngostroboscopic examination of treatment effects in patients with chronic hyperthrophic larynges. *Otolaryngol. Pol.* **2008**, *62*, 680–685. (In Polish) [CrossRef] [PubMed]
25. Kim, B.S.; Shin, J.H.; Kim, K.Y.; Lee, Y.S.; Kim, K.R.; Tae, K. Change of Acoustic Parameter and Voice Handicap Index after Laryngeal Microsurgery. *J. Korean Soc. Laryngol. Phoniatr. Logop.* **2008**, *19*, 142–145. (In Korean)
26. Kluch, W.; Olszewski, J. The use of laryngostroboscopy in diagnostics and results evaluation of treatment of patients with organic lesions in the larynx. *Otolaryngol. Pol.* **2009**, *63*, 11–15. (In Polish) [CrossRef] [PubMed]

27. Kim, S.T.; Jeong, G.E.; Kim, S.Y.; Choi, S.H.; Lim, G.C.; Han, J.H.; Nam, S.Y. The effect of voice therapy in vocal polyp patients. *Phon. Speech Sci.* **2009**, *1*, 43–49. (In Korean)
28. Choi, J.I.; Yeo, J.O.; Jin, S.M.; Lee, S.H. Result of voice analysis after laryngeal microsurgery for vocal polyp in elderly. *J. Korean Soc. Laryngol. Phoniatr. Logop.* **2011**, *22*, 47–51. (In Korean)
29. Petrović-Lazić, M.; Babac, S.; Vuković, M.; Kosanović, R.; Ivanković, Z. Acoustic voice analysis of patients with vocal fold polyp. *J. Voice* **2011**, *25*, 94–97. [CrossRef]
30. Ju, Y.H.; Jung, K.Y.; Kwon, S.Y.; Woo, J.S.; Cho, J.G.; Park, M.W.; Park, E.H.; Baek, S.K. Effect of voice therapy after phonomicrosurgery for vocal polyps: A prospective, historically controlled, clinical study. *J. Laryngol. Otol.* **2013**, *127*, 1134–1138. [CrossRef]
31. Schindler, A.; Mozzanica, F.; Maruzzi, P.; Atac, M.; De Cristofaro, V.; Ottaviani, F. Multidimensional assessment of vocal changes in benign vocal fold lesions after voice therapy. *Auris Nasus Larynx* **2013**, *40*, 291–297. [CrossRef]
32. Choe, H.; Jung, K.Y.; Kwon, S.Y.; Woo, J.S.; Park, M.W.; Baek, S.K. The usefulness of CO_2 laser-assisted phonomicrosurgery using a computer-guided scanner in broad-based vocal polyp. *Korean J. Otorhinolaryngol.-Head. Neck Surg.* **2013**, *56*, 511–515. (In Korean) [CrossRef]
33. Wang, C.T.; Huang, T.W.; Liao, L.J.; Lo, W.C.; Lai, M.S.; Cheng, P.W. Office-based potassium titanyl phosphate laser-assisted endoscopic vocal polypectomy. *JAMA Otolaryngol. Head. Neck Surg.* **2013**, *139*, 610–616. [CrossRef] [PubMed]
34. Karasu, M.F.; Gundogdu, R.; Cagli, S.; Aydin, M.; Arli, T.; Aydemir, S.; Yuce, I. Comparison of effects on voice of diode laser and cold knife microlaryngology techniques for vocal fold polyps. *J. Voice* **2014**, *28*, 387–392. [CrossRef]
35. Lin, L.; Sun, N.; Yang, Q.; Zhang, Y.; Shen, J.; Shi, L.; Fang, Q.; Sun, G. Effect of voice training in the voice rehabilitation of patients with vocal cord polyps after surgery. *Exp. Ther. Med.* **2014**, *7*, 877–880. [CrossRef] [PubMed]
36. Wang, C.T.; Liao, L.J.; Huang, T.W.; Lo, W.C.; Cheng, P.W. Comparison of treatment outcomes of transnasal vocal fold polypectomy versus microlaryngoscopic surgery. *Laryngoscope* **2015**, *125*, 1155–1160. [CrossRef] [PubMed]
37. Mizuta, M.; Hiwatashi, N.; Kobayashi, T.; Kaneko, M.; Tateya, I.; Hirano, S. Comparison of vocal outcomes after angiolytic laser surgery and microflap surgery for vocal polyps. *Auris Nasus Larynx* **2015**, *42*, 453–457. [CrossRef]
38. Petrovic-Lazic, M.; Jovanovic, N.; Kulic, M.; Babac, S.; Jurisic, V. Acoustic and perceptual characteristics of the voice in patients with vocal polyps after surgery and voice therapy. *J. Voice* **2015**, *29*, 241–246. [CrossRef]
39. Zhang, Y.; Liang, G.; Sun, N.; Guan, L.; Meng, Y.; Zhao, X.; Liu, L.; Sun, G. Comparison of CO2 laser and conventional laryngomicrosurgery treatments of polyp and leukoplakia of the vocal fold. *Int. J. Clin. Exp. Med.* **2015**, *8*, 18265–18274.
40. Lee, Y.C.; Na, S.Y.; Kim, H.J.; Yang, C.W.; Kim, S.I.; Byun, Y.S.; Jung, A.R.; Ryu, I.Y.; Eun, Y.G. Effect of postoperative proton pump inhibitor therapy on voice outcomes following phonomicrosurgery for vocal fold polyp: A randomized controlled study. *Clin. Otolaryngol.* **2016**, *41*, 730–736. [CrossRef]
41. Zhuge, P.; You, H.; Wang, H.; Zhang, Y.; Du, H. An Analysis of the effects of voice therapy on patients with early vocal fold polyps. *J. Voice* **2016**, *30*, 698–704. [CrossRef]
42. Barillari, M.R.; Volpe, U.; Mirra, G.; Giugliano, F.; Barillari, U. Surgery or rehabilitation: A randomized clinical trial comparing the treatment of vocal fold polyps via phonosurgery and traditional voice therapy with "voice therapy expulsion" training. *J. Voice* **2017**, *31*, 379.e13–379.e20. [CrossRef] [PubMed]
43. You, H.; Zhuge, P.; Wang, H.; Zhang, Y.; Du, H. Clinical observation of the effect of voice training on patients with vocal cordpolyps after phonomicrosurgery. *Biomed. Res.* **2017**, *28*, 3874–3879.
44. Lin, Y.H.; Wang, C.T.; Lin, F.C.; Liao, L.J.; Lo, W.C.; Cheng, P.W. Treatment outcomes and adverse events following in-office angiolytic laser with or without concurrent polypectomy for vocal fold polyps. *JAMA Otolaryngol. Head. Neck Surg.* **2018**, *144*, 222–230. [CrossRef]
45. Sahin, M.; Gode, S.; Dogan, M.; Kirazli, T.; Ogut, F. Effect of voice therapy on vocal fold polyp treatment. *Eur. Arch. Otorhinolaryngol.* **2018**, *275*, 1533–1540. [CrossRef]
46. Oh, D.J.; Kim, S.Y.; Choi, I.H.; Han, H.M.; Byeon, H.K.; Jung, K.Y.; Baek, S.K. The usefulness of postoperative direct voice therapy in vocal polyps. *Korean J. Otorhinolaryngol.-Head. Neck Surg.* **2018**, *61*, 686–691. (In Korean) [CrossRef]
47. Wang, H.; Zhuge, P.; You, H.; Zhang, Y.; Zhang, Z. Comparison of the efficacy of vocal training and vocal microsurgery in patients with early vocal fold polyp. *Braz. J. Otorhinolaryngol.* **2019**, *85*, 678–684. [CrossRef]
48. Prasad, S.; Raychowdhury, R.; Roychoudhury, A. Assessment of pre and postoperative voice quality in cases of vocal fold polyp. *Inter. J. Otorhinolaryngol. Head. Neck Surg.* **2020**, *6*, 352–358. [CrossRef]
49. Kim, S.W.; Kim, S.Y.; Cho, J.K.; Jin, S.M.; Lee, S.H. Reliability of OperaVOXTM against multi-dimensional voice program to assess voice quality before and after laryngeal microsurgery in patient with vocal polyp. *J. Korean Soc. Laryngol. Phoniatr. Logop.* **2020**, *31*, 71–77. (In Korean) [CrossRef]
50. Ma, J.; Fang, R.; Zhen, R.; Mao, W.; Wu, X.; He, P.; Wei, C. A 532-nm KTP laser for vocal fold polyps: Efficacy and relative factors. *Ear Nose Throat J.* **2021**, *100*, 87S–93S. [CrossRef]
51. Lee, Y.; Park, H.J.; Bae, I.H.; Kwon, S.; Kim, G. The usefulness of multi voice evaluation for measuring voice recovery after endolaryngeal phonomicrosurgery in patients with vocal fold polyps. *J. Voice* **2021**, *in press*. [CrossRef]
52. Kang, D.W.; Kim, S.I.; Noh, J.K.; Jeong, S.J.; Lee, Y.C.; Ko, S.G.; Eun, Y.G. Voice outcome after cold knife surgery according to the characteristics of vocal fold polyp. *J. Voice* **2021**, *in press*. [CrossRef] [PubMed]

53. Barsties v. Latoszek, B.; Watts, C.R.; Neumann, K. The effectiveness of voice therapy on voice-related handicap: A network meta-analysis. *Clin. Otolaryngol.* **2020**, *45*, 796–804. [CrossRef] [PubMed]
54. Barsties v. Latoszek, B.; Watts, C.R.; Schwan, K.; Hetjens, S. The maximum phonation time as marker for voice treatment efficacy: A network meta-analysis. *Clin. Otolaryngol.* **2023**, *48*, 130–138. [CrossRef] [PubMed]
55. Lee, Y.S.; Lee, D.H.; Jeong, G.E.; Kim, J.W.; Roh, J.L.; Choi, S.H.; Kim, S.Y.; Nam, S.Y. Treatment efficacy of voice therapy for vocal fold polyps and factors predictive of its efficacy. *J. Voice* **2017**, *31*, 120.e9–120.e13. [CrossRef]
56. Gilbert, M.R.; Gartner-Schmidt, J.L.; Rosen, C.A. The VHI-10 and VHI item reduction translations-are we all speaking the same language? *J. Voice* **2017**, *31*, 250.e1–250.e7. [CrossRef]
57. Björck, G.; Hertegård, S.; Ekelund, J.; Marsk, E. Voice rest after vocal fold polyp surgery: A Swedish register study of 588 patients. *Laryngoscope Investig. Otolaryngol.* **2022**, *7*, 486–493. [CrossRef]
58. King, R.E.; Novaleski, C.K.; Rousseau, B. Voice Handicap Index changes after microflap surgery for benign vocal fold lesions are not associated with recommended absolute voice rest duration. *Am. J. Speech Lang. Pathol.* **2022**, *31*, 912–922. [CrossRef]
59. Chi, H.W.; Cho, H.C.; Yang, A.Y.; Chen, Y.C.; Chen, J.W. Effects of different voice rest on vocal function after microlaryngeal surgery: A systematic review and meta-analysis. *Laryngoscope* **2023**, *133*, 154–161. [CrossRef]

Disclaimer/Publisher's Note: The statements, opinions and data contained in all publications are solely those of the individual author(s) and contributor(s) and not of MDPI and/or the editor(s). MDPI and/or the editor(s) disclaim responsibility for any injury to people or property resulting from any ideas, methods, instructions or products referred to in the content.

MDPI AG
Grosspeteranlage 5
4052 Basel
Switzerland
Tel.: +41 61 683 77 34

Journal of Clinical Medicine Editorial Office
E-mail: jcm@mdpi.com
www.mdpi.com/journal/jcm

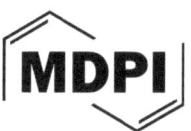

Disclaimer/Publisher's Note: The title and front matter of this reprint are at the discretion of the Guest Editor. The publisher is not responsible for their content or any associated concerns. The statements, opinions and data contained in all individual articles are solely those of the individual Editor and contributors and not of MDPI. MDPI disclaims responsibility for any injury to people or property resulting from any ideas, methods, instructions or products referred to in the content.

www.ingramcontent.com/pod-product-compliance
Lightning Source LLC
LaVergne TN
LVHW072356090526
838202LV00019B/2561